Porphyrins in Tumor Phototherapy

Porphyrins
in Tumor
Phototherapy

Edited by

Alessandra Andreoni
and
Rinaldo Cubeddu

The Polytechnic Institute of Milan and
National Research Council
Milan, Italy

Plenum Press • New York and London

Library of Congress Cataloging in Publication Data

International Symposium on Porphyrins in Tumor Phototherapy (1983: Milan, Italy)
   Porphyrins in tumor phototherapy.

   "Proceedings of the International Symposium on Porphyrins in Tumor Phototherapy,
held May 16–28, 1983, in Bruzzano, Milan, Italy"—T.p. verso.
   Includes bibliographical references and index.
   1. Photochemotherapy—Congresses. 2. Cancer—Radiotherapy—Congresses. 3. Por-
phyrin and porphyrin compounds—Therapeutic use—Congresses. 4. Hematopor-
phyrin—Therapeutic use—Congresses. 5. Laser coagulation—Congresses. I. Andreoni,
Alessandra. II. Cubeddu, Rinaldo. III. Title. [DNML: 1. Porphyrins—Therapeutic use—
Congresses. 2. Photochemotherapy—Congresses. 3. Neoplasms—Therapy—Congresses.
WB 480 I61p 1983]
RC271.P43I58 1983   616.99′40631   84-3371
ISBN 0-306-41630-1

Proceedings of the International Symposium on Porphyrins in Tumor
Phototherapy, held May 16–28, 1983, in Bruzzano, Milan, Italy

© 1984 Plenum Press, New York
A Division of Plenum Publishing Corporation
233 Spring Street, New York, N.Y. 10013

PREFACE

This book contains the contributions of the participants to
the International Symposium on Porphyrins in Tumor Phototherapy held
in Bruzzano (Milano), Italy on May 26-28, 1983.

The contributions are written as extended papers to provide a
broad and representative coverage of the use of porphyrins in tumor
phototherapy and diagnosis.

In the last few years, this technique has received increasing
interest for its potential applications in clinical oncology. In
fact, 1,500 patients have been already treated by this therapy which
has been tested in more than 100 clinical centres. Among the reported
cases, a significant therapeutic effectiveness was found in some early
stage cancers of lung, esophagus and stomach.

The development of this therapy requires interdisciplinary
studies from such diverse fields as physics, chemistry, biology,
pharmacology, and experimental and clinical oncology. The contents
of the book reflect the character of this research and deal with all
the problems, from fundamental to clinical, that still require to be
analysed and understood for a better evaluation of the potential of
this therapy.

The first chapter of the book deals with photophysics and
photochemistry of hematoporphyrin derivative and its components,
with the aim of defining the parameters for the best therapeutic
effectiveness. The interactions of porphyrins with model systems,
cellular structures and cells are examined in the second chapter with
reference to both the drug excitation and emission properties and
to the photosensitization mechanisms and targets. The subjects of
the third chapter are pharmacokinetics, characterization of the
photo-induced damage at the histological level, and evaluation of
the therapeutic effects on both transplanted and spontaneous animal
tumors. The fourth chapter is devoted to light dosimetry, instrumentation and fluorescent properties of hematoporphyrin derivative
in vivo for detection and characterization of tumors. In particular,
an apparatus for the localization of small lung tumors is described.

The last chapter reports on clinical experiences with both direct and endoscopic procedures. Applications of the therapy to bronchial, lung and gastrointestinal cancers, bladder carcinomas, and ocular tumors are discussed.

Many aspects of this complex subject area still need to be clarified: the selectivity of porphyrins for tumors, the best light delivery in tissues, and the mechanisms of tumor necrosis. This book, providing an updated review of the latest developments, hopefully will be a valuable aid to scientists working in this interdisciplinary field or intending to enter it.

We wish to thank the Technical Program Committee of the Symposium, the Centro di Elettronica Quantistica e Strumentazion Elettronica (Milano) and the Centro per le Emocianine ed altre Metalloporfirine (Padova) for supporting the organization of the meeting. We also acknowledge the cooperation and support of the following institutions:
Italian National Research Council (C.N.N.R.)
C.N.N.R. Special Project on High-Power Lasers: Medical Applications
Istituto Nazionale Tumori of Milano
Italian Society for Laser Surgery and Biomedical Applications
We are grateful to Coherent, Inc. for its sponsorship.

                                        Alessandra Andreoni

                                        Rinaldo Cubeddu

CONTENTS

Chapter 1

Physics and Chemistry of Porphyrins and Related Compounds

EXCITED STATE PROPERTIES OF HAEMATOPORPHYRIN

R. Brookfield[*], M. Craw[+], C.R. Lambert[+], E.J. Land[†],
R. Redmond[+], R.S. Sinclair[+], T.G. Truscott[+]

[*]Davy Faraday Laboratory, The Royal Institution, London
[+]Chemistry Dept., Paisley College, Paisley, Scotland
[†]Paterson Laboratories, The Christie Hospital and Holt
   Radium Institute, Manchester

INTRODUCTION

The active component of 'haematoporphyrin derivative ' (HpD)
is probably some aggregate involving both haematoporphyrin (Hp)
and hydroxyethylvinyldeuteroporphyrin (HVD) at least as far as
selective accumulation in tumours is concerned.   Subsequent
monomerisation in the cell could occur with the aggregate acting
as a 'pool' of Hp and HVD so that it is of interest to examine
the photophysical properties of such molecules in environments
where they may be expected to be monomers as well as in environments
where aggregation occurs.   In this paper we describe the photophysical properties of Hp in acetone, various detergents, methanol-
water mixtures, phosphate buffers and aqueous alkali as well as
preliminary results using phosphatidyl choline (PC) vesicles and
white blood cells.   The major part of the work concerns the study
of the lowest excited triplet state of Hp by laser flash photolysis
(347 nm excitation).   In some environments such excitation causes
monophotonic photo-ionisation so that both the radical cation and
anion of Hp can be produced

$$Hp \xrightarrow{h\nu} Hp^{\cdot +} + e^- \tag{1}$$

$$Hp + e \rightarrow Hp^{\cdot -} \tag{2}$$

and a minor aspect of the paper describes a study of such radical
ions using nano-second pulse radiolysis to generate the ions.   In
addition we also report preliminary studies on the first excited

3

singlet state of Hp in phosphate buffers using a time-resolved
fluorescence technique.

MATERIALS AND METHODS

Haematoporphyrin was obtained from Sigma and was recrystallised
from methanol before use.   Some results were compared with those
obtained using highly purified Hpα kindly supplied by Professor R.
Bonnett and were found to be similar.   The pulse radiolysis[+][1],
time resolved fluorescence[2] and laser flash photolysis[3] techniques
have been described previously.

For the determination of the triplet-singlet extinction
coefficient ($\Delta\varepsilon_T$) the so-called complete conversion method was used
in which the laser intensity is increased until there is no further
increase in the transient optical density obtained (ΔOD_T^{max}) - we
may then write

$$\Delta OD_T^{max} = \Delta\varepsilon_T \, C \, \ell \tag{3}$$

where ℓ is the path length (assumed to be 1 cm) and C is the
concentration of solute.   However if some of the haematoporphyrin
does not yield triplets (e.g. aggregated haematoporphyrin) the value
of $\Delta\varepsilon_T$ obtained will be too low.   Thus, for example, if we have a
relatively simple situation in which we have an equilibrium between
Hp which produces triplet states on excitation (monomer) and Hp which
does not yield the triplet state (such as aggregates) and half of the
Hp is aggregated then the $\Delta\varepsilon_T$ obtained will be only a half of the
value for the monomer.   Indeed the measurement of $\Delta\varepsilon_T$ may well give
a good indication of the degree of aggregation in the system.

Values of the quantum yield of triplet formation (Φ_T) were
obtained by a comparative technique[4] using anthracene as standard.
With both low laser intensities and low absorbance at the excitation
wavelength (347 nm) it can be shown that:-

$$\Phi_T^{Hp} = \Phi_T^S \cdot \frac{\Delta OD_T^{Hp}}{\Delta OD_T^S} \cdot \frac{\Delta\varepsilon_T^S}{\Delta\varepsilon_T^{Hp}} \cdot \frac{OD_g^S}{OD_g^{Hp}} \tag{4}$$

where Φ_T^S, ΔOD_T^S, $\Delta\varepsilon_T^S$ and OD_g^S are the triplet quantum yield, triplet-
singlet optical density, triplet-singlet extinction coefficient and
ground state optical density (at 347 nm) of the standard respectively
and OD_g^{Hp} is the ground state optical density of the Hp (at 347 nm)

[+] Pulse radiolysis of aqueous solutions generates both oxidising
    species (OH·) and reducing species (e⁻).   Chemical methods are
    used to selectively produce solute radical cations or anions.

which lead to triplets (monomer).   Clearly there are problems in
using this relationship since we do not have a value for $\Delta\varepsilon_T^{Hp}$ nor
for OD_g^{Hp}.   However, unlike for the determination of $\Delta\varepsilon_T^{Hp}$ the errors
tend to cancel out in the determination of Φ_T and for the simple
equilibrium situation described above depend only on the ratio of
the ground state extinction coefficients of the Hp monomer and
aggregate at the laser excitation wavelength (347 nm).   Indeed, for
the above example which shows an error of a factor of two in $\Delta\varepsilon_T^{Hp}$,
we estimate an error of only 20% in Φ_T^{Hp}

Table 1.   Triplet Decay Rate Constants (k_1) and Second-Order
Oxygen Quenching Rate Constants (k_Q) [a]

Environment	[Hp] μM	$10^4 k_1 (s^{-1})$ argon	$10^5 k_1 (s^{-1})$ air	$10^6 k_1 (s^{-1})$ oxygen	$10^9 k_Q$ ($M^{-1}s^{-1}$)
SDS (10^{-2}M)	[8]	3.2	6.1	2.4	2.0
(7×10^{-2} M)	[8]	3.0	4.8	2.7	1.8
TX-100 (3.3 mM)	[8]	1.2	3.9	1.2	1.4
(33 mM)	[8]	1.3	4.1	1.4	1.3
CTAB (1.5 mM)	[8]	3.4	3.9	–	1.3
(15 mM)	[8]	2.6	4.8	1.9	1.6
Liposome I	[5]	5.5	1.0	1.2	1.0
	[14]	3.6	–	1.7	1.2
Liposome II	[5]	6.0	0.9	1.4	1.0
	[14]	4.0	–	–	–
Phosphate buffer pH 7.4	[5]	2.5	4.1	–	1.4
	[8]	2.6	4.8	–	1.7
	[14]	2.8	4.4	–	1.5
90% Methanol 10% Water	[5]	1.9	–	65	1.4
	[11]	2.4	11.6	–	1.7
	[14]	2.1	9.5	–	1.5

[a] $[O_2]$ in air saturated methanol/water assumed to be 6.2×10^{-3}M.
In all other environments $[O_2]$ in air saturated system assumed
to be 2.7×10^{-4}M.

RESULTS AND DISCUSSION

We have previously reported the triplet-triplet spectra of several porphyrins including protoporphyrin, coproporphyrin, TPPS[*], and Hp[5,6,7]. Little or no difference is observed in the spectral shapes and we have now extended this to Hp in several environments including various concentrations of the detergents Triton X-100, CTAB and SDS as well as in methanol/water mixtures and acetone. In general very similar difference spectra are obtained with the minor changes being related to the changes in the ground state absorption spectra. We have also generated the radical ion spectra of Hp, Hp monoacetate, Hp diacetate, Hp disuccinate and Na$_4$TPPS and, at least in the range 450-750 nm, there is little difference in spectra obtained[6,7].

Table 1 reports the triplet decay first-order rate constants (k_1) in argon, air and oxygen saturated environments, together with the oxygen quenching second-order rate constants (k_Q). This latter parameter is only a rough estimate because the effect of detergent and liposome on oxygen concentration was ignored. Nevertheless the fact that variation in detergent concentrations had little or no effect on k_Q implies that any error in these values is small. In general we obtained k_Q values of $1-2 \times 10^9$ M^{-1}s^{-1} for all systems studied. Similar values in alcohol/water and formamide/water mixtures have been reported by Reddi et al[8]. These workers have also shown that in the detergent environments only about one-third of the triplets quenched by oxygen lead to the production of singlet ($^1\Delta$g) oxygen.

The $\Delta\varepsilon_T$ values obtained by the complete conversion technique are reported in Table 2. For the organic or mainly organic solvents the values obtained lie in the range 15,000-17,000 M^{-1}cm^{-1}. As the water content in the methanol/water system increases or in phosphate buffers (pH $\sim$ 7) we obtain substantially lower (concentration dependent) values for $\Delta\varepsilon_T$. We believe that in these mainly aqueous environments the Hp is extensively aggregated and that such aggregates yield little or no triplet, so that the complete conversion technique for determining $\Delta\varepsilon_T$ results in low values for the Hp monomer. In detergents it is generally accepted that Hp is monomeric and the $\Delta\varepsilon_T$ values we obtain are higher than in aqueous solvents although somewhat lower than in methanol and acetone. Poisson statistics imply significant multiple occupancy of micelles for Hp in 0.2% Triton X-100 so that the reduction in $\Delta\varepsilon_T$ for this system may be related to some Hp....Hp interaction within a micelle.

---

[*] tetrasodium salt of meso-tetraphenylporphyrin-tetrasulphuric acid.

Table 2.   Haematoporphyrin Triplet Extinctions

Environment	$\Delta\varepsilon_T$ (λ_{nm}) $M^{-1}cm^{-1}$
SDS $(10^{-2}M)$	10,700 (440)
$(7\times10^{-2}M)$	10,200 (440)
TX-100 (0.2%)	11,370 (440)
(2.0%)	14,600 (440)
CTAB (1.5 mM)	15,000 (440)
(15 mM)	14,100 (440)
Liposome I *	4123 (440)
Liposome II *	3800 (440)
Phosphate Buffer pH 7.4	8300 (420)
90% Methanol 10% Water	15,000 (440)
Acetone	17,250 (440)
White Blood Cells	$\sim$ 4000 (450)
Photofrin I in 1.5 mM CTAB	$\sim$ 12,000 (450)

* Phosphatidyl choline liposomes were prepared by the method of Suwa et al.[11] such that Hp was incorporated into the internal phase (Liposome I) or was in the external buffer (Liposome II).

As noted in Table 2 liposome I concerns an environment in which the Hp is incorporated in the phosphatidyl choline vesicle while liposome II refers to equivalent concentrations but with the Hp in the external buffer – both preparations being made without sonication as described by Grossweiner et al[9]. The values of $\Delta\varepsilon_T$ obtained ($\sim$ 4000 $M^{-1}cm^{-1}$) for both liposome environments imply a significant proportion of the Hp yield no triplet state, that is, much Hp in such vesicles is probably aggregated or at least interact to give no triplets. These results are in agreement with the conclusions drawn by Grossweiner et al. (1982) based on the mechanism of photosensitised lysis of the liposomes. Future work

Table 3.   Hp Triplet Optical Densities (ΔOD_T) as a Function of
                Alkali Concentration

$10^2 \, \Delta OD_T$	2.3	2.1	1.8	1.7	1.2
[NaOH] (M)	10^{-4}	10^{-3}	10^{-2}	10^{-1}	1.0

[Hp] was 10 µM

will extend our studies to sonicated liposome environments which
may lead to less aggregation of the Hp.   Table 2 also gives
preliminary data obtained for Hp (12 µM) in white blood cells (WBC)
and photofrin I in CTAB.   For the WBC environment we obtain $\Delta \varepsilon_T$
values which are the same as those in the liposomes, implying
significant aggregation or interaction of Hp in this environment
while for the therapeutically used drug photofrin I in CTAB our
values imply that the Hp (or Hp dimer) is not aggregated.   Future
work will concern studies of Photofrin I and II in various
environments including cells.

Table 3 reports the values of the ΔOD_T for Hp in various
aqueous alkali solutions.   Above 1M we observed degradation so the
data is limited to the range 10^{-4}-1M NaOH.   While these results
are incomplete because no determinations of $\Delta \varepsilon_T$ or Φ_T were made they
may imply increasing aggregation of Hp with increasing alkali
strength.   Since the preparation of HpD for therapeutic use
involves dissolution in 10^{-1}M NaOH as one of the steps and the
active component for cell-accumulation involves aggregates it may
well be worth investigating the value of higher alkali
concentrations for the preparation of HpD.

Time resolved fluorescence studies of Hp in different solvent
systems have been reported by Andreoni and co-workers[10].   In mainly
aqueous environments they report two exponential components in the
fluorescence decay which they relate to monomeric ($\sim$ 15 ns) and
dimeric ($\sim$ 3.8 ns) species.   We have also studied the Hp
fluorescence decay in phosphate buffer (see Table 4) and obtain a
similar result for the slow component as shown in Table 4 .   Our
preliminary data imply a somewhat faster decay ($\sim$ 1.7 ns) for the
second component which, at this stage, we cannot assign to
dimerisation or aggregation.   The relatively long singlet lifetime
for monomeric Hp implies that oxygen may increase the triplet yield
via enhanced intersystem crossing and we have studied the triplet
yield as a function of argon and air saturation of 90% methanol as

Table 4.   Fluorescence Decay Time Constants for Hp in Britton-
            Robinson Buffer at pH 7.0

[Hp]	τ_1
(μM)	(ns)
1.3	14.8
10.5	14.7
21	14.9

Buffer: 0.04M H_3PO_4 + 0.04M H_3BO_3 + 0.04M $CH_3.COOH$
           Made up with 0.2M NaOH to pH 7.0 (calibrated
           with standard phosphate buffer).

Table 5.   Typical Values of the Quantum Yield of Triplet
            Formation (Φ_T) for Haematoporphyrin[+] in various
            Solvent Environments

Environment[*]	Φ_T
90% Methanol, 10% Water (argon saturated)	0.8
90% Methanol, 10% Water	1.0
SDS (10^{-2}M)	0.9
TX-100 (3.3×10^{-2}M)	0.8
CTAB (1.5×10^{-2}M)	0.9
Acetone	1.0

[*] Air saturated except where stated

[+] 8 μM

the solvent.   Some typical results are given in Table 5.   These results may imply some benefit if the oxygen concentration could be increased in the in vivo situation.   Table 5 also gives other Φ_T values obtained in various environments (air saturated).   In general most values are near unity.

ACKNOWLEDGEMENTS

     We thank Dr. M.A.J. Rodgers for useful discussions and Dr. Reddi and co-workers for details of their pre-publication results. We are very grateful to Professor Bonnett for the supply of the highly purified Hpα.   The single-photon-counting apparatus for time-resolved fluorescence studies was kindly made available by Professor Sir George Porter.   RB, MC and RR wish to acknowledge the SERC for financial support and CRL thanks SED for a studentship. We also thank MRC for financial support.

REFERENCES

1. J.P. Keene, J. Sci. Instr. 41:493 (1964).
2. R.A. Lampert, L.A. Chewter, D. Phillips, D.V. O'Connor, A.J. Robert, and S.R. Meech, Anal. Chem. 55:68 (1983).
3. J. McVie, R.S. Sinclair, and T.G. Truscott, J. Chem. Soc. Faraday Trans. II 74:1870 (1978).
4. R. Bensasson, C.R. Goldschmidt, E.J. Land, and T.G. Truscott, Laser intensity and the comparative method for determination of triplet quantum yields, Photochem. Photobiol. 28:277 (1978).
5. R. Bonnett, A.A. Charalambides, E.J. Land, and R.S. Sinclair, J. Chem. Soc. Faraday I 76:852 (1980).
6. R. Bonnett, R.J. Ridge, E.J. Land, R.S. Sinclair, D. Tait, and T.G. Truscott, J. Chem. Soc. Faraday I 78:127 (1982).
7. R. Bonnett, C. Lambert, E.J. Land, P.A. Scourides, R.S. Sinclair, and T.G. Truscott, Photochem. Photobiol. in press.
8. E. Reddi, G. Jori, M.A.J. Rodgers, and J.P. Spikes, Flash photolysis studies of hemato-and copro-porphyrins in homogeneous and microheterogeneous aqueous dispersions, Photochem. Photobiol. in press.
9. L.I. Grossweiner, A.S. Patel, and J.B. Grossweiner, Type I and type II mechanisms in the photosensitized lysis of phosphatidylcholine liposomes by Hematoporphyrin, Photochem. Photobiol. 36:159 (1982).
10. A.Andreoni, R. Cubeddu, S. De Silvestri, G. Jori, P. Laporta and E. Reddi, Time-resolved fluorescence studies of Hematoporphyrin in different solvent systems, Z. Naturforsch. 38c:83 (1983).
11. K. Surya, T. Kimura, and A.P. Suwa, Reactivity of singlet molecular oxygen with cholesterol in a phospholipid membrane matrix. A model for oxidative damage of membranes, Biochim. Biophys. Res. Commun. 75:785 (1977).

FLUORESCENCE PROPERTIES OF HpD AND ITS COMPONENTS

Alessandra Andreoni and Rinaldo Cubeddu

Centro Elettronica Quantistica e Strumentazione
Elettronica del C.N.R., Istituto di Fisica del Politecnico
Milano, Italy

INTRODUCTION

Hematoporphyrin (Hp) and related compounds, in particular Hematoporphyrin Derivative (HpD), are increasingly used in tumor phototherapy. HpD was shown to differ respect to Hp for a higher percentage of non-fluorescent aggregated species when dissolved in
aqueous solutions[1]. Moreover these species, which can be separated,
for example, by gel filtration from HpD, have been shown to have a
higher therapeutic activity[2].

The emission properties of porphyrins have been characterized
in view of their possible use in tumor diagnosis. However, it was
recently reported the existence "in vivo" of a new emission band
peaked at 580 nm [3]. This band was detected by observing the fluorescence excited at 405 nm of a solid tumor in a mouse that was
previously injected intravenously with HpD. Afterwards the same
band was found for Hp in buffer solutions[4], for HpD in physiological
anoxic solutions[5], and in cells after incubation with HpD [6]. On the
basis of these findings, the formation of this new band seems to be
important in the mechanisms of uptake and retention of HpD components.

In this paper we describe the emission properties under both
cw and pulsed excitation in aqueous solutions of various HpD components that differ in the amount of stable aggregated species and
in their therapeutic activity. The results show that the formation
of the 580 nm band requires the presence of both monomers and stable
aggregates and is irreversible. Furthermore it presents the following properties: (i) its shape follows that of Hp but is shifted of
about 35 nm to the blue, (ii) the excitation spectrum is peaked at

11

405 nm, (iii) the fluorescence decay time constant is ∿ 2.6 ns.
The comparison of these features with the emission properties of Hp
indicates the existence of a new molecular species, possibly orig-
inating from a binding of monomers to polymeric porphyrins.

EXPERIMENTAL

The following substances were investigated: (i) Hematoporphyrin
(Hp), (ii) Hematoporphyrin Derivative (HpD), (iii) the most aggregated fraction (GF) obtained by polyacrilamide gel filtration with Bio-
-Gel P-10 and (iv) Photofrin II (PII). Hematoporphyrin, free base,
from Porphyrin Products (Logan, Utah, USA), was dissolved and characterized as described elsewhere[7]. HpD is the substance marketed
by Oncology Research and Development (Cheektowaga, N.Y., USA) as
Photofrin. The fraction GF was kindly provided by Dr. F. Zunino
(Istituto Nazionale Tumori, Milano, Italy) who measured also the
w/v (weight to volume) concentration of the samples. Finally, Photofrin II was obtained from Oncology Research and Development.
Being the chemical composition of most substances undetermined, all
solutions to be investigated were made at the w/v concentration of
1.25 $\mu g/cm^3$ in water.

The absorption spectra were taken by a Perkin-Elmer 554 UV-VIS
spectrophotometer with 2 nm-slit using matched quartz cuvettes of
1 cm optical pathway. The emission and excitation spectra were measured by a Perkin-Elmer 650-40 spectrofluorometer with 5 nm-slits in
both the excitation and observation monochromators. Both emission
and excitation spectra were not corrected for either the lamp spectrum, nor monochromator and photomultiplier responses.

The excitation source for the time-resolved fluorescence was
a dye laser pumped by an atmospheric-pressure nitrogen laser[8]. A
10^{-3} M solution of α-NPO [2-(1-Naphthyl)-5 phenyloxazole] in ethanol
was used as the lasing medium. The laser could be tuned either at
395 nm or at 405 nm as required during the experiments. The dye
laser provided pulses of 150 ps duration (FWHM, full width at half
maximum) with peak power of ∿ 50 KW at a repetition rate of up to
100 Hz. The solutions to be measured were contained in a 1 cm^2
cross-section cell and their emission was observed at 90° through
either a Kodak Written nr. 22 cut-off filter or Corion SS 580-00 or
Karl Zeiss IF 615 interference filters. The single-photon timing
technique was used for the measurements of fluorescence lifetimes.
The fluorescence was detected by a single-photon semiconductor photodiode operating in non-proportional avalanche multiplication.
The detector had a junction area of ∿ 50 μm diameter, with uniform
breakdown over it, and was biased above the breakdown voltage. The
avalanche quenching necessary for generating single-photon pulses
was obtained using an active-quenching method that allows the detector to be operated with well controlled parameters and deadtimes

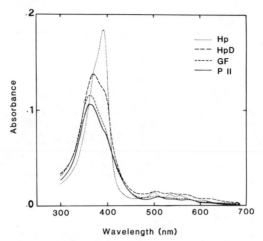

Fig. 1.   Absorption spectra of fresh solutions of Hp, HpD, GF and
          PII (1.25 μg/ml in water).

of less than 20 ns. A time-to-pulse-height converter and a multi-
channel pulse-height analyzer (MCA) were used to measured the delay
distribution of detected single photons with respect to reference
start pulses, synchronized with the laser pulses. The start pulses
were obtained by using a beam splitter and a Hp 4220 photodiode,
associated to fast electronic circuitry. The full-width at half-
-maximum (FWHM) response of the detection apparatus was ∿ 70 ps [9].
The experimental data were then transferred from the MCA memory to
a Tektronix 4051 graphic system for processing and plotting.

RESULTS AND DISCUSSION

     The absorption spectra of fresh solutions of Hp, HpD, GF and
PII are shown in Fig. 1. They are indicative of different degrees
of aggregation of the four substances. In fact, while the absorption peak for Hp is at 395 nm (i.e. the monomer absorption peak[10]),
the spectrum for HpD and, more markedly, those for GF and PII show
an increase in absorption at 365 nm (i.e. the aggregate absorption
peak[10]). This difference in the degree of aggregation of the four
solutions is confirmed by the emission spectra in Fig. 2 that were
taken under excitation at 405 nm, where the solutions present similar values of absorbance. In fact, the lower fluorescence intensity, which is found, for instance, for PII as compared with Hp (by
a factor of ∿ 9), accounts for the large amount of non-fluorescent
aggregated species present in the former substance[1,10,11]. All the
spectra in Fig. 2 exhibit the classical Hp fluorescence with dis-

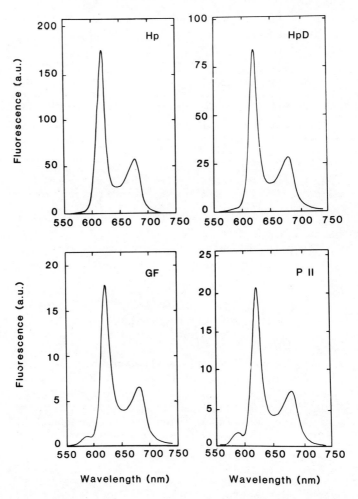

Fig. 2. Emission spectra of 1.25 µg/ml water solutions of Hp, HpD, GF and PII under excitation at 405 nm.

tinct major peaks at 615 nm and 675 nm. Furthermore a minor peak at 580 nm is barely visible in the spectra of both GF and PII solutions.

For a more complete characterization of the emission properties, the time-resolved fluorescence of the four solutions was measured through cut-off filters (> 565 nm) under pulsed excitation at 405 nm.

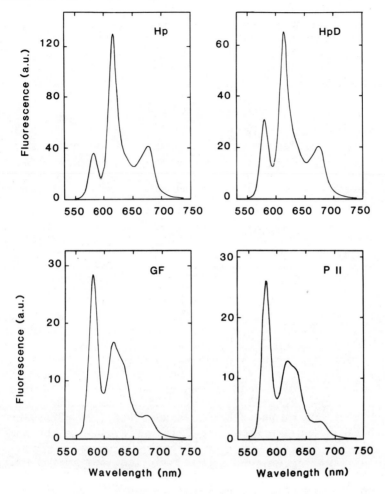

Fig. 3. Emission spectra of 1.25 μg/ml water solutions of Hp, HpD,
         GF and PII after 48 hours incubation at 37°C under exci-
         tation at 405 nm.

All experimental decay curves could be fitted by two exponential
components whose time constants and relative amplitudes are listed
in Table 1. While the time constants are almost the same, the relative amplitude of the fast component increases from Hp to PII, for
which a value of 25.9% is found.

    In order to simulate the temperature conditions in which the
580 nm band was reported to occur "in vivo" or "in vitro" [3-6], the

Table 1. Fluorescence Decay Time Constants (τ_1 and τ_2) and Relative
          Amplitudes (A_1 and A_2) for 1.25 μg/ml Fresh Solutions of
          Hp, HpD, GF and PII under Excitation at 405 nm and Observ-
          ed at λ > 565 nm.

	τ_1 (ns)	A_1 (%)	τ_2 (ns)	A_2 (%)
Hp	14.43	88.7	2.98	11.3
HpD	14.45	79.6	2.93	20.4
GF	14.18	76.4	3.10	23.6
PII	14.04	64.1	3.10	25.9

same solutions were kept at 37°C in the dark for 48 hours. Figure
3 shows the resulting emission spectra measured at room temperature
after the incubation period and excited at 405 nm. It can be seen
that the 580 nm peak is greatly increased at the expenses of the
two other peaks (at 615 nm and 675 nm) particularly for GF and PII.
Furthermore, the growing of the 580 nm fluorescence is associated
with that of a secondary peak around 635 nm. For all solutions the
excitation spectra of the 580 nm- and 615 nm- emissions were found
to be peaked at 405 nm and 395 nm, respectively, in agreement with
other authors[4,5] and are shown for PII in Fig. 4. In the same figure the emission spectra, excited at both 405 nm and 395 nm, are
also reported for comparison. These modifications in the emission
spectra were found not only to be irreversible but also to proceed
slowly even at room temperature. For instance, starting from the
situation depicted in Fig. 3, the GF and PII solutions after a few
days at room temperature in the dark presented a complete disappear-
ance of the 615 nm and 675 nm bands. Figure 5 shows the excitation
spectrum of the 580 nm fluorescence for an aged PII solution super-
imposed to its absorption spectrum. Since the two spectra are almost coincident, a single modified molecular species must be present
in this solution.

The experimental results seem to suggest that two different
molecular species contribute to the spectra in Fig. 3, one being
responsible for the classical emission (with peaks of 615 nm and
675 nm) and the other for the shifted emission (with peaks at 580 nm
and 635 nm). The data obtained from the time-resolved measurements
give further support to this interpretation. The fitting parameters
of the experimental fluorescence decays for the PII solution incubated 48 h at 37°C under excitation at 405 nm and 395 nm are summa-

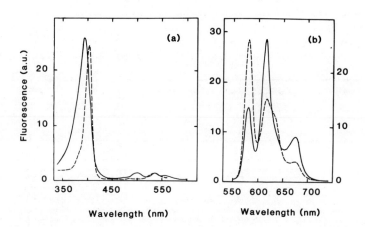

Fig. 4.   Excitation (a) and emission (b) spectra of 1.25 µg/ml water
          solution of PII after 48 hours incubation at 37°C.
          (a): observation at 580 nm (– – – –) and 615 nm (———) ;
          (b): excitation at 405 nm (– – – –, left vertical scale) and
          395 nm (———— , right vertical scale).

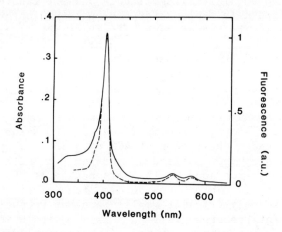

Fig. 5.   Absorption spectrum (———— , left vertical scale) and
          excitation spectrum (– – – – , right vertical scale) observed
          at 580 nm of an aged 1.25 µg/ml aqueous solution of PII.

Table 2.   Fluorescence Decay Time Constants (τ_1 and τ_2) and Relative
Amplitudes (A_1 and A_2) for a 1.25 µg/ml Water Solution of
PII after 48 Hours Incubation at 37°C.

Excitation	Observation	τ_1 (ns)	A_1 (%)	τ_2 (ns)	A_2 (%)
	λ > 565 nm	14.71	11.3	2.58	88.7
405 nm	IF 580	–	–	2.51	100.0
	IF 615	14.56	17.6	2.66	82.4
	λ > 565 nm	14.86	28.7	2.75	71.3
395 nm	IF 580	–	–	2.48	100.0
	IF 615	14.80	37.9	2.74	62.1

rized in Table 2.   The relative amplitudes of the two components
depend on both the excitation and the emission wavelengths.   In particular, under excitation at 405 nm, only the fast component is observed at 580 nm, while the maximum relative amplitude of the slow
component is found for excitation at 395 nm and observation at
615 nm.   Note that the relative intensities of the peaks at 580 nm
and 615 nm in Fig. 4, being measured under cw excitation, are proportional to both the initial amplitudes and the fluorescence decay-
time values reported in Table 2 for the spectrum-integrated measurements.   It is possible therefore to attribute the fluorescence-decay
time constant of $\sim$ 2.6 ns to the molecular species emitting at 580 nm
and the time constant of $\sim$ 14 ns to the monomeric form of Hematoporphyrin.   These attributions are confirmed by the measurements on a
fresh Hp solution where, observing the emission at 615 nm, a single slow
decay of 14.29 ns was found and that on the aged PII solution where
only the fast decay component could be observed, as reported in
Table 3.   Figure 6 shows, for comparison, the emission spectra of
these solutions under excitation at 405 nm.   The two spectra are
very similar in shape but shifted of $\sim$ 35 nm.   A shift was also
found in the absorption spectra that are peaked at 395 nm and
405 nm, respectively.   This behaviour is often observed when a dye
molecule binds to polymeric materials[12] and was recently reported,
in particular, for Uroporphyrin I[13].   This molecule in pH 7.4 buffer solution, where it exists entirely in monomeric form, has the absorption peak at approximately 389 nm, while that for Uroporphyrin
covalently bound to amino-terminal agarose gel shifts to approximately 402 nm.   According to this behaviour, our results suggest

Table 3. Fluorescence Decay Time Constants (τ_1 and τ_2) and Relative Amplitudes (A_1 and A_2) for 1.25 µg/ml Water Solutions of Fresh Hp and Aged PII under Excitation at 405 nm.

		τ_1 (ns)	A_1 (%)	τ_2 (ns)	A_2 (%)
fresh Hp	$\lambda > 565$ nm	14.43	88.7	2.98	11.3
	IF 580	NM [a]	–	NM	–
	IF 615	14.29	100.0	–	–
aged PII	$\lambda > 565$ nm	–	–	2.61	100.0
	IF 580	–	–	2.41	100.0
	IF 615	–	–	2.57	100.0

[a] NM: not measurable

that the species emitting at 580 nm originate from monomers chemically bound to polymeric structures of porphyrins. In fact GF and PII, which have been reported to contain the highest percentages of aggregates very stable in aqueous solutions[11], resulted to exhibit the fastest growing of the 580 nm band. Also the presence of a certain amount of monomers turned out to be required to produce this species. This can be argued from the absorption spectrum of the aged PII solution in Fig. 5 that shows the behaviour typical of a monomeric solution compared with that in Fig. 1 of the corresponding fresh solution. Furthermore, we have found that an increase in the porphyrin concentration, which decreases the relative amount of monomers, slowed and limited its formation. A similar result was also reported for HpD in physiological solution[14]. This is also in agreement with the enhancement of the 580 nm emission obtained for the solutions incubated at 37°C. In fact, temperatures above 35°C were found to produce a conversion of aggregates due to hydrofobic interaction to monomers in Hp buffer solutions[10].

The experimental data indicate that the formation of the 580 nm band is favoured in solutions of porphyrins with the highest therapeutic efficiency. The similarity between our results and the HpD fluorescence changes reported to occur both "in vitro" and "in vivo", suggest that a binding of monomers to aggregates or other polymeric structures may also happen in cells following the drug uptake process.

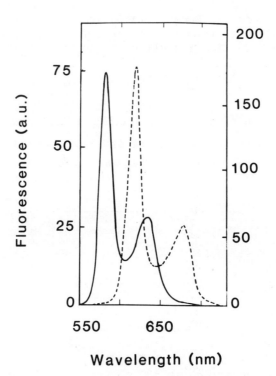

Fig. 6.   Emission spectra of an aged PII solution (———, left ver-
          tical scale) and a fresh Hp solution (- - - - , right verti-
          cal scale) under excitation at 405 nm. The concentration
          is 1.25 µg/ml in water.

REFERENCES

1. A. Andreoni, R. Cubeddu, S. De Silvestri, P. Laporta, G. Jori,
    and E. Reddi, Hematoporphyrin Derivative: experimental evi-
    dence for aggregated species, Chem. Phys. Lett. 88:33 (1982).
2. T. J. Dougherty, D. G. Boyle, K. R. Weishaupt, B. A. Henderson,
    W. R. Potter, D. A. Bellnier, and K. E. Wityk, Photoradia-
    tion therapy; clinical and drug advances, in: "Porphyrin
    Photosensitization", D. Kessel and T. J. Dougherty, eds.,
    Plenum Press, New York-London (1983).
3. A. J. M. van der Putten, and M. J. C. van Gemert, Hematopor-
    phyrin Derivative fluorescence spectra "in vitro" and in
    animal tumor, in: "Proceedings of Laser '81 Opto-Electronik,
    München, West Germany" (1981).

4. A. Pasqua, A. Poletti, and S. M. Murgia, Ultrafiltration tech-
    nique as a tool for the investigation of Hematoporphyrin ag-
    gregates in aqueous solutions, Biol. Med. Environm. 10:287
    (1982).
5. F. Docchio, R. Ramponi, C. A. Sacchi, G. Bottiroli, and I.
    Freitas, Fluorescence studies of biological molecules by
    laser irradiation, in: "New Frontiers in Laser Medicine and
    Surgery", K. Atsumi, ed., Excerpta Medica, Amsterdam-Oxford-
    -Princeton (1983)
6. M. W. Berns, M. Wilson, P. Rentzepis, R. Burns, and A. Wile,
    Cell biology and Hematoporphyrin Derivative (HpD), Lasers
    in Surgery and Medicine 2:261 (1983).
7. S. Cannistraro, G. Jori, and A. Van de Vorst, Photosensitiza-
    tion of amino acids by di-cyan-hemin: kinetic and EPR stud-
    ies, Photochem. Photobiol. 27:517 (1978).
8. R. Cubeddu, S. De Silvestri, and O. Svelto, Subnanosecond am-
    plified spontaneous emission pulses by a nitrogen-pumped
    dye laser, Opt. Commun. 34:460 (1980).
9. S. Cova, A. Longoni, A. Andreoni, and R. Cubeddu, A semicon-
    ductor detector for measuring ultraweak fluorescence decays
    with 70 ps FWHM resolution, IEEE J. Quantum Electron. QE-19:
    :630 (1983).
10. A. Andreoni, R. Cubeddu, S. De Silvestri, G. Jori, P. Laporta,
    and E. Reddi, Time-resolved fluorescence studies of Hemato-
    porphyrin in different solvent systems, Z. Naturforsch.
    38c:83 (1983).
11. T. J. Dougherty, W. R. Potter, and K. R. Weishaupt, The struc-
    ture of the active component of Hematoporphyrin Derivative,
    in: "Porphyrins in Tumor Phototherapy", A. Andreoni and R.
    Cubeddu, eds., Plenum Press, New York-London (1983).
12. J. S. Bellin, Photophysical and photochemical effects of dye
    binding, Photochem. Photobiol. 8:383 (1968).
13. J. D. Spikes, B.F. Burnham, and J. C. Bonner, Photosensitizing
    properties of free and bound Uroporphyrin I, in: "Porphy-
    rins in Tumor Phototherapy", A. Andreoni and R. Cubeddu,
    eds., Plenum Press, New York-London (1983).
14. G. Bottiroli, I. Freitas, F. Docchio, R. Ramponi, and C. A.
    Sacchi, The time-dependent behaviour of Hematoporphyrin
    Derivative in saline: a study of spectral modifications,
    to be published.

THE STRUCTURE OF THE ACTIVE COMPONENT OF HEMATOPORPHYRIN DERIVATIVE

T. J. Dougherty, W. R. Potter and K. R, Weishaupt*

Roswell Park Memorial Institute, *Oncology Research and Development
Buffalo, New York; *Cheektowaga, New York

INTRODUCTION

Photoradiation therapy (PRT) for local treatment of malignant tumors utilizing hematoporphyrin derivative (Hpd) as photosensitizing drug is undergoing clinical trials in several centers in the U. S. and abroad. This therapy is based on the localization and retention of Hpd in most tumors, as well as its photodynamic action which likely generates singlet oxygen at least as a first step. The only drug toxicity encountered to date in over 1500 patients receiving Hpd has been a generalized photosensitivity which requires patients to avoid bright light, especially sunlight, for 30 days or more. While this toxicity is avoidable it presents a drawback to utilizing PRT for early stage disease in ambulatory and active patients.

Hpd is known to be a mixture of porphyrins first prepared by Schwartz by the mixture formed by acetic acid–sulfuric acid treatment of hematoporphyrin (Lipson, 1960). Several known porphyrins have been identified in this hydrolysis mixture, namely hematoporphyrin (Hp), hydroxyethylvinyldeuteroporphyrin (HVD), and protoporphyrin (proto). In addition, several investigators have noted an additional porphyrin of unknown structure found to be the material primarily responsible for photosensitizing activity of the Hpd mixture both in vitro and in vivo (Moan and Sommers, 1981; Berenbaum, et al., 1982; Kessel and Chow, 1983). In 1981 we described a gel filtration procedure to isolate this material in relatively pure form and showed that it was the component of Hpd solely responsible for in vivo photosensitization (Dougherty, et al., 1983). We now report the structure of this material.

23

MATERIALS AND METHODS

Hematoporphyrin derivative (Hpd) under the trade name, Photofrin, was obtained from Oncology Research and Development, Inc.,
Cheektowaga, New York. This material is supplied as 5.0 mg/ml in
sterile saline at pH 7.2-7.4.

The Hpd solution was applied directly to a gel filtration
column (Bio-Gel P-10, 100-200 mesh, Bio-Rad, Richmond, California)
using distilled water (pH 7-8) as eluent. As previously described,
this allowed the separation of a dark brown colored aggregate fraction
(Fraction A) which eluted at the exclusion limit of the column well
separated from the other fractions (Dougherty, et al., 1983). This
same material was also purchased from Oncology Research and Development, Inc. under the trade name, Photofrin II, supplied in sterile
saline, 2.5 mg/ml, pH 7.2-7.4. This material was identical to that
separated by gel filtration by visible spectrometry, HPLC (see
below) and biologic activity (see below). Its purity ranged from
80 to 90% with hydroxyethylvinyldeuteroporphyrin as the major contaminant. The methyl esters of the porphyrins were obtained by treating
the free base forms (isolated from solution by adjusting the pH to
3.5) in tetrahydrofuran ethyl ether with diazomethane at ice bath
temperature. Diazomethane was generated from N-Methyl-N'-nitro-N-
nitrosoquanidine obtained from Aldrich Chemical Co., Inc., Milwaukee,
Wisconsin.

High performance liquid chromatography (HPLC) was carried out
using a reverse phase column (Altex Model 110 ultrasphere, 4.6 x
150 mm) with Constametric pump (the Anspec Co., Inc., Ann Arbor,
Michigan) and visible light detection at 405 nm (AN-203 detector,
the Anspec Co.). The eluent consisted of two solvent systems; A,
containing equal volumes of water, tetrahydrofuran and methanol and
pH adjusted to 5.7-5.8 with acetic acid and 1 N sodium hydroxide
solution and B, tetrahydrofuran, water (9:1 by volume). Samples were
injected into the column (20 µl) either in aqueous solutions or in
solvent A. Solvent A was run at 1 ml/min for 20-30 min and then
solvent B was run at the same rate until no additional peaks eluted
(approximately 10 min). Under these conditions, Hp, the two HVD
structural isomers, and proto, were eluted at approximately 2.2 min,
4.4 min, 5.2 min and 18-20 min respectively. The final material was
eluted at approximately 5 min after changing to solvent B. The corresponding dimethyl esters eluted with the same pattern, each peak
being eluted slightly later than the free base forms. The fraction
eluted by solvent B corresponded to Fraction A isolated from Hpd by
gel filtration described above. These HPLC conditions were chosen
since none of the known porphyrins were aggregated in solvent A
(determined spectrophotometrically). However, Fraction A remained
largely aggregated in solvent A (Soret absorption ∼ 365 nm) and was
not eluted until solvent B was used in which it was primarily dis-
aggregated (Soret absorption ∼ 400 nm).

The relative proportions of each material eluted by HPLC was determined by measuring the area under the curves and correcting for relative absorption at 405 nm; Hp, HVD and proto absorption at 405 nm was determined in solvent A and that for Photofrin II or Fraction A (gel fractionation) in solvent B. Hp, HVD and proto were identified by correspondence of elution time, HPLC and thin layer chromatography (silicon plates, 80/20/1.5, benzene, methanol, water) compared to authentic samples. Hp and HVD were obtained from Porphyrin Products, Logan, Utah, and proto from Fluka, AG (Germany).

Nuclear magnetic resonance spectroscopy (^{13}C) was carried out at 25.2 MHz by the NIH facility at Syracuse University, Syracuse, New York. Proton magnetic response were obtained at 200 MHz by the NIH facility at Carnegie-Mellon Institute in Pittsburgh, Pennsylvania. Fast atom bombardment mass spectrometry was carried out by the NIH facility at Johns Hopkins University, Baltimore, Maryland.

RESULTS

The visible spectrum of Fraction A showed a typical non-metallic porphyrin pattern (etio type) in water or organic solvents. In water absorption occurs at 620 nm<570 nm<535 nm <500 nm <<365 nm (Soret).

Hydrolysis of Fraction A

Acid: A 2 ml sample of Fraction A (or Photofrin II) (2.5 mg/ml) was mixed with 2 ml of 1 N hydrochloric acid, protected from light, and kept at room temperature. A similar sample was kept at 37°, and a third was heated in a water bath at approximately 80° under nitrogen. All samples produced a similar mixture of products although at different rates. Forty minutes at 80° C was sufficient to hydrolyze all of the porphyrin and produce a mixture of equal parts of Hp and HVD, determined by HPLC following neutralization. The same proportions of Hp and HVD were produced at 37° and room temperature although the latter required approximately 2 to 3 weeks for completion. Conversion of HVD to Hp or vice versa was insignificant in this time period for all three conditions (separate experiments with Hp and HVD were carried out as above). Similar treatment of protoporphyrin produced a small amount (10-20%) of HVD and a trace of Hp (<10%).

Base: Two ml portions of Fraction A (2.5 mg/ml) were dissolved in 2 ml 1 N sodium hydroxide solution, protected from the light and stored at room temperature. The sample was periodically analyzed by HPLC (after neutralization) over a period of four weeks. No changes were detected.

Neutral Hydrolysis: A sample of Fraction A (2.5 mg/ml) pH 7.2-7.4 was heated at 120° for 15 min in an autoclave. This sample

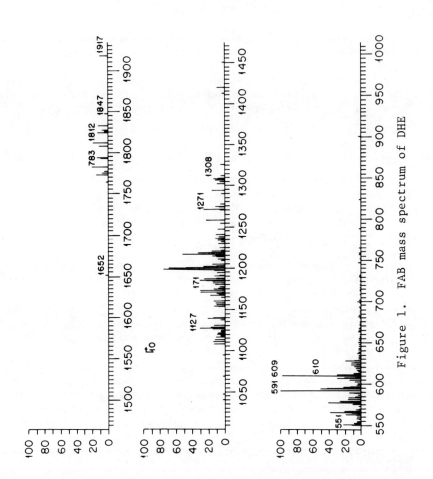

Figure 1. FAB mass spectrum of DHE

produced small amounts of Hp and HVD but appeared not to undergo hydrolysis. Attempts to subsequently hydrolyze this sample in acid as above indicated that it was essentially insoluble in 1 N hydrochloric acid whereas prior to this procedure it had been completely soluble.

Fast Atom Bombardment (FAB) Mass Spectrometry

Figure 1 demonstrates a typical spectrum obtained from the methyl ester of Fraction A. The major peaks at 591 and 609 mass numbers correspond to the dimethyl esters of protoporphyrin and HVD respectively and are present in approximately equal amounts. A small amount of Hp dimethyl ester appears at a mass number of 627. In the higher mass range the major peaks at 1199 and 1200 mass numbers represent 7-8% of the base peaks (591, 609). Numerous other high mass peaks are also apparent. Many of the smaller mass peaks (e.g. 149, 181) correspond to the thioglycerol in which the sample was mixed for the spectral analysis. The free base form of Fraction A yielded essentially the same pattern, but all peaks were markedly less intense than those of the methyl ester. Essentially no mass peaks above HVD and proto were observed in the free base spectrum.

NMR Spectra

^{13}C: The methyl ester of Fraction A was dissolved in deuterated chloroform (50 mg/ml) for ^{13}C-NMR spectroscopy (Figure 2). The ^{13}C-NMR spectrum of the dimethyl ester of Hp was obtained in a similar way for comparison. Peaks were identified as follows (δ, ppm, referred to tetramethylsilane); 11.48, CH3, 21.7, - CH2 CH2 CO2 CH3, 25.9, CH3 CHOH, 27.9, CH3-CHO-, 36.8, - CH2 CH2 CO2 CH3, 51.7, CH2 CH2 CO2 CH3, 65.3, CH3 CHOH, 68.4, CH3 CH O-, 94 to 100 methine carbons, 132 to 150 pyrrole carbons, and 173.6, -CH2 CH2 CO2 CH3. Chloroform appears at δ = 77 and its inverted image near 124. The small peaks at 121 ppm and 131 ppm may be assigned to -CH = CH2 and are likely due to HVD and proto impurity which accounted for approximately 15% of the sample. Except for the carbons at 27.9 and 68.4, the same absorbances were found in Hp dimethyl ester. The relative proportions, however, were different for the hydroxyethyl groups at 25.9 and 65.3 ppm in Fraction A compared to Hp which represent only one group per porphyrin moiety (e.g. per four methine carbons). The peaks at 27.9 and 68.4 ppm appear to have the same relative areas as those assigned to the hydroxyethyl groups. Because of an apparent wide difference in relaxation times the proportions of each type of carbon atom are difficult to establish with accuracy. In order to improve the situation, a 10 second delay was used between the accumulated scans. Under these conditions the ratio of areas was 4:2:1:1:2:2:1:1:3:9:2 in increasing ppm. Clearly the ratio of methine to pyrrole carbons should be 4:16, not 3:9 as found. Thus, even with a long delay between scans, ratios were inexact. When similar spectra were attempted with the free base form of Fraction A in DMSO-d_6, the

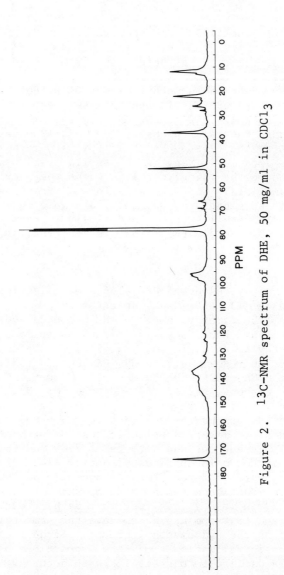

Figure 2.   13C-NMR spectrum of DHE, 50 mg/ml in CDCl$_3$

peaks at 27.9 and 68.4 ppm were not apparent. The spectrum between 60 and 70 ppm was scanned with a 30 sec delay indicating that the absorbances at 65.3 and 68.4 ppm were of approximately equal areas.

^{1}H-NMR: Proton NMR spectra were complicated by the inability to obtain samples completely free of water which obscured the spectra from 3–4 ppm. The spectrum of the methyl ester of Fraction A in deuterated chloroform, however, revealed multiple peaks in the range of 1.85 to 2.36 ppm (major peaks appeared at 1.85 ppm, broad, 2.05, 2.2, 2.28 and 2.36 ppm, sharp). These absorbances were not discernable in the spectrum of the free base in DMSO-d_6 (30 μg/ml) which showed a single small peak at 2.16 ppm. Hematoporphyrin free base under the same conditions provided the expected spectrum with a sharp doublet at 2.13 and 2.17 ppm attributed to the methyl protons of the hydroxyethyl groups. Other absorbances apparent in the proton NMR spectra of Fraction A free base were found at approximately –4 ppm, broad, N–H, 3.8 ppm, multiplet, aromatic CH$_3$, 4.3 ppm, broad, –$\underline{CH_2}$ CH$_2$ CO$_2$H, 6.2–6.5, broad doublet, CH$_3$ $\underline{CH}$OH and CH$_3$ $\underline{CH}$O – and possibly –CH = $\underline{CH_2}$, 10.2 to 10.8 ppm, broad multiplet, methine protons and 12.2 ppm CO$_2$ $\underline{H}$. The CO$_2$ $\underline{H}$, methine, CH$_3$ $\underline{CH}$OH, and CH$_3$ CH–O– (combined) and –$\underline{CH_2}$ CH$_2$ CO$_2$ $\underline{H}$ protons were in ratio of 1:2:1:2.

Effect of Concentration on Formation of Fraction A

The usual procedure for basic hydrolysis of the acetate mixture resulting from reaction of Hp with acetic acid–sulfuric acid to produce the Hpd product mixture requires a 1 h reaction at room temperature of one part acetate mixture to 50 parts 0.1 N sodium hydroxide. This produces a mixture of porphyrins containing 40–50% Fraction A (Dougherty, et al., 1983). However, we have found that if the hydrolysis was carried out with a lower concentration of acetate in the alkaline solution, the proportion of Fraction A in the final product mixture decreased to essentially zero, when the proportion of acetate mixture to 0.1 N sodium hydroxide was 1:2500. Under these conditions the only detectable products by HPLC were Hp and HVD in ratio of approximately 2:1. Elemental analysis of Fraction A in either free base form or as the sodium salt yielded varying results because of the inability to remove all the water. We estimate that even after drying, the sample contained 5–7% water. The carbon to nitrogen ratio was found to be 7.38:1 by weight.

DISCUSSION

The structure(s) most consistent with these data are those of the ether(s) formed by linkage through the hydroxyethylvinyl groups of hematoporphyrin, Figure 3. Since there are three different ways to link the molecules, i.e. the hydroxyl groups on the two 8-, the two 3- or one 8- and one 3-hydroxyethylvinyl groups, three structural isomers are possible, each with four chiral centers. The three

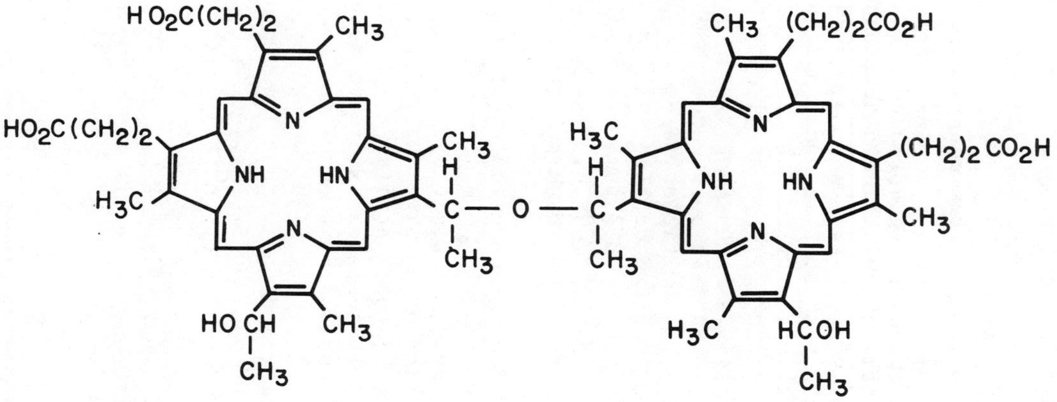

Bis-1-[8-((1-hydroxyethyl) deuteroporphyrin-3-yl] ethyl ether

Figure 3. Structure of Hpd-Active Component.

structural isomers are: bis-1-[3-(1-hydroxyethyl)-deuteroporphyrin-8-yl] ethyl ether, bis-1-[8-(1-hydroxyethyl)-deuteroporphyrin-3-yl] ethyl ether and 1-[3-(1-hydroxyethyl)-deuteroporphyrin-8-yl]-1'-[8-(1-hydroxyethyl)-deuteroporphyrin-3-yl] ethyl ether. We propose the common name dihematoporphyrin ether (DHE).

The decrease in formation of Fraction A with decreasing concentrations of acetate during hydrolysis is consistent with a bimolecular reaction involving the porphyrin acetates and/or intermediate hydrolysis products. It may indicate the necessity of a pre-formed non-covalent dimer properly aligned to allow for the formation of the ether by trapping of the intermediate carbonium ion (or other intermediate) by the hydroxyethyl group of the adjacent molecule. It has been previously reported that the porphyrin acetates can form ethers if ethyl alcohol is present during chromatography (Clezy, et al., 1980).

The acid hydrolysis to produce equal parts of Hp and HVD is consistent with the usual reaction path of ethers (Equation 1). The resistance to basic hydrolysis is also consistent with the ether structure.

The fast atom bombardment mass spectra analysis of the methyl esters indicates a small mass peak corresponding to DHE at 1236 (M +1) and 1237 (M + 2). However, the major peaks in this range appear at 1199, 1200 and 1201 (7-8% of the base peaks) corresponding to the loss of two water molecules. The larger mass peaks correspond to the addition of various numbers of water molecules. It thus appears that under the conditions of the analysis, the ether undergoes dehydration followed by cleavage with H transfer as indicated.

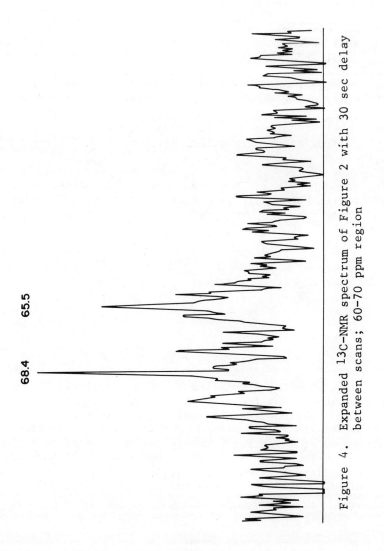

Figure 4. Expanded 13C-NMR spectrum of Figure 2 with 30 sec delay between scans; 60-70 ppm region

Other peripheral
groups deleted

Proto   HVD

Attempts to obtain mass spectra without fast atom bombardment
were completely unsuccessful resulting only in a large number of
small mass peaks. Initial ^{13}C-NMR spectra obtained for the free base
of Fraction A in DMSO-d_6 indicated all the required structural
elements of the ethers but did not reveal the necessary 'new' structure containing the ether link. Since this was considered possibly
due to slow relaxation and/or aggregation, the methyl ester was prepared and ^{13}C-NMR spectra obtained in CDCL$_3$ at a slow accumulation
rate, i.e., with a 10 sec delay between scans. Spectra obtained in
this way revealed the ether structure with the expected absorptions
occurring at 27.9 ppm and 68.4 ppm for – C(CH$_3$)–O and – C(CH$_3$)–O
respectively. A slight downfield shift for the ether structures
compared to the corresponding alcohol structures (i.e. –C(CH$_3$)–OH)
is predictable (Levy, 1983). Quantitative information is difficult
to obtain from ^{13}C-NMR because of the wide variation in relaxation
times. However, in order to verify that there were equal numbers of
ether structures and alcohol structures as required for DHE, the
scans were run with a 30 sec delay and expanded to observe the area
in the 60-70 ppm range. Within the margin of error and noise it
appeared that there was an equal number of ether carbons and alcohol
carbon atoms (Figure 4).

The ^{1}H NMR spectrum demonstrated the necessary structures but
was not definitive since it was not possible to remove all the water
from the samples thus producing a spectrum in which the absorptions
near water were at least partly obscured. However, as in the ^{13}C
spectrum, the proton NMR spectrum of the free base in DMSO-d_6 did not
reveal the protons of the methyl group attached to the ether group.
A portion of the spectrum obtained for the methyl ester in CDCL$_3$ is
shown in Figure 5, which revealed a complex set of methyl absorptions
which probably result from the multiple isomeric structures possible
for the ether and alcohol structures. In general, the proton spectra
are much more sensitive to structural modifications than are the ^{13}C
spectra which appeared to be relatively uncomplicated.

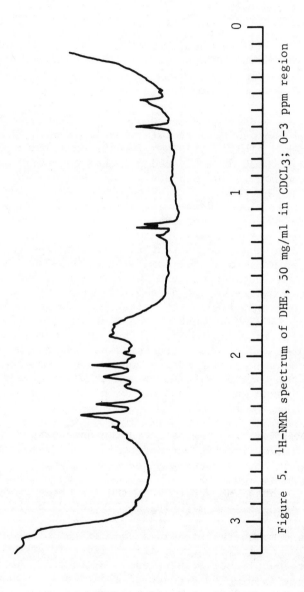

Figure 5.   1H-NMR spectrum of DHE, 50 mg/ml in CDCL3; 0-3 ppm region

Fraction A (DHE) was not stable when heated in aqueous solution (120°, 15 min) as evidenced by its insolubility in 1 N hydrochloric acid after this procedure. This may indicate an oxidative process or possibly formation of polymeric structures. When tested in this manner, the material also lost its ability to photosensitize the SMT-F tumor system used as a standard in our laboratory (Dougherty, et al., 1983).

Finally, the elemental analysis provided a carbon to nitrogen ratio of 7.38:1 compared with a calculated ratio of 7.29 to 1.

ACKNOWLEDGMENTS

We would like to acknowledge the considerable assistance of Dr. George Levy and associates at Syracuse University who ran the 13C-NMR spectra and assisted in interpretation, as well as Dr. R. L. Stephens at Carnegie-Mellon Institute who provided the proton NMR spectra, and to Dr. James Yergy of Johns Hopkins University, who was very helpful in determining and interpreting the FAB mass spectral data.

1. M. C. Berenbaum, R. Bonnett and P. O. Scourides, In vivo biological activity of the components of hematoporphyrin derivative. Br. J. Cancer 45:571 (1982).
2. P. S. Clezy, T. T. Hai, R. W. Henderson and L. Thuc, The chemistry of pyrrolic components XLV. Hematoporphyrin derivative diacetate as the main product of the reaction of hematoporphyrin with a mixture of active and sulfuric acid. Aust. J. Chem. 33:585 (1980).
3. T. J. Dougherty, D. G. Boyle, K. R. Weishaupt, B. A. Henderson, W. R. Potter, D. A. Bellnier and K. E. Wityk, Photoradiation therapy – Clinical and drug advances, in: "Porphyrin Photosensitization," D. Kessel and T. J. Dougherty, eds., Plenum Publishing Corp., New York (1983).
4. D. Kessel and T. Chow, Tumor-localizing components of the porphyrin preparation hematoporphyrin derivative. Can. Res. 43:1994 (1983).
5. G. Levy, Private communication (1983).
6. R. L. Lipson, The photodynamic and fluorescent properties of a particular hematoporphyrin derivative and its use in tumor detection. Master's Thesis, University of Minnesota (1960).
7. J. Moan and S. P. Sommer, Fluorescence and absorption properties of the components of hematoporphyrin derivative. Photobiochem. Photobiophys. 3:93 (1981).

PHOTOPHYSICAL AND PHOTOSENSITIZING PROPERTIES OF PHOTOFRIN II

A. Poletti, S.M. Murgia, A. Pasqua, *E. Reddi and *G. Jori

Dipartimento di Chimica, Università di Perugia and

*Istituto di Biologia Animale, Centro C.N.R. Emocianine
Padova (Italy)

INTRODUCTION

Photofrin II is a newly developed Hematoporphyrin Derivative
(Oncology Research & Development), which is widely used in the
phototherapy of tumors owing to its optimal tumor-localizing properties and ability to photosensitize the killing of the tumor cells
upon visible light-irradiation[1]. As known, the mechanism and efficiency of porphyrin photosensitization is dependent on several parameters, including the chemical structure of the porphyrin, its
aggregation state and the nature of the microenvironment[2-5]. Therefore, we decided to perform a detailed investigation on the photophysical and photosensitizing properties of Photofrin II, using
experimental conditions which mimic specific situations occurring
in vivo.

MATERIALS AND METHODS

Photofrin II (PF), at a nominal concentration of 2.5 mg/ml,
was kindly supplied by Prof. T.J. Dougherty. Human serum albumin
(HSA) (fraction V, Sigma) and tryptophan (Trp) (Merck) were used
without further purification. Sodium dodecyl sulphate (SDS) and
cetyltrimethylammonium bromide (CTABr) were obtained from Fluka
and purified as reported by M. Murgia et al.[6].

The photophysical and photosensitizing experiments were performed in the following media: neat aqueous solution, binary mixtures containing either 10% or 90% aqueous methanol (MeOh), aqueous
dispersions of 2% SDS or 0.25% CTABr, and aqueous solutions of HSA
(protein/PF ratio about 100/1 w/w). All the solutions were buffered at pH 7.4 with 0.05 M phosphate.

The laser photolysis experiments were performed on PF solutions in the range 25-50 mg/l, using the apparatus and techniques previously described[4] with the doubled emission (λ = 347 nm) of the pulse ruby laser as the excitation line. The output of the photomultiplier (Hamamatzu R928) was monitored by a digital oscillograph (Tektronix mod. 468) interfaced with a Cromemco Z2D computer system, equipped with an Epson MX80 printer and a Watanabe WX4671 plotter. Very low oscillographic signals were improved by means of a home--made filter-bias unit.

In photosensitizing experiments, 10 ml of the PF solution containing 20 μM Trp or 75 μM HSA were exposed to the light of four 250 watt incandescent bulbs (continuous emission above 380 nm). The solutions were air-equilibrated and maintened at 20 $\pm$ 1°C by water circulating in a jacket surrounding the test tube. At timed intervals, aliquots of the irradiated solutions were withdrawn and assayed for the residual Trp concentration by a spectrophotofluorimetric procedure[7].

The absorption spectra were monitored with a Perkin-Elmer 752 spectrophotometer using PF concentration in the range 2.5-25 mg/l. Fluorescence measurements were carried out with a Perkin-Elmer MPF 44 instrument equipped with a spectrum correction accessory (Rhodamine B as quantum counter), using a PF concentration in the range 0.025-25 mg/l.

RESULTS

Fig. 1 shows the absorption and emission spectra of PF (25 mg/l) in the different media. For the MeOH/H_2O (9:1, v/v) binary mixture the excitation spectrum in the Soret region is also reporeted. All the emission spectra were obtained using the 397 nm excitation line.

Table 1 collects the maxima wavelengths of the absorption and emissione bands of PF in the various solutions with ε and R (fluorescence yield relative to water) values, respectively. Since the spectral behaviour of PF in MeOH/H_2O (1:9, v/v) is very similar to that observed in neat aqueous solutions, the data for this mixture are not reported. The absorption and emission spectra were unaffected by dilution up to 2.5 and 0.025 mg/ml, respectively. A blue shift of the Soret band can be observed only for aqueous solutions. Moreover by more 200-fold dilution of the solution in 90% MeOH, the 670 nm emission peak of PF tends to desappear.

Fig. 2 shows the differential absorption spectrum (excited state minus ground state absorptions) of the transients produced after laser excitation of PF (2.5 mg/ml) in 90% MeOH solution. The spectrum is not appreciably affected by changing the medium as it may be seen in Table 1. In pure aqueous 10% MeOH solutions no appre-

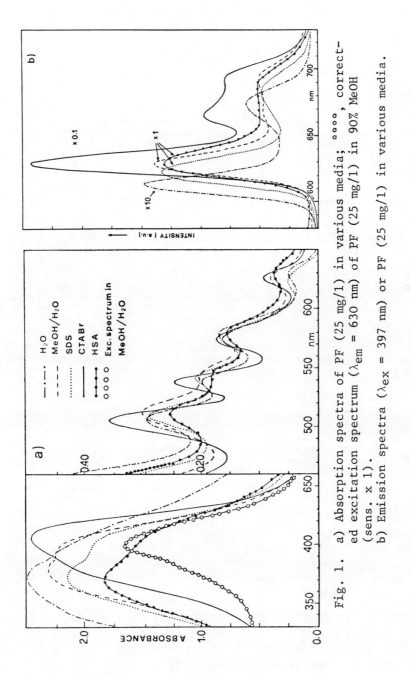

Fig. 1. a) Absorption spectra of PF (25 mg/l) in various media; °°°°, correct—
ed excitation spectrum (λ_{em} = 630 nm) of PF (25 mg/l) in 90% MeOH
(sens. x 1).
b) Emission spectra (λ_{ex} = 397 nm) or PF (25 mg/l) in various media.

Table 1. Photophysical Properties of PF (25 mg/1) in the ground and Excited States.

Medium	Absorption λ_{max} (nm)	$\varepsilon^{a)}$	Fluorescence λ_{max} (nm)	$R^{b)}$	T-T λ_{max} (nm)	Absorption Decay $k \cdot 10^3 (s^{-1})$
H_2O	$372^{c)}$	102.0	615	1.0		
	390sh		675			
	513	12.4				
	542	8.2				
	578	7.0				
	629	2.2				
SDS	372	88.0	623	9.0	320	
2%	395sh		685		450	4.7
	509	11.2			895	
	542	8.6				
	574	7.2				
	624	3.5				
CTABr	380sh		630	55.0	320	
0.25%	407	98.0	665		450	0.8
	506	14.6	693		890	
	539	10.0				
	574	7.2				
	626	4.0				
MeOH/H_2O	380	94.0	630	9.5	320	
90%	394sh		670		450	25.0
	507	12.0	694		895	
	539	8.2				
	576	6.8				
	627	3.4				
HSA Protein/PF 100/1 w/w	371	75.0	629	3.0		
	395sh		685			
	511	10.3				
	541	7.4				
	578	6.3				
	630	3.1				

$^a\varepsilon$ = O.D./1 mg ml^{-1};
^bR = I/I(H_2O);
^{c}364 nm for dilution more than 200-fold.

ciable transient signal has been observed after laser excitation.

Table 1 also shows the decay rate constants of the triplet observed at 450 nm. Similar decay rate constants were obtained for the absorptions at 320 nm and 890 nm. It has been found that this transient is strongly quenched by oxygen in all the investigated solutions with a biomolecular rate constant of about $2 \times 10^9 M^{-1} s^{-1}$.

As already found for other porphyrins[7], Trp is photooxidized according to first-order kinetics upon visible light-irradiation of solutions of the amino acid containing PF. The first-order rate constants as deduced from the slopes of the semi-logarithmic plots: ln[Trp] vs. time are shown in Table 2. Clearly, the nature of the reaction medium and the concentration of the PF are of major importance in determining the efficiency of Trp photooxidation. The data for HSA-PF system refer to the photooxidation of the single tryptophyl residue which is present in the protein molecule.

DISCUSSION

The spectroscopic data indicate that Photofrin II is strongly aggregated in neat aqueous solution; the aggregation state is only scarcely affected by dilution. The addition of compounds, such as HSA, ionic surfactants and organic solvents, which are known to disrupt porphyrin aggregates[3-9], induces spectral changes that are also indicative of PF deaggregation: e.g., absorption spectral pattern in the Soret region points out a red shift, which is especially

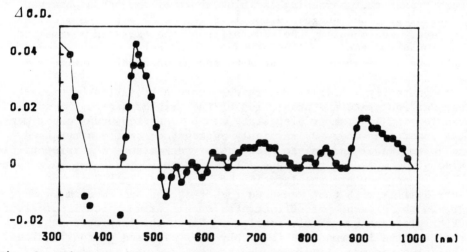

Fig. 2.   Differential absorption spectrum of the transients of PF
          (25 mg/1) in 90% MeOh solution.

Table 2.   First-order Rate Constants for the PF-sensitized Photooxidation of 20 μM Trp in Different Reaction Media.

Reaction medium [a]	PF mg/ml	Rate constant $k \cdot 10^3$ (s^{-1})
Aqueous solution	250.0	< 0.05
	8.7	0.23
2% aqueous SDS	8.7	0.39
75 μM aqueous HSA	250.0	0.14
	8.7	2.43
10% aqueous MeOH	250.0	< 0.05
	8.7	0.47
90% aqueous MeOH	250.0	11.04
	8.7	3.95

[a]All solutions were buffered at pH 7.4 with 0.05 M phosphate.

pronounced in the presence of CTABr micelles; also in the spectral
region above 500 nm, the absorption bands undergo significant per-
turbations; the sharpening and blue shift of the bands observed in
CTABr dispersions suggest a complexation of PF with the micellar
surface. Analogously, the red shifts of the emission maxima and
the enhancement of the fluorescence yield caused by the deaggregat-
ing substances are consistent with the above conclusions.

Apparently, there is a straighforward correlation between PF
aggregation state and properties of the triplet state. No appreciable signals from triplet state can be detected under experimental conditions where PF is highly aggregated; on the other hand,
in 90% methanol and in the presence of surfactants a triplet-triplet
absorption spectrum closely similar with that of HP[8] can be measured. In particular, the lifetime of PF triplet in 90% methanol is
very similar with that measured for HP in the same medium[9]. However, in the presence of surfactants, the lifetime values typical of
PF triplet are remarkably smaller[8]. Since the triplet state is
the reactive intermediate in porphyrin-sensitized photooxidations,
the above reported findings suggest that the photooxidizing efficiency of PF is controlled by the nature of the reaction medium.

In actual fact, the kinetic data reported in Table 2 demonstrate that PF is a very poor photosensitizer in media such as neat aqueous solution or 10% methanol, where the porphyrin is aggregated. The enhancement of the reaction rate constant obtained by dilution of neat PF aqueous solutions (from 250 to 8.7 mg/l) is related with a partial deaggregation of the porphyrin. The greatest photosensitizing efficiency is observed in 90% methanol, notwithstending the lower reactivity of the triplet porphyrin or $^1O_2$ (generated by electronic energy transfer to ground $^3O_2$) toward Trp in media of low dielectric constants[10]. Therefore, it appears that PF must undergo a large reduction in the degree of aggregation in order to act as a photosensitizer. We are presently performing studies in vivo in order to correlate the above findings with the phototherapeutic properties of PF.

REFERENCES

1. Bulletin "Photoradiation Technical Information" Jan. 4, 1983, published by Oncology Research & Development Inc., Cheecktowaga, N.Y., the sample was supplied by Prof. T.J. Dougherty.
2. D. Kessel and E. Rossi, Determinations of porphyrin-sensitized photooxidation characterized by fluorescence and absorption spectra, Photochem. Photobiol. 35:83 (1982).
3. G. Jori, E. Reddi, L. Tomio, and F. Calzavara, Factor governing the mechanism and efficiency of porphyrin-sensitized photooxidations in omogeneous solutions and organized media, in: "Porphyrin Photosensitation", D. Kessel and T.J. Dougherty, ed., Plenum Press, New York (1983).
4. A. Poletti, S.M. Murgia, and S. Cannistraro, Laser flash photolysis of the Hematoporphyrin- βcarotene system, Photobiochem. Photobiophys. 2:167 (1981).
5. A. Pasqua, A. Poletti, and S.M. Murgia, Ultrafiltration techniques as a tool for the investigation of Hematoporphyrin aggregates in aqueous solution, Med. Biol. Envir. 10:286 (1982).
6. S.M. Murgia and A. Poletti, Laser photolysis of methylene blue in aqueous micellar systems, Photobiochem. Photobiophys. 5:53 (1983).
7. E. Rossi, A. Van de Vorst, and G. Jori, Competition between the singlet oxygen and electron transfer mechanism in the porphyrin-sensitized photooxidation of L-tryptophan and tryptamine in aqueous micellar dispersions, Photochem. Photobiol. 34:447 (1981).
8. S.M. Murgia, A. Pasqua, and A. Poletti, Laser flash photolysis studies on Hematoporphyrin IX in aqueous and micellar systems, Med. Biol. Envir. 10:278 (1982).
9. S.M. Murgia, A. Pasqua, and A. Poletti, Laser photolysis study of the Hematoporphyrin IX-L-tryptophan system in solvent mixtures at different polarity, Chem. Phys. Lett. (1983) in press.
10. E. Reddi and M.A. Rodgers, unpublished results.

ON THE PURIFICATION OF HEMATOPORPHYRIN IX AND ITS ACETYLATED

DERIVATIVES

Daniel Brault, Christine Bizet and Olavio Delgado

Laboratoire de Biophysique, INSERM U.201, CNRS ERA 951
Muséum National d'Histoire Naturelle
61, Rue Buffon, 75005 Paris, France

INTRODUCTION

Hematoporphyrin IX (Hp, Fig. 1a) and especially the related product known as "Hematoporphyrin Derivative or HpD" have been the most used compounds in tumor diagnostic and phototherapy as outlined during this symposium. Also, hematoporphyrin is one of the most common photosensitizer. This situation is disquieting because of the general uncertainty about the purity of hematoporphyrin [1]. The major impurities of the commercial product are 8(3)-(1-hydroxyethyl)-3(8)-vinyldeuteroporphyrin (HVD, 2 isomers, Fig. 1b), protoporphyrin (PP, Fig. 1c) and unidentified brown impurities.

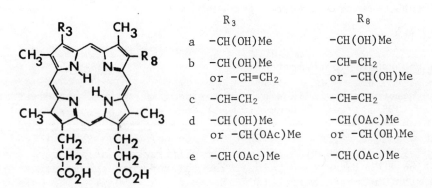

	R_3	R_8
a	$-CH(OH)Me$	$-CH(OH)Me$
b	$-CH(OH)Me$ or $-CH=CH_2$	$-CH=CH_2$ or $-CH(OH)Me$
c	$-CH=CH_2$	$-CH=CH_2$
d	$-CH(OH)Me$ or $-CH(OAc)Me$	$-CH(OAc)Me$ or $-CH(OH)Me$
e	$-CH(OAc)Me$	$-CH(OAc)Me$

Fig. 1. Structure of Hematoporphyrin IX (a) and related compounds.

HpD preparation[2] involves treatment of commercial Hp with
acetic acid which leads to the partial formation of mono and
diacetylated hematoporphyrin MAHp, DAHp (Fig. 1d, 1e). However,
the preparation of the HpD solutions used in clinical studies
involves the dissolution of the acetylated hematoporphyrin in
0.1 N NaOH followed by neutralisation[2]. As shown by HPLC studies[4-6]
the acetylated derivatives do not survive and, actually, in addition to Hp, HpD solutions contain HVD and PP, i.e. the usual
impurities of commercial Hp but in somewhat increased amounts.
However, HVD and PP were found to have no therapeutical activity.
The better efficiency of HpD as compared to crude Hp has been
tentitatively attributed to aggregated forms[7] but other contaminants
might be involved. In addition, HpD solutions prepared in various
laboratories have been reported to differ from one another in
therapeutical activity[8].

This situation emphasizes the interest in using purified Hp
to prepare HpD. This might make it possible to answer the important
question : does the "activation" of hematoporphyrin via the ace-
tylation-hydrolysis procedure involve Hp itself, other contaminant
porphyrins or other impurities present in various amounts in crude
hematoporphyrin ? Except the method of Momenteau et al.[9] which
consists of chromatography of Hp on sephadex gel, Hp purification
involves carboxylic chain esterification, chromatography and
hydrolysis in sequence[3]. Due to Hp instability,uncertainty often
remains on purity, and storage must be avoided.

MATERIALS

Hematoporphyrin IX was obtained as its dihydrochloride form
from Sigma. Silica gel 60, 230-400 mesh (Merck) was used for
column chromatography. Elution was performed through gravity with
an eluent flow rate of 1-2 ml/min. Detection was made by photo-
metric measurements at 498 nm with a 1 mm optical cell. TLC analysis were performed using silica gel 60 on plastic sheets (Merck).
Solvents were of analytical grade.

RESULTS

Hematoporphyrin purification

Hematoporphyrin IX dihydrochloride (200 mg) was dissolved in
water (375 ml) and acetone (100 ml) the solution was extracted
with chloroform (1 x 375 ml) and the chloroformic phase washed
with water (2 x 250 ml, pH must be kept below pH $\simeq$ 5.5). This
step allows elimination of polar impurities seen as a spread brown
spot on TLC plates (see below). The chloroformic phase was extracted with phosphate buffer (10^{-2} M, pH : 7.5, 250 ml). The porphyrin contained in the aqueous phase was extracted with a ethyl
acetate/ethyl formiate mixture (8/2, v/v). After aqueous washing,

the organic solution was concentrated. Addition of isooctane afforded precipitation of pre-purified hematoporphyrin (Yield ≃ 50 %)
which was usually found to contain less than 5 % HVD and no PP.
Further purification of hematoporphyrin involved chromatography
on silica gel. The pre-purified Hp (12 mg) dissolved in the eluent
solvent was put on a 2.5 x 45 cm column and eluted with acetone/
ethyl acetate/water (17/13/7, v/v/v). The elution profile is
shown in Fig. 2a. The eluted fractions were added with water and
ethyl formiate. The organic phase was washed with water, dried
over sodium sulfate,concentrated and the porphyrin precipitated
by using isooctane.

The purified Hp moved as a single spot (R_F = 0.62) on silica
gel TLC plates using the acetone/ethyl acetate/water mixture,
when HVD and PP gave distincts spots (R_F = 0.67 and 0.71, respectively) and other brown impurities remained spread over R_F ≃ 0.51 -
0.59. The NMR spectra of purified Hp agreed with literature data
and do not show any contamination. Other contaminant porphyrins
were identified from comparison with authentic samples.

Acetylated hematoporphyrin

Acetylation of purified hematoporphyrin was performed using
acetic acid containing 5 % sulfuric acid as described elsewhere[4].

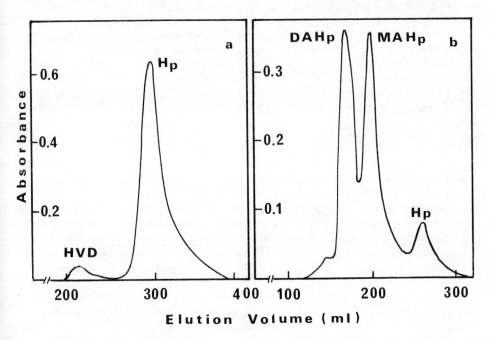

Fig. 2. Chromatography of pre-purified Hp (a) and acetylated Hp (b).
        Elution profiles.

The resulting material essentially contains monoacetylated and diacetylated hematoporphyrin and unreacted hematoporphyrin. As shown in Figure 2b, these compounds are well separated on a silica gel column using acetone/ethyl acetate/water (17/13/7, v/v/v). The identification of the mono- and diacetate derivatives was easily made on the basis of the dependence of their ratio on the acetylation reaction time. The result shown in Figure 2b corresponds to 15 min. reaction time at 20°C. The mono- and diacetylated derivatives were isolated as solid as described for hematoporphyrin. Identification was confirmed by NMR spectra.

Analysis of acetylated hematoporphyrin can also be made using TLC with the same solvent mixture. R_F values were found to be 0.66 and 0.69 for mono- and diacetate derivatives, respectively.

CONCLUSION

The chromatography system we described allows the separation of closely related porphyrins. Due to the poor solubility of the porphyrins in the eluent mixture, it is restricted to small scale preparations. But, this solvent mixture avoid side reactions which have been reported to occur to some extent in presence of alcools . Elution through gravity does not make it possible to isolate individual isomers (see Figure 1), but improvement through the use of HPLC techniques is under study.

We also found that hematoporphyrin derivative can be characterized by TLC using our system. As it involves normal phase chromatography, contrary to most of the systems described so far, additional informations might be obtained.

Finally, hematoporphyrin can be purified in a simple way which might be of help in answering the above mentionned question.

REFERENCES

1. R.K. Di Nello and C.K. Chang, in: "The Porphyrin" Vol. 1, Academic Press, New York (1978).
2. T.J. Dougherty, G. Lawrence, J.H. Kaufman, D. Boyle, K.R. Weishaupt, and A. Goldfarb, Photoradiation in the treatment of recurrent breast carcinoma, J. Natl. Cancer Inst. 62:231 (1979).
3. P.S. Clezy, T.T. Hai, R.W. Henderson, and L.V. Thuc, The chemistry of pyrrolic compounds 45. Hematoporphyrin Derivative, Austral. J. Chem. 33: 585 (1980).
4. R. Bonnett, R.J. Ridge, P.A. Scourides, and M.C. Berenbaum, On the nature of Hematoporphyrin Derivative, J. Chem. Soc. Perkin I. 3135 (1981).

5. P.A. Cadby, E. Dimitriadis, M.G. Grant, and A.D. Ward, Separa-
    tion and analysis of Hematoporphyrin Derivative components
    by high-performance liquid chromatography, J. Chromatogr.
    231:273 (1982).
6. J. Moan, T. Christensen, and S. Sommer, The main photosensitiz-
    in components of Hematoporphyrin Derivative, Cancer Lett.
    15:161 (1982).
7. T.J. Dougherty, D.G. Boyle, K.R. Weishaupt, B.A. Henderson,
    W.R. Potter, D.A. Bellnier, and K.E. Wityk, Photoradiation
    therapy; clinical and drug advances, in: "Porphyrin Photo-
    sensitization", D. Kessel and T.J. Dougherty, ed., Plenum
    Press, New York-London (1983).
8. T.J. Dougherty, Variability in Hematoporphyrin Derivative pre-
    paration, Cancer Res. 42:1188 (1982).
9. M. Momenteau, C. Ropars, and M. Rougee, J. Chim. Phys. Chim.
    Biol. 65:1635 (1968).

PHOTOSENSITIZING PROPERTIES OF PORPHYRINS IN MODEL CELL SYSTEMS

John D. Spikes

Department of Biology
University of Utah
Salt Lake City, Utah 84112 USA

INTRODUCTION

A large amount of work has been done on the photophysics, photochemistry and photosensitizing properties of porphyrins in aqueous solutions. Even so, much remains to be learned about porphyrin-sensitized photooxidation reactions (photodynamic effects) in simple systems. In particular, the dependence of the mechanisms and efficiencies of the reactions on porphyrin structure, the aggregation state of the porphyrin, the properties of the reaction medium and the chemical structure of the substrate being photooxidized must be studied in more detail.[1] It is difficult at present to usefully extrapolate much of the wealth of information available on the photosensitizing behavior of porphyrins in homogeneous solution to the cellular situation. First, the cell membrane poses a differential barrier to the penetration of different porphyrins from the external solution because of its hydrophobic core, and perhaps because of its charge. Further, cells are not homogeneous bags of fluid; both the membrane and the interior are made up of an enormous number of microregions with widely different chemical-physical properties. Because of these localized differences, porphyrins will tend to bind non-covalently or dissolve in particular microenvironments, depending on their properties. This can change the photochemical properties of the porphyrin from those observed in solution. For example, the quantum yield of porphyrin triplet formation and the triplet lifetime can be altered, the lifetimes of the photo-generated singlet oxygen and other reactive species could be changed, and the relative participation of Type I (free radical) and Type II (singlet oxygen) mediated pathways could be shifted.

Further, the concentration of oxygen and the availability and
chemical nature of substrates could be very different in different
subcellular sites. Localized porphyrins would be expected to
sensitize selective damage to certain regions and structures of the
cell on illumination.

As a result of this complex situation, it is difficult to
establish in detail the patterns of photodynamic damage in
mammalian cells and to define the particular photochemical lesions
which lead to cell death. One preliminary approach to the
investigation of these complexities is to study the photosensitizing behavior of porphyrins in model systems which simulate
in very simplified ways some of the properties of living cells.[2,3]
Several of the models which are now being studied will be discussed
here including porphyrins bound non-covalently and covalently to
macrobiomolecules and particles, porphyrins in aqueous detergent
micelle systems, and porphyrins incorporated into the membranes of
bilayered phospholipid vesicles termed liposomes; some comments
will also be made on the use of a "semi-model" system involving
porphyrins in isolated red blood cell membranes.

PHOTOSENSITIZING BEHAVIOR OF BOUND PORPHYRINS

Many types of photosensitizers bind to certain kinds of
biomolecules in solution and might therefore be expected to bind to
the same types of molecules in vivo. Thus the in vitro examination
of the photochemical behavior of bound porphyrins may be useful in
the interpretation of photosensitization studies with cells. Many
porphryins bind non-covalently to proteins, and a number of reports
have been made on the photochemistry of such complexes. Bound
porphyrins sensitize only those susceptible amino acid residues
(cysteine, histidine, methionine, tryptophan, tyrosine) located in
the immediate vicinity of the binding site on the protein since
both Type I and II photoprocesses have only a very small effective
radius of action. Thus bound porphyrins can be used as probes of
the three-dimensional structure of proteins in solution.[4]
Hematoporphyrin forms a 2:1 sensitizer-protein complex with the
enzyme lysozyme. On illumination of the complex, one methionine in
the enzyme (methionine-12) is photooxidized and the enzyme activity
is reduced by 50%; the other methionine residue in the enzyme
molecule is not affected.[5] Many porphyrins bind strongly to serum
albumins. Under physiological conditions, hematoporphyrin binds to
a specific site on the human serum albumin (HSA) molecule to give a
1:1 complex. The binding site is less than 2 nm from the single
tryptophan residue in the molecule. Illumination of the complex
photooxidizes this residue with significantly greater efficiency
than the photooxidation of a tryptophan derivative (N-acetyl
tryptophan amide) by hematoporphyrin free in solution.[6] This
increased efficiency of photooxidation of moieties in macro-

molecules by sensitizers bound to the macromolecule has been observed in a number of other cases.[2] Other workers have shown that bound hematoporphyrin is an efficient sensitizer for tryptophan residues in both HSA and bovine serum albumin (BSA); the reaction is faster with BSA, which has two tryptophan residues in the molecule. The rate of photooxidation of tryptophan residues in serum albumins is increased approximately 8-fold in going from H_2O to D_2O as solvent, suggesting that singlet oxygen is the dominant photooxidizing intermediate. Hematoporphyrin bound to serum albumins is photobleached thirty times faster than hematoporphyrin in solution.[7] The efficiency of protein bound porphyrins as photodynamic sensitizers for molecules in solution in the medium outside of the porphyrin-protein complex is not known. However, the porphyrin might be expected to act as a photosensitizer in this situation since it has been shown that illumination of the tetra-(4-sulfonato-phenyl)porphine-HSA complex in aqueous solution generates singlet oxygen, some of which escapes from the complex into the surrounding solvent.[8]

     The photosensitizing behavior of protein-bound porphyrins has also been studied extensively using hemoproteins, which have a heme (iron protoporphyrin IX) moiety firmly, but not covalently, bound to a specific site on the protein. In general, hemoproteins are not light sensitive since the heme iron is in the high spin form which very rapidly quenches the photogenerated triplet state of the porphyrin. However, some hemoproteins such as catalase are photo-oxidized on illumination at wavelengths absorbed by the heme, suggesting that in these cases the heme iron is in a low spin state. The usual strategy for carrying out photosensitization studies with hemoproteins is to remove the heme from the molecule and replace it with a sensitizing porphyrin (either a metal-free porphyrin or one containing a diamagnetic metal such as zinc) which binds at the same site. For example, native myoglobins have the heme iron in the high spin state and thus are not light sensitive. Addition of protoporphyrin IX, a metal-free sensitizing porphyrin, to apomyoglobin gives a 1:1 porphyrin-protein complex; illumination of this under aerobic conditions results in the destruction of histidine-93 in the protein, which is known to be located in the heme-binding site of the protein.[9] Analogous studies have been carried out with similar results using other hemoproteins including leghemoglobin and horseradish peroxidase. Quantitative use of this technique permits identifying those susceptible amino residues located in or near the heme-binding site of the hemoprotein.[1] Thus studies with hemoproteins show again that porphyrins can be effective sensitizers for the photooxidation of amino acid residues located in the protein molecule to which they are bound.

     In one case, a porphyrin covalently bound to a protein has been shown to be an effective photosensitizer for other molecules.

In this work hematoporphyrin was covalently coupled to monoclonal antibodies (gamma globulin) toward a tumor specific antigen from a particular type of sarcoma cell. The coupled porphyrin is still photodynamically active toward external substrates as shown by the ability of the porphyrin-protein conjugate to sensitize the photodynamic hemolysis of red blood cells; in fact, the coupled porphyrin is slightly more efficient than free hematoporphyrin in this reaction. Further, the conjugate shows specific phototoxicity for the tumor cell type used in generating the antibody, both in vitro and in vivo.[10] Hematoporphyrin bound covalently to chloromethylated styrene-divinylbenzene copolymer beads retains some photosensitizing activity.[11] In recent studies, we (J. D. Spikes, B. Burnham and J. C. Bommer, unpublished experiments) have found that uroporphyrin remains a very effective photosensitizer when covalently bound to beads of an agarose gel. With aqueous 2 mM furfural alcohol at pH 7.4 as substrate, the quantum yield for oxygen uptake during illumination is 0.22 with uroporphyrin and 0.18 with the agarose-coupled porphyrin. With cysteine as substrate under the same conditions, the quantum yields are 0.062 and 0.065, respectively. Laser flash kinetic studies show that the natural porphyrin triplet half lives (as measured under nitrogen) are the same (approximately 900 usec) for both the free and the covalently bound uroporphyrin. The bimolecular rate constant for oxygen quenching of the porphyrin triplet is significantly greater for free uroporphyrin (1.2×10^9 1 mol^{-1} sec^{-1}) than for the conjugate (3.1×10^8 1 mol^{-1} sec^{-1}).

In summary, porphyrins bound to proteins and particulate materials often exhibit as high, or even higher, photosensitizing efficiencies than the same porphyrins free in solution. These observations are relevant to the situation in mammalian cells where porphyrins bound to the cell membrane have been shown to sensitize photodamage to the cell much more efficiently than porphyrins free in the external medium.[12,13]

PHOTOSENSITIZING BEHAVIOR OF PORPHYRINS IN AQUEOUS DETERGENT MICELLE SYSTEMS

Amphipathic molecules (also termed detergents, soaps, surfactants, etc.) possess both water soluble (hydrophilic) and water insoluble (hydrophobic) groups. If an aqueous solution of such a molecule is prepared at concentrations above a certain level, termed the critical micellar concentration, the molecules aggregate to form dynamic, roughly spherical structures known as micelles. These are made up of approximately one hundred detergent monomers with the hydrophobic fatty acid chains of the molecules pointing inward and entwined to form a core and with the hydrophilic groups at the outer surface forming a layer in contact with the aqueous medium. The hydrophilic groups can be negatively

or positively charged, or neutral, depending on the chemical
structure of the detergent. Micelles are used as very simple
models of cell membraneous structures since they possess external
hydrophilic and internal hydrophobic regions. Lipid soluble
sensitizers and substrates can be solubilized in micelles, and many
kinds of photochemical studies have been carried out with reactants
dissolved in micellar preparations.[14] However, the discussion here
will be restricted to porphyrin-sensitized photooxidations of
biomolecules in such systems; only a few studies of this type have
been reported.

Hematoporphyrin is incorporated (as a monomer) into sodium
dodecyl sulfate (SDS = anionic), cetyltrimethylammonium bromide
(CTAB = cationic) and Triton-100 (neutral) micelles. When these
preparations are illuminated, triplet porphyrin is formed with
about the same quantum yield and shows essentially the same
properties (spectrum, natural decay rate, etc.) as hematoporphyrin
in homogeneous aqueous media. Further, the quantum yield of the
hematoporphyrin-sensitized formation of singlet oxygen is
approximately the same in SDS and CTAB micelles in D_2O as for the
porphyrin dissolved in D_2O alone.[15]

Photodynamic studies with porphyrins have been carried out in
micellar preparations of anionic, cationic or neutral detergents;
substrates can be located within the micelles or in the external
solvent, depending on their solubility properties and charge.
Further, mixed experiments can be done with the porphyrin located
in one set of micelles and the substrate in another in order to
examine interactions across phase boundaries and at a distance.
Such arrangements simulate the situation in cells where it might be
expected that the porphyrin could be localized in one micro-
compartment and the substrate in another. Along these lines,
detailed studies have been made recently of the hematoporphyrin-
sensitized photooxidation of indole derivatives in aqueous micellar
preparations at pH 10.[6,16,17] The negatively charged derivative,
tryptophan, dissolves in the aqueous medium and also penetrates
into positively charged CTBA micelles but not into negatively
charged SDS micelles or neutral Triton X-100 micelles. The
uncharged indole, tryptamine, dissolves in the medium and also
penetrates into all three types of micelles. The experimental
results are somewhat complicated; however they do show that the
micelle incorporated hematoporphyrin can sensitize the
photooxidation of substrates located in the same micelle, in the
external aqueous medium, and in other micelles (in some cases).
Hematoporphyrin photooxidizes indole derivatives via competing Type
I (electron transfer from triplet porphyrin) and Type II (singlet
oxygen mediated) pathways; the relative participation depends on
the reaction conditions. Singlet oxygen oxidizes substrates in the
micelle in which it is photogenerated and also diffuses out and

oxidizes substrates located in the external medium and in other
micelles. Photogenerated electrons can also diffuse out of
micelles and oxidize substrates located in the solvent or
incorporated into other cationic or neutral micelles; however
incorporation of substrates into anionic micelles almost completely
protects them from attack by photogenerated electrons.

PHOTOSENSITIZING BEHAVIOR OF PORPHYRINS IN LIPOSOMAL SYSTEMS

Liposomes are very small, bilayered phospholipid vesicles.
The core of the liposomal membrane is highly hydrophobic since it
is composed of the hydrocarbon tails of the fatty acid moieties of
the phospholipid molecules, and thus has properties in common with
the core of cell membranes. For this reason, liposomes have been
used extensively as models for some aspects of cell membrane
behavior. Highly sonicated liposomes have overall diameters in the
25-40 nm (250-400 A) range and therefore do not scatter visible
light strongly. Suspensions of such liposomes are sufficiently
transparent to be used for quantum yield measurements and flash
photolysis studies. Water soluble porphyrins and substrates can be
entrapped within liposomes, and lipid soluble porphyrins and
substrates can be incorporated into the liposomal membranes during
preparation. If hematoporphyrin (which is fairly lipid soluble and
occurs in monomeric form in the liposomal membrane) and cholesterol
are incorporated into liposomal membranes, subsequent illumination
results in efficient photooxidation of the cholesterol by a singlet
oxygen mechanism.[18] The cholesterol is photooxidized several times
more rapidly when illumination is carried out at temperatures above
the phase transition temperature of the phospholipid used in the
preparation of the liposomes. This probable results from an
increased rate of diffusion of the photochemically generated
singlet oxygen in the more fluid membrane.[19] Hematoporphyrin in
the external aqueous medium is a very inefficient sensitizer for
the membrane incorporated cholesterol, even though singlet oxygen
is known to diffuse through liposomal membranes. These results
with liposomes parallel the situation in cells where it appears
that the sensitizer must be bound to or incorporated into the cell
membrane in order to effectively sensitize the photooxidation of
membrane components.[12,13] Protoporphyrin also sensitizes the
photooxidation of lipophilic substrates in liposomal systems
including 9,10-dimethylanthracene and diphenylfurane.[20]

Liposomes prepared from egg lecithin (which is composed of
unsaturated phosphatidyl cholines) and with membrane-incorporated
hematoporphyrin are lysed on illumination in a process reminescent
of the photodynamic hemolysis of red blood cells. Lysis presumably
results from the porphyrin-sensitized photooxidation of the
unsaturated side chains of the phospholipid; liposomes prepared
from saturated phospholipids such as dipalmitoylphosphatidyl

choline are not photosensitive. Mechanistic studies with the
unsaturated liposomes show that photosensitized lysis occurs by a
Type II singlet oxygen pathway at low hematoporphyrin
concentrations; with high concentrations of porphyrin in the
membranes, lysis occurs by a Type I process which does not require
the presence of oxygen. Crude hematoporphyrin derivative
incorporated into the liposomal membranes gives the same results as
hematoporphyrin.[21] Water soluble porphyrins in the external medium
sensitize liposome photolysis with only very low efficiencies.

Both hematoporphyrin in aqueous solution and hematoporphyrin
dimethyl and dipalmitoyl esters incorporated into the membranes of
dipalmitoylphosphatidylcholine liposomes sensitize the photooxidation of molecules such as cysteine, histidine, methionine,
tryptophan, tyrosine and the enzyme lysozyme in aqueous solution.
The quantum efficiencies of photooxidation are essentially the same
with the porphyrin in solution and with the membrane incorporated
porphyrin esters. In both cases the yields are increased
significantly in D_2O and decreased by azide suggesting that the
reactions are mediated by singlet oxygen; singlet oxygen generated
in the liposomal membranes would presumably have to diffuse out of
the membrane in order to react with large molecules in solution
such as the enzyme.[22,23] Metal-free porphyrins, like most good
photodynamic sensitizers, have fairly long triplet lifetimes. For
example, hematoporphyrin at 80 uM in pH 7.4 aqueous phosphate
buffer has a triplet halflife of approximately 60 usec in nitrogen;
the triplet is quenched efficiently by oxygen so that the halflife
in air is only 1.5 usec. The triplet halflife of hematoporhyrin
dimethyl ester incorporated into the membranes of dipalmitoylphosphatidylcholine liposomes is 100 usec in nitrogen and 2.7 usec
in air.[23] Liposomes with membrane-incorporated porphyrin esters
are also good sensitizers for the photodynamic killing of mammalian
cells. If such liposomes are added to cultures of HeLa cells, for
example, they are rapidly taken up and appear to localize in the
lysosomes of the cells; the cells are then rapidly killed on
illumination.[22,23]

PHOTOSENSITIZING BEHAVIOR OF PORPHYRINS IN RED BLOOD CELL MEMBRANES

Mammalian red blood cells have been used extensively as "semi-
model" systems for the study of porphyrin-sensitized photoeffects
on biomembranes. Illumination of red blood cells in the presence
of many kinds of porphyrins results in damage to the cell membrane
which eventually leads to the colloid osmotic rupture of the cell
membrane (photodynamic hemolysis). There is still some argument
over the mechanism of photohemolysis.[24] Perhaps most investigators
feel that protein damage is the principal cause of hemolysis,[25] but
others feel that the photooxidation of membrane lipids is
involved.[26] Mature mammalian red blood cells are useful biological

models for membrane studies since the cells do not contain nuclei or much in the way of the usual cytoplasmic organelles. Red blood cells can be processed to give resealed "ghosts" in which essentially only the plasma membrane of the cell remains; selected molecules of different molecular weight, charge, etc. can be entrapped within the membranes during preparation. The leakage of such marker molecules as a result of photodynamic treatment can then be measured. Recent work has shown that trapped sodium ions start diffusing out of protoporphyrin-sensitized membranes almost immediately after the start of illumination, whereas there is a considerable delay before the efflux of a larger molecule (glucose-6-phosphate) begins. The photooxidative mechanism involved in the release of the markers appears to be different in the two cases since the antioxidant butylated hydroxytoluene (which inhibits the porphyrin-sensitized photooxidation of membrane lipids) blocks glucose-6-phosphate leakage but has no effect on the efflux of sodium ion. Sodium ion loss probably results from photodynamic damage to membrane proteins involved in the control of the passive permeability of the red blood cell membrane to small cations.[27]

SUMMARY

Several of the principal model systems presently being used in preliminary attempts to interpret the mechanisms involved in the porphyrin-sensitized photodynamic killing of cells have been briefly reviewed including bound porphyrins, porphyrins in detergent micelles, porphyrins incorporated into liposomal membranes, and porphyrins in resealed membranes isolated from mammalian red blood cells. All of these experimental approaches are in very early stages of development. Hopefully, as additional work is done in these areas, the resulting information will improve our understanding of porphyrin-sensitized phototoxic processes in cells, tissues and organisms.

The preparation of this manuscript was supported in part by NIH Biomedical Research Support Grant No. RR07092 and by the University of Utah Research Fund.

REFERENCES (space permits listing only a few basic references; these may be consulted for more detailed bibliographies)

1. G. Jori and J.D. Spikes, The photobiochemistry of porphyrins, in: "Topics in Photomedicine", K. C. Smith, ed., Plenum Publishing Corp., New York, in press.
2. G. Jori and J.D. Spikes, Photosensitized oxidations in complex biological structures, pp. 441-457 in: "Oxygen and Oxy-Radicals in Chemistry and Biology," M. A. J. Rodgers and E. L. Powers, eds., Academic Press, New York (1981).

3. J.D. Spikes, Photosensitization in mammalian cells, pp. 23-49
    in: "Photoimmunology", J. A. Parrish, Margaret Kripke and
    W. L. Morison, eds., Plenum Publishing Corp., New York
    (1983).
4. G. Jori and J.D. Spikes, Mapping the three-dimensional
    structure of proteins by photochemical techniques,
    Photochem. Photobiol. Rev. 3:193 (1978).
5. G. Jori, G. Galiazzo and E. Scoffone, Photodynamic action of
    porphyrins on amino acids and proteins. III. Further
    studies on the hematoporphyrin-sensitized photooxidation
    of lysozyme, Experientia 27:379 (1971).
6. G. Jori, E. Reddi, L. Tomio and F. Calzavara, Factors
    governing the mechanism and efficiency of porphyrin-
    sensitized photooxidations in homogeneous solutions and
    organized media, Adv. Exptl. Biol. Med. 160:193 (1983).
7. P. Richard, A. Blum and L.I. Grossweiner, Hematoporphyrin
    photosensitization of serum albumin and subtilisin BPN',
    Photochem. Photobiol. 37:287 (1983).
8. M.A.J. Rodgers, Time resolved studies of 1.27 um luminescence
    from singlet oxygen generated in homogeneous and
    microheterogeneous fluids, Photochem. Photobiol. 37:99
    (1983).
9. M.R. Mauk and A.W. Girotti, Photooxidation of the
    protoporphyrin-apomyoglobin complex, Biochemistry 12:3187
    (1973).
10. D. Mew, C-K. Wat, G.H.N. Towers and J.G. Levy,
    Photoimmunotherapy: Treatment of animal tumors with
    tumor-specific monoclonal antibody-hematoporphyrin
    conjugates, J. Immunol. 130:1473 (1983).
11. A.P. Schaap, A.L. Thayer, E.C. Blossey and D.C. Neckers,
    Polymer-based sensitizers for photooxidations, J. Am.
    Chem. Soc. 97:3741 (1975).
12. K. Kohn and D. Kessel, On the mode of cytotoxic action of
    photoactivated porphyrins, 28:2465 (1979).
13. S. Sandberg and I. Romslo, Porphyrin-induced photodamage at
    the cellular and subcellular level as related to the
    solubility of the porphyrin, Clin. Chem. Acta 109:193
    (1981).
14. B.A. Lindig and M.A.J. Rodgers, Molecular excited states in
    micellar systems, Photochem. Photobiol. 31:617 (1980).
15. E. Reddi, G. Jori, M.A.J. Rodgers and J.D. Spikes, Flash
    photolysis studies of hemato-and copro- porphyrins in
    homogeneous and microheterogeneous aqueous dispersions,
    Photochem. Photobiol. (in press).
16. C. Sconfienza, A. Van de Vorst and G. Jori, Type I and Type II
    mechanisms in the photooxidation of L-tryptophan and
    tryptamine sensitized by hematoporphyrin in the presence
    and absence of sodium dodecyl sulphate micelles,
    Photochem. Photobiol. 31:351 (1980).

17. E. Rossi, A. Van de Vorst and G. Jori, Competition between
    singlet oxygen and electron transfer mechanisms in the
    porphyrin-sensitized photooxidation of L-tryptophan and
    tryptamine in aqueous micellar dispersions, Photochem.
    Photobiol. 34:447 (1981).
18. K. Suwa, T. Kimura and A.P. Schaap, Reactivity of singlet
    molecular oxygen with cholesterol in a phospholipid
    membrane matrix. A model for oxidative damage of
    membranes, Biochem. Biophys. Res. Commun. 75:785 (1977).
19. K. Suwa, T. Kimura and A.P. Schaap, Reaction of singlet oxygen
    with cholesterol in liposomal membranes. Effect of
    membrane fluidity on the photooxidation of cholesterol,
    Photochem. Photobiol. 28:469 (1978).
20. T. Parasassi and S. Scarpa, Photodynamic reactions in
    dimyristoyl-L-alpha-phosphatidylcholine (DMPC) liposomes,
    Inorg. Chim. Acta, 66:137 (1982).
21. L.I. Grossweiner, A.S. Patel and J.B. Grossweiner, Type I and
    Type II mechanisms in the photosensitized lysis of
    phosphatidylcholine liposomes by hematoporphyrin,
    Photochem. Photobiol. 36:159 (1982).
22. J.D. Spikes, A preliminary comparison of the photosensitizing
    properties of porphyrins in aqueous solution and liposomal
    membranes. Adv. Exptl. Med. Biol. 160:181 (1983).
23. J.D. Spikes, W. Matis and M.A.J. Rogers, The photochemical
    behavior of porphyrins in solution and incorporated into
    liposomal membranes, Studia Biophys. (in press).
24. J.P. Pooler and D.P. Valenzeno, Dye-sensitized photodynamic
    inactivation of cells, Med. Phys. 8:614 (1981).
25. J. Van Steveninck, T.M.A.R. Dubbelman and H. Verweij,
    Photodynamic membrane damage, Adv. Exptl. Med. Biol.
    160:227 (1983).
26. A.A. Lamola and F.H. Doleiden, Cross-linking of membrane
    proteins and protoporphyrin-sensitized photohemolysis,
    Photochem. Photobiol. 31:597 (1980).
27. A.W. Girotti and M.R. Deziel, Photodynamic action of
    protoporphyrin on resealed erythrocyte membranes:
    mechanisms of release of trapped markers, Adv. Exptl. Med.
    Biol. 160:213 (1983).

PHOTOSENSITIZING PROPERTIES OF FREE AND BOUND UROPORPHYRIN I

John D. Spikes*, Bruce F. Burnham** and
Jerry C. Bommer**
*Department of Biology, University of Utah, Salt Lake
City, Utah 84112 USA and **Porphyrin Products, Inc.
Logan Utah 84321 USA

INTRODUCTION

Most studies of the sensitized photooxidation of biomolecules
have been carried out with the sensitizer in solution or, as in the
case of many porphyrins, in the form of small aggregates suspended
in the medium.[1] Cells, however are not homogeneous; they consist
of a wide variety of microenvironments with different physical-
chemical properties. Thus most photosensitizers added to cellular
systems, depending on their properties, would be expected to
dissolve in particular microregions of the cells or bind to
cellular macromolecules such as proteins, nucleic acids or
carbohydrates.[2] This could change the sensitizer properties, the
efficiency of photosensitization and the sensitizing mechanism.[2,3]
Thus it is difficult to carry over information on photosensitizers
as obtained in solution to the cellular-organismal level. One
preliminary approach to this problem is to examine the photochemical behavior of photosensitizer molecules bound to surfaces to
simulate the possible intracellular situation. The present paper
describes a preliminary comparison of the photosensitizing
properties of uroporphyrin I in aqueous solution and bound
covalently to beads of an agarose gel. Uroporphyrin I was selected
for this study since, unlike most of the porphyrins used as
sensitizers for biological systems, it appears to exist entirely in
monomeric form in aqueous buffer.[1]

MATERIALS AND METHODS

Uroporphyrin I dihydrochloride (uro) was provided by Porphyrin
Products, Inc., Logan, Utah, and the Affi-Gel 102 and the water
soluble carbodiimide coupling agent (EDAC) were obtained from Bio-

Rad Laboratories, Richmond, California. Affi-Gel 102 is an amino
terminal agarose gel with a 6-atom hydrophilic spacer arm and a
bead size of 80-180 microns. Uro was attached covalently to the
gel at room temperature by adding 4x10 mg quantities of uro
dissolved in 1:1 dimethylformamide:pyridine (V/V) to a 50 ml packed
volume of the gel suspended in the same solvent.[4] After each
addition of uro, 100 mg amounts of EDAC were added to the
mixture. The pH was adjusted to 4.7 with 1 N HCl and was
continually monitored. These additions were carried out at hourly
intervals for four hours. Finally, the reaction mixture was
stirred in the dark overnight. A parallel control experiment in
which the coupling agent was omitted was carried out
simultaneously. The reaction product was separated by
centrifugation and then washed with ten volumes each of dimethyl-
formamide, ethanol, 5 N HCl, 2 N KOH, and water. The final product
was dark reddish-purple in color; this material will be termed
urogel. The control material prepared without the coupling agent
was white, indicating that no significant amount of uro was
directly adsorbed to the gel. Urogel of smaller particle size was
obtained by sonication in buffer under nitrogen at 25 degrees using
a model W-375 (375 watt) sonicator from Heat Systems-Ultrasonics,
Inc., Plainview, New York.

Quantum yields of oxygen uptake during the uro and urogel
sensitized photooxidation of substrates were measured using a
recording membrane-type oxygen electrode system; reaction mixtures
were illuminated in air at 25 degrees with stirring by a 500 watt
slide projector provided with appropriate interference filters.[5]
Unless otherwise indicated, the reaction mixtures were 2 mM in
substrate, 0.22 mM in oxygen (air saturated) and 0.125 M in sodium
phosphate buffer at pH 7.4, and were either 5 μM in uro or
contained 1.25 mg/ml urogel. Hydrogen peroxide accumulation in the
illuminated reaction mixtures was determined by measuring the
oxygen evolved following the addition of catalase.

RESULTS AND DISCUSSION

The urogel beads settled out of suspension quite rapidly which
made it difficult to do light absorption measurements. Sonicated
urogel had a much smaller particle size and remained in suspension
reasonably well. A standard 30 minute sonication time was used;
the photosensitizing efficiency of the urogel was increased
approximately 50% at this point. Centrifugation studies indicated
the complete absence of free uro in the sonicated material. The
absorption peak of uro in pH 7.4 buffer was at approximately
398 nm, while that for uro covalently bound to the gel shifted to
approximately 402 nm. Such a shift of the spectral peak to longer
wavelengths is often observed when dyes bind to polymeric
materials.[6]

An examination was made of the kinetics of the photooxidation of furfuryl alcohol as sensitized by uro and urogel. Furfuryl alcohol was used for this initial survey because its rate of photooxidation is independent of pH; thus any observed dependence of reaction rates on pH must result from effects on the photosensitizer. The quantum yields of oxygen uptake during the photooxidation of furfuryl alcohol with both sensitizers was independent of incident light intensity over the range 0.3-3 mWatts/cm^2. As the concentration of furfuryl alcohol was increased from 0.4-20 mM, the quantum yield of oxygen uptake increased from 0.056 to 0.34 with uro as sensitizer; at standard conditions (2 mM furfuryl alcohol), the yield was 0.22. With urogel, the yields increased from 0.037-0.32 over the same concentration range; at 2 mM furfuryl alcohol the yield was 0.18. The quantum yields also increased progressively with increasing sensitizer concentration; the yields could not be determined accurately at high urogel concentrations because of light scattering by the sensitizer. With both uro and urogel, there was relatively litle change in the quantum yields as the oxygen concentration was reduced from 0.22 mM (air saturation) to one-tenth that value; at lower concentrations the yields dropped fairly rapidly. There was essentially no change in the quantum yields of oxygen uptake for the photooxidation of furfuryl alcohol with either sensitizer over the pH range 5-11; at lower pH values, the yields decrease. Both uro and urogel seemed stable from pH 5-11. There was also no significant change in yields over the temperature range 10-50 degrees. Hydrogen peroxide accumulation in the reaction mixtures during illumination was measured with furfuryl alcohol as substrate. The peroxide yields (moles hydrogen peroxide accumulating/moles oxygen consumed) with uro as sensitizer were 0.20, 0.81 and 0.57 at pH 5, 7.4 and 11, respectively; the corresponding yields with urogel were 0.28, 0.78 and 0.29. Effects of sodium azide concentration on the yields were examined. With urogel as sensitizer, the yield was decreased 50% at 1.2 mM azide and with urogel at 0.92 mM. Inhibition at these low azide concentrations suggests the possible participation of singlet oxygen in the photooxidation mechanism as has often been observed with porphyrin photosensitizers.[7]

In addition to the studies with furfuryl alcohol, a few preliminary measurements were made of the quantum yields of oxygen uptake during the sensitized photooxidation of selected amino acids as a function of pH. With uro, the yields at approximately pH 5, 7.4 and 10 with the different amino acids were, respectively,: cysteine (0.0019, 0.062, 0.27), histidine (0.0083, 0.13, 0.17), methionine (0.030, 0.037, 0.050), tryptophan (0.037, 0.083, 0.13), and tyrosine (0.0010, 0.044, 0.089). With urogel they were: cysteine (0.0015, 0.065, 0.23), histidine (0.0058, 0.079, 0.12), methionine (0.021, 0.028, 0.032), tryptophan (0.049, 0.068, 0.089), and tyrosine (0.0016, 0.0031, 0.064). These data show the same pattern of pH dependence as observed with some other porphyrins;[7] the sharp increase in photochemical yields with cysteine, histidine and tyrosine with increasing pH somewhat parallels the increase in ionization of the side chains of these amino acids as pH is increased.

It is difficult to compare precisely the results with uro and urogel as photodynamic sensitizers since uro is in true solution and the uro in urogel is bound covalently to large particles of agarose; thus a sensitizer concentration in the usual sense cannot be determined for urogel. However, the data presented above show that the kinetics of the photooxidation reactions as sensitized by uro and urogel are very similar; further, uro bound to the agarose is stil a very effective photodynamic sensitizer for those substrates examined. Schaap et al.[8] found that rose bengal bound covalently to chloromethylated styrene-divinylbenzene copolymer beads was still an effective photosensitizer in organic solvent. However, similarly bound chlorophyllin and hematoporphyrin were very inefficient in sensitizing photooxidation reactions. In the present case, it may be that the porphyrin remains an efficient photosensitizer even when bound because it is separated from the agarose surface by a 6-atom spacer arm.

In summary, the present work shows that uro bound covalently to agarose beads is a very efficient photosensitizer. In studies with other types of immobilized sensitizers it has been found that they are often as efficient photochemically and sometimes more photostable than the same sensitizers in solution.[8] Of importance, bound sensitizers can be removed from the illumination system rapidly and conveniently by filtration or centrifugation. In contrast, dissolved sensitizers must be removed by more difficult and time consuming processes such as gel filtration, dialysis, etc.

This work was supported in part by NIH Biomedical Research Support Grant No. RR07092 and the University of Utah Research Fund. We thank Doug Evans for skillful technical assistance.

REFERENCES

1. E. Reddi, E. Rossi, and G. Jori, Factors controlling the efficiency of porphyrins as photosensitizers of biological systems to damage by visible light, Med. Biol. Environ. 9:337 (1981).
2. G. Jori and J. D. Spikes, Photosensitized oxidations in complex biological structures, pp. 441-457 in: "Oxygen and Oxy-Radicals in Chemistry and Biology", M. A. J. Rodgers and E. L. Powers, eds., Academic Press, New York (1981).

3. R. C. Straight, Photophysical, photochemical and photodynamic
    properties of bound sensitizers, Program Amer. Soc. Photobiol.
    10:90 (1982) (and references therein).
4. P. Cuetrecasas and C. B. Anfinsen, Affinity chromatography,
    pp. 345-378 in: "Methods in Enzymology", Vol. 22, W. B.
    Jacoby, ed., Academic Press, New York (1971).
5. F. Rizzuto and J. D. Spikes, The eosin-sensitized photo-
    oxidation of substituted phenylalanines and tyrosines,
    Photochem. Photobiol. 25:465 (1977).
6. J. S. Bellin, Photophysical and photochemical effects of dye
    binding, Photochem. Photobiol. 8:383 (1968).
7. G. Jori and J. D. Spikes, The photobiochemistry of porphyrins,
    in: "Topics in Photomedicine", K. C. Smith, ed., Plenum
    Publishing Corp., New York, in press.
8. A. P. Schapp, A. L. Thayer, E. C. Blossey, and D. C. Neckers,
    Polymer-based sensitizers for photooxidation. II, J. Am.
    Chem. Soc. 97:3741 (1975).

CHEMICAL AND BIOLOGICAL STUDIES ON HAEMATOPORPHYRIN DERIVATIVE:

AN UNEXPECTED PHOTOSENSITISATION IN BRAIN

R. Bonnett,* M.C. Berenbaum,** and H. Kaur*

*Chemistry Department   **Pathology Department
 Queen Mary College   St. Mary's Hospital Medical
 London E1 4NS   School, London W2 1PG

INTRODUCTION

The porphyrins are a group of heteroaromatic compounds possessing the parent skeleton shown in structure (1). Although it can be oxidised and reduced, this skeleton in general shows considerable stability. It is characterised by an absorption spectrum possessing a very strong band (the Soret band) at about 400 nm, and (generally) four further bands in the region 500 nm to 600 nm. The electronically excited state (S_1) of the porphyrin system follows two pathways, radiative and (initially) non-radiative. The radiative pathway generates the ground state by energy emission (characteristically a red fluorescence, a very sensitive test for the porphyrin system in the absence of a co-ordinated transition metal ion), while intersystem crossing generates the triplet state, which is capable of sensitising the formation of singlet oxygen.

The first effect has been used in tumour localisation studies: the second effect is believed to contribute to the photodestruction of tumours.

The photodestructive effect ("photodynamic action") of porphyrins in mammals was first observed by workers in Germany in the early years of this century.[1,2] One of the problems has always been in the administration of porphyrins: the porphyrin nucleus is relatively large and hydrophobic, and hence (unless functional groups which confer water solubility are purposely introduced) the porphyrins tend to be sparingly soluble in water. It was to overcome this that in 1960 Lipson and Baldes[3] described the preparation cryptically known as "haematoporphyrin derivative". They treated

67

haematoporphyrin (2) with sulphuric acid in acetic acid to give a
solid material: they referred to this as "haematoporphyrin
derivative", and this name is retained here.   Before use, it was
treated with alkali.   This treatment is now known to cause chemical
changes in the solid derivative, and hence we refer to the material
prepared for injection as "alkali-treated haematoporphyrin
derivative".   The observation was made that this preparation was
preferentially localised in tumour tissue,[4] and hence the way was
open to a photosensitised destruction of tumours.   This development,
which now seems so obvious, did not in fact occur until 1972, when
Diamond et al.[5] described the use of haematoporphyrin.   Alkali-
treated haematoporphyrin derivative was first employed in this way
in 1975 by two groups[6],[7] and since then a considerable and world-
wide interest in this novel approach has developed.

HAEMATOPORPHYRIN DERIVATIVE

Our interest has been to determine the chemical nature of
haematoporphyrin derivative, to separate the components and
identify them, and to find out which are the most effective
components by developing a biological assay in vivo.   It became
obvious that haematoporphyrin derivative was a complex and
variable mixture.   Part of the variation was due to the fact that
haematoporphyrin, commercially available as the dihydrochloride,
was itself often far from pure.   But even when satisfactory
samples of haematoporphyrin were employed in the preparation,
several components were detected in the product, and some of these
were rather sensitive compounds.

The components of haematoporphyrin derivative were separated
by preparative high pressure liquid chromatography.[8]   This gave
the products as dicarboxylic acids, suitable for biological assay.
(In an independent approach, Clezy and his colleagues have
separated the dimethyl esters).[9]   The composition of a typical
mixture is shown in Table 1.   The main component was haematoporphyrin diacetate (3).   The other components which were recognised
were the monoacetate (mixed isomers, 4, 5); the isomeric hydroxyethyl vinyl deuteroporphyrins (6, 7); the isomeric acetoxyethyl
vinyl deuteroporphyrins (8, 9); and protoporphyrin (10).   Hence
the reactions occurring were acetylation and elimination processes,
as shown in Scheme 1.

Alternative and more satisfactory routes have been developed
for the preparation of some of these compounds.   These are shown
in Scheme 2.   It should be noted in passing that the acetates and
alcohols being studied here are pseudo-benzylic systems: the
carbocation (11) is readily formed, and all the reactions shown in
Scheme 1 are reversible.   Hence these substances require careful
manipulation.

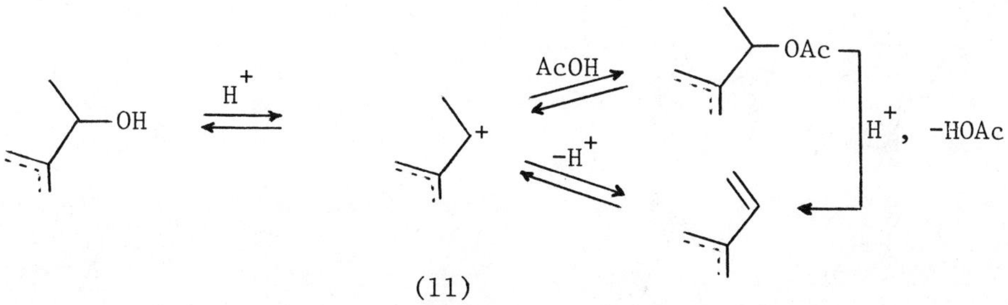

(11)

Scheme 1

Table 1.   Composition of a typical sample of haematoporphyrin
           derivative (analytical reverse phase hplc)[8]

Porphyrin	Retention volume (ml)	Relative Abundance (%)
Haematoporphyrin (2)	7.0	5.1
Haematoporphyrin monoacetate (4/5)	9.3	22.4
Isomeric hydroxyethyl (6)	13.0	1.4
vinyl deuteroporphyrin (7)	13.5	1.8
Haematoporphyrin diacetate (3)	14.5	60.3
Isomeric acetoxyethyl (8)	20.0	2.7
vinyl deuteroporphyrin (9)	21.0	4.8
Protoporphyrin (10)	31.5	1.4

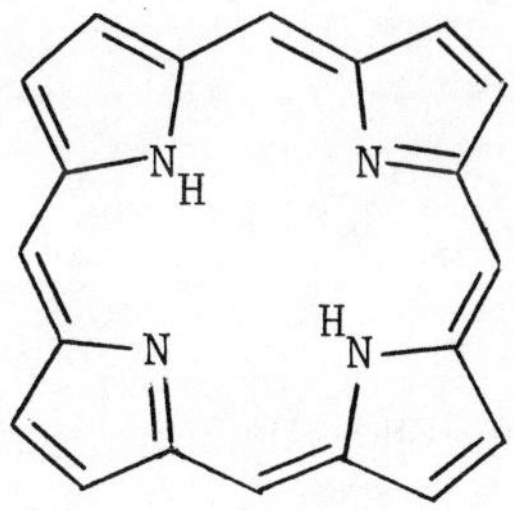

(1) Porphyrin

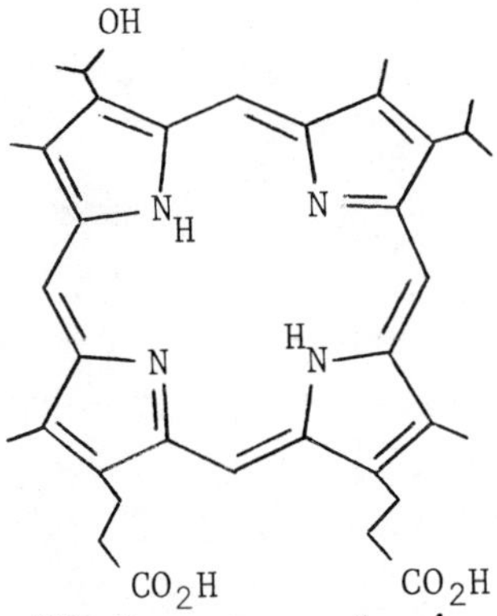

(2) Haematoporphyrin

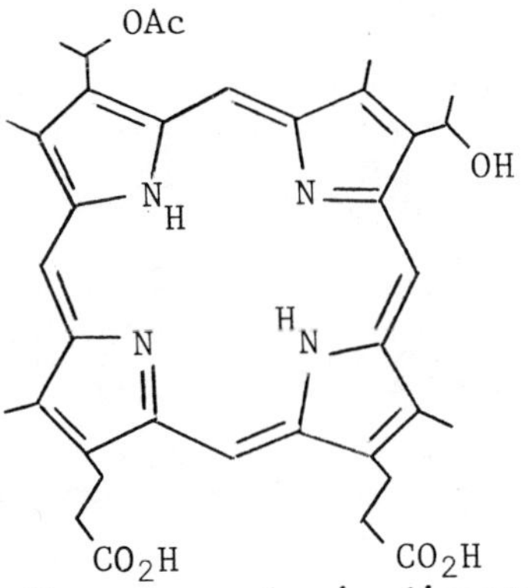

(3) Haematoporphyrin diacetate

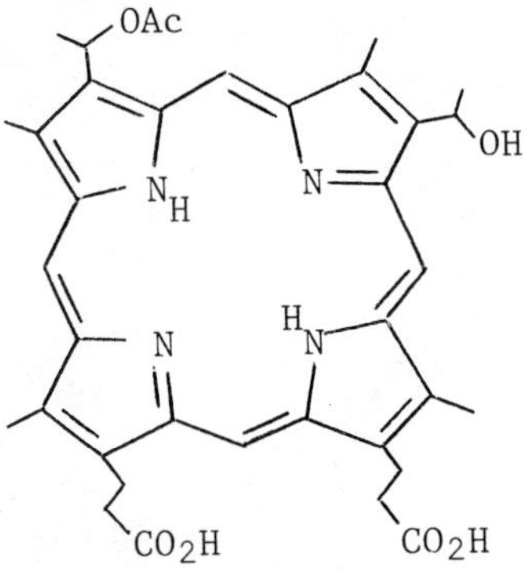

(4) Haematoporphyrin monoacetate
(5) Isomer, OH and OAc inter-
    changed

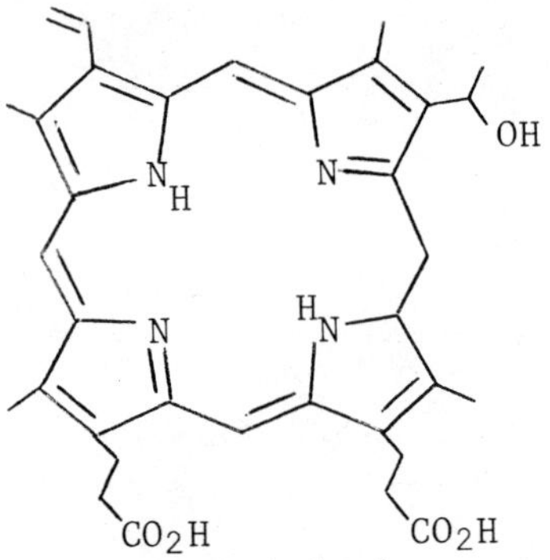

(6) Hydroxyethylvinyl
    deuteroporphyrin
(7) Isomer, $-CH=CH_2$ and $-CHOHMe$
    interchanged

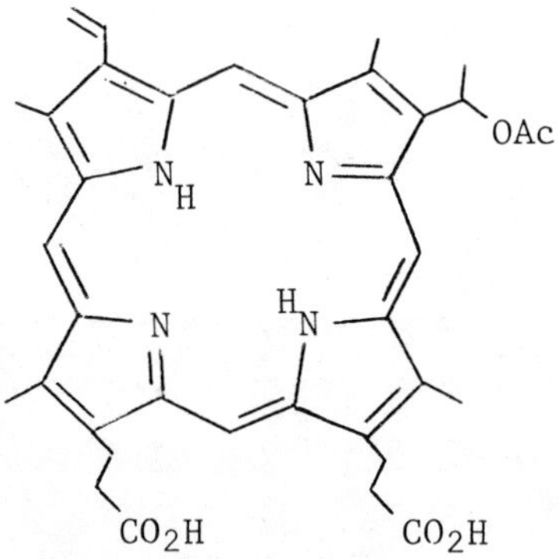

(8) Acetoxyethylvinyl
    deuteroporphyrin
(9) Isomer, $-CH=CH_2$ and $-CHOAcMe$
    interchanged

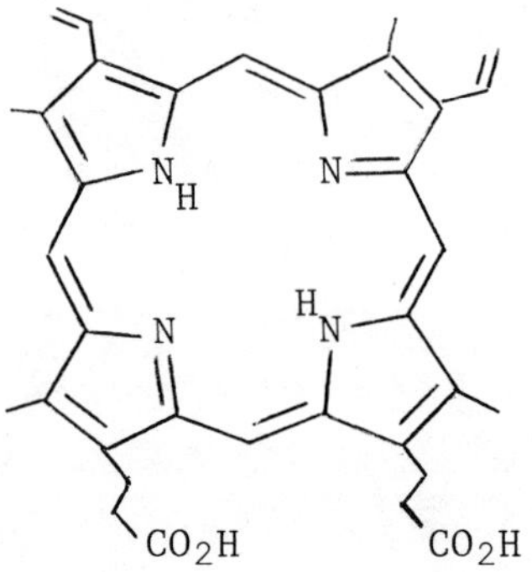

(10) Protoporphyrin

Figure 1.   Structures of porphyrins related to haematoporphyrin

$$2 \cdot 2HCl \xrightarrow[4°C, 72h, N_2]{AcOH-Ac_2O-HCl} \quad 3 \ (87\%)$$

$$2 \cdot 2HCl \xrightarrow[20°C, 4h, N_2]{Ac_2O-Py} \quad 3 \ (81\%)$$

$$2 \cdot 2HCl \xrightarrow[\text{(ii) Hplc}]{\text{(i) AcOH-HCl} \atop 4°C, 72h, N_2} \quad 4/5 \ (30\%)$$

$$2 \cdot 2HCl \xrightarrow[\text{(ii) Hplc}]{\text{(i) } 65°C, DMF, 1h, N_2 \text{ flush}} \quad 6 \ (12\%) + 7 \ (13\%)$$

$$6 \xrightarrow[20°C, 4h, N_2]{Ac_2O-Py} \quad 8 \ (85\%)$$

$$7 \xrightarrow[20°C, 4h, N_2]{Ac_2O-Py} \quad 9 \ (88\%)$$

Scheme 2.   Alternative routes to the main components of
haematoporphyrin derivative.[9]

A biological assay for tumour photonecrosis has been
developed.[10]   In essence this is as follows.   The test porphyrin,
dissolved in dimethyl sulphoxide – sodium bicarbonate – phosphate
buffer saline, is injected intravenously into a mouse with a
tumour implant, the dose being 6.2×10^{-5} mol/kg.   After 24 hours
the tumour is irradiated with heat-filtered white light under
standard conditions.   After a further 24 hours, Evan's blue is
injected, and the animals are killed 2 hours later.   The tumours
are excised, fixed, and sectioned vertically to the skin surface,
and the depth of photonecrosis, as judged by lack of staining, is
measured with a stereomicroscope fitted with a micrometer eyepiece.
Six animals are used in each assay.   Although it is quite possible
that this procedure may somewhat underestimate damage (since some
damage may have occurred in the tissue which is still able to
sustain capillary flow) we believe that it provides a satisfactory
and direct test of biological activity of porphyrin photosensitisers
and, indeed, of tumour-directed photonecrotic agents in general.

The results of the biological assay were clear cut: haematoporphyrin (2), the hydroxyethyl vinyl isomers (6/7), and protoporphyrin (10) were apparently inactive.   The acetates (3, 4/5,
8/9) were all active (Table 2).

The idea that the acetates were the active components was an
attractive one: but the problem turned out to be much more complex

Table 2. Photonecrotic activity of porphyrin acetates

Porphyrin		Activity[a]	
		Expt 1	Expt 2
Haematoporphyrin	(2)	0 (6)	0 (4)
Haematoporphyrin diacetate	(3)	0.72 ± 0.46 (6)	0.78 ± 0.21 (5)
Haematoporphyrin monoacetates	(4/5)	1.02 ± 0.29 (6)	0.66 ± 0.34 (6)
Acetoxyethyl vinyl deuteroporphyrin	(8/9)	0.86 ± 0.64 (5)	1.11 ± 0.24 (6)

[a]Given as depth of necrosis (± s.d.) as a function of that
 obtained with HpD (assumed mean mol. wt. = 650).
[b]Number of animals.

than this. Firstly, the porphyrins were prepared in solutions
containing base (sodium bicarbonate) over a period of 30 minutes
or so at room temperature, and these conditions cause changes
involving the acetoxy functions. Secondly, when the solution of
haematoporphyrin diacetate in the dimethyl sulphoxide – sodium
bicarbonate-buffer was injected less than a minute after
dissolution, it showed no apparent activity: after 3 hours the
solution was fully active. (Because of this, we routinely make
injections 3 hours after solution preparation in the standard test).

     Evidently hydrolysis and elimination reactions were occurring,
the same reactions that are known to occur with HpD when it is
"activated" by alkali treatment (0.1 M NaOH, 1h, 20°C). The
difficulty is that this treatment apparently leads to haematoporphyrin (2), the hydroxyethyl vinyl isomers (6, 7) and protoporphyrin (10).[11] These products are not unexpected, but they do
not show activity in our biological assay. Hence we postulated
that another type of substance must be formed but was not being
detected in the hplc analysis.

     Two possibilities appeared reasonable:

(i) The presence of haematoporphyrin sulphates (e.g. 2, 4, 5, 6,
7 with $-OSO_3H$ in place of $-OH$) in haematoporphyrin derivative.
These would be derived from the sulphuric acid present in the

HOAc-HSO₄ used to make HpD. On treatment with base these would give sodium salts, which as amphipathic molecules, would have detergent properties and might assist in the transport of less soluble porphyrins. While this idea has not been ruled out, we have discovered no evidence to support it. The very polar first fraction from the reverse phase hplc, which might be expected to contain any haematoporphyrin sulphate derivatives found, does not show biological activity. Moreover this idea does not account for the activation of pure haematoporphyrin diacetate in DMSO-NaHCO₃-buffer during 30 minutes or so.

(ii) The presence of dimeric/oligomeric substances which because of their high molecular weights, did not emerge from the column. Evidence in support of this idea came from experiments in which alkali-treated HpD was subjected to preparative reverse phase chromatography. After the elution of the known products (2, 6, 7, 10) the spent column was eluted with powerful elutriants, which brought off a further porphyrin fraction (fraction D) which showed high biological activity.

We have suggested that the active substance may be a covalently bonded dimeric (or oligomeric) structure with ether or ester linkages,[10,12] and we are now engaged in a combined chemical and biological study designed to solve this problem. It seems clear that the haematoporphyrin acetates are precursors of the active constituent, and one approach has been to study the chemical reactions of these substances which are likely to lead to dimers and oligomers. To take an example, the thermal treatment of haematoporphyrin diacetate in 2,4,6-trichlorobenzene at 210°C for 4 hours leads to a product which contains substances which appear to be different from protoporphyrin on hplc, and which are possibly condensation oligomers. However, the product, although soluble in DMSO, is only very sparingly soluble in water, and in this respect is very unlike alkali-treated HpD. It is also inactive in the biological test, and is evidently not what we are looking for.

BRAIN PHOTOSENSITISATION

About two years ago, we began to investigate the problem of using sensitisation with HpD and other porphyrins in the treatment of tumours in what, at first sight, would appear to be an ideal site, i.e. the central nervous system. Human gliomas are sensitised by porphyrins in vitro[13] and, while brain tumours fluoresce after systemic administration, normal brain does not, except at a few restricted sites, as noted below.[14] Phototherapy might thus be a highly suitable treatment for brain tumours, especially for glioblastoma, where the results of conventional therapy are poor. We were surprised to find, however, that mice given HpD (40 mg/kg, which is equivalent on a surface area basis to 3 mg/kg in man) and

illuminated through the intact cranium with red light (630 nm, 18-
20 mW/cm^2 for 10-12 minutes, or 11-13 Joules/cm^2) generally died
within 24 hours, and this was the case whether the mice carried an
intracerebral tumour transplant or were normal.   There was a
striking increase in vascular permeability in the illuminated
area, as shown by penetration of intravenously injected Evan's blue,
(Figure 2).   We also found that cerebral photosensitivity could be
produced in rats and, in these, a craniotomy with mobilisation of
the cranial vault before exposure to light prevented damage.   We
think, therefore, that the cause of death is a rapid rise of intracranial pressure due to cerebral oedema.   Oedema seems to be of
the vasogenic rather than the cytotoxic type (although coexistence
of the two types cannot at present be excluded) because cytotoxic
oedema is not accompanied by increased vascular permeability.[15]

    Damage was not limited to oedema formation.   In animals that
survived, examination one week after illumination showed neuronal
necrosis in the illuminated areas of brain.

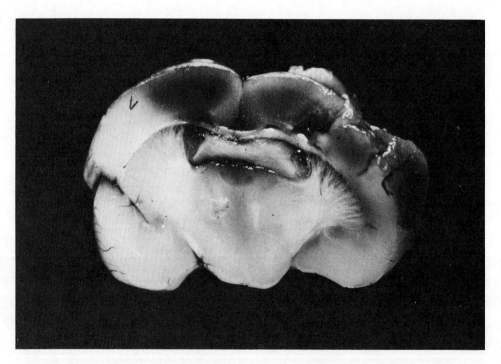

Figure 2.   Brain of mouse given HpD (40 mg/kg), illuminated
            24 hours later, and given Evan's blue 3 hours after
            illumination. Note deep staining of illuminated
            region of cerebrum, especially white matter.

We do not find it easy to explain these findings. The possibility that photosensitisation is due to porphyrins persisting in the circulation is unlikely because we could produce the lesion even 2-3 weeks after injection of HpD.

It is possible that porphyrins, especially lipophilic porphyrins can, despite the general belief to the contrary, pass the intact blood-brain barrier and persist in extra-vascular sites, particularly myelin sheaths, in amounts insufficient to produce visible fluorescence but nevertheless sufficient to cause lethal photosensitisation. The dimers which we have postulated[10],[12] to be the active constituents of HpD _in vivo_ might be expected to behave in this way.

Little work has been done on the extent to which porphyrins enter normal brain tissue. Low levels have been reported by Gomer and coworkers,[16] but measurements were not made beyond 72 hours and were not corrected for porphyrins that would still be present intravascularly at the time of measurement. Moreover, the blood-brain barrier is known to be deficient in a few areas, i.e. the choroid plexuses and some small paraventricular sites such as the area postrema and the pituitary stalk.[17] The barrier can also be circumvented to some extent by uptake of materials at peripheral axon endings followed by retrograde transport to cranial nerve nuclei.[18] Entry at these points might account for the low concentrations of porphyrins found after systemic injection, and it is possible therefore that the bulk of the brain, which is insulated by a normal blood-brain barrier, it essentially closed to porphyrin entry. (The lesions we observed were not due to porphyrin entry into paraventricular sites or cranial nerve nuclei as these sites were not damaged - increased vascular permeability was limited to the illuminated parts of the cerebrum and cere-bellum). Thus there is at present no good evidence that photo-sensitivity is due to porphyrins crossing the normal blood-brain barrier in small amounts.

Further, if photosensitivity is due to porphyrins retained in extravascular sites (and the myelin sheath would be a strong candidate), it is difficult to see why the oedema should so clearly be due to damage to vascular endothelium. We have incidentally found that a highly polar porphyrin, tetraphenylporphyrin tetra-sulphonate, which is even less likely than the constituents of HpD to pass the blood-barrier in significant amounts, is also effective in photosensitising the brain.

The alternative to sensitisation being due to porphyrins crossing the blood-brain barrier is that they do not cross, but are retained for long periods within the vascular endothelium. The possibility of covalent linkage to cell constituents is relevant here, but we have no direct evidence of retention by cerebral vessels, and our investigations are continuing.

MECHANISTIC CONSIDERATIONS

To conclude on a general mechanistic note. Although the
basic laws of photobiology are the same as those of photochemistry
there is, in photobiology, an additional parameter – evolution.
This makes it necessary to distinguish between two sorts of
process. First there are the photobiological processes which have
evolved to fulfil a precise function. Photosynthesis and vision
are examples here. These processes are under structural and/or
metabolic control: the mechanistic pathway may have many steps,
but generally a single main pathway exists.

The other class of photobiological processes is not under
metabolic control, and photodynamic action – including the
processes described in the present paper – is an example here.
The photosensitiser has arisen adventitiously, and there is no
purpose-made structure to determine the course of the photochemically initiated event, nor is there an enzyme system
specifically designed to deal with the products of photochemical
reactions. The excited species, or reactive molecules derived
from it, can react with a variety of target molecules in the cell.
Hence the reaction is expected to be able to follow several
alternative pathways. We should not expect a single route.

These ideas have been expressed elsewhere in a general way[19]
and can be summarised in the following postulate for photobiology.

"Those photoreactions in living systems which have evolved
under metabolic control in a structured system (e.g. photosynthesis, vision) essentially follow one main chemical pathway,
giving the biologically desirable result.

Those photoreactions in living systems which are not under
metabolic control (e.g. photodynamic effects) are expected to be
much more complex since cells offer a variety of targets for the
excited species produced and for the reactive intermediates
generated from them."

There is much evidence that <u>one</u> of the routes followed with
porphyrin photosensitisers <u>in vivo</u> leads to the formation of
singlet oxygen, thus:

$$\text{Por} \xrightarrow{h\nu} \text{Por}(S_1) \xrightarrow{\text{ISC}} \text{Por}(T_1) \xrightarrow{{}^3O_2} {}^1O_2 + \text{Por}(S_o)$$

The singlet oxygen is then able to react with one of a number of
molecules (tryptophan, histidine, unsaturated lipid, cholesterol).
One method for studying photosensitization in cells has involved

photohaemolysis. Photohaemolysis is the photoinitiated rupture of
erythrocytes in the presence of sensitisers with the liberation of
haemoglobin: it was discovered in the early years of this century
by workers employing eosin[20] and porphyrins.[21]   It has attracted
a good deal of attention recently, and there is good evidence for
the involvement of singlet oxygen here.[22]

       In collaborative work with Professor I.A. Magnus, Dr. S.
Chandra has recently carried out experiments on the effectiveness
of haematoporphyrin and its relatives in photohaemolysis. Results
are recorded in Table 3.

Table 3. Photohaemolysis of erythrocytes sensitised with various
          porphyrins.

Porphyrin	Molarity/10^2 nM	% Photohaemolysis after 3h[a]
Protoporphyrin (10)	3.7	81
	5.6	93
Haematoporphyrin diacetate (3)	4.6	48
	7.6	70
Haematoporphyrin monoacetate (4/5)	4.5	15
	7.6	51
Haematoporphyrin (2)	8.4	22
	12.6	23
HpD	7.2	11
	9.6	33
TPPSS[b]	7.8	6
	19.2	13

[a]The photohaemolysis curves show an induction period, and it is
 difficult to make precise comparisons. Nevertheless this
 parameter allows broad distinctions between activities to be made.
[b]meso-Tetra(p-hydroxysulphonylphenyl)porphyrin tetrasodium salt.

Clearly the photohaemolysis experiment is not a satisfactory model for the activity of porphyrins in tumour photonecrosis. Haematoporphyrin and its relatives fall in the mid range of activity: protoporphyrin (which does not photosensitise tumours in our assay, possibly partly because of solubility reasons) is very effective in photohaemolysis while TPPSS, which is effective in our biological assay, is a very poor photosensitiser for photohaemolysis.

Photohaemolysis has a useful role, though, in directing attention to the possible ways in which porphyrins interact with membranes, since it is the disruption of the latter which allows the haemoglobin finally to leak out. A molecule like protoporphyrin may be regarded as an amphipathic system, and the nonpolar end might be expected to become incorporated into the lipid part of the membrane as shown in Figure 3. We may add to this model the known fact that oxygen is more soluble in organic solvents than it is in water by (approximately) an order of magnitude (Table 4). Hence the partition of oxygen will tend to concentrate oxygen in the lipid bilayer. As a result the latter, containing both porphyrin and ground state oxygen, will be a favoured site for the formation of singlet oxygen. The disruption of the membrane may therefore be understood in terms of the reaction of this reactive species with the target molecules (particularly cholesteryl and unsaturated lipid residues) which are essential constituents of the membrane.

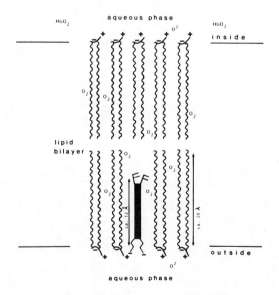

Figure 3.   Proposed incorporation of amphipathic porphyrins in lipid bilayer portion of membrane (see text)[23].

Table 4. Solubility of oxygen in various solvents[a]
(Landholt-Bornstein, 1923, 1931)

Solvent	Temperature 0°	Bunsen absorption coefficient[b]
H_2O	20	0.0310
	35	0.6244
PhH	19	0.163
$CHCl_3$	16	0.205
MeOH	20	0.237
Et_2O	20	0.415

[a]From Landholt-Bornstein Physikalisch-Chemisches Tabellen, Springer, Berlin (1923), p.765 and (1931) 2nd Supplement, Part 1, p.484.
[b]Volume of oxygen (reduced to STP) which dissolves at the stated temperature in one volume of the solvent when the partial pressure of the gas is 760 nm.

ACKNOWLEDGEMENT

We are grateful to the Medical Research Council and the University of London Research Fund for the financial support of this work.

1. W. Hausmann, The sensitising action of haematoporphyrin, Biochem. Z. 30: 176 (1911)
2. F. Meyer-Betz, Investigations on the biological (photodynamic) action of haematoporphyrin and other derivatives of blood and bile pigments, Dtsch. Arch. Klin. Med. 112: 476 (1913).
3. R.L. Lipson and E.J. Baldes, The photodynamic properties of a particular haematoporphyrin derivative, Arch. Dermatol. 82: 508 (1960).
4. R.L. Lipson, E.J. Baldes, and A.M. Olsen, The use of a derivative of haematoporphyrin in tumour detection, J. Natl. Cancer Inst. 26: 1 (1961).
5. I. Diamond, A.F. McDonagh, C.B. Wilson, S.L.Granelli, S. Nielsen and R. Jaenicke, Photodynamic therapy of malignant tumours, Lancet ii: 1175 (1972).
6. J.F. Kelly, M.E. Snell, and M.C. Berenbaum, Photodynamic destruction of human bladder carcinoma, Br. J. Cancer, 31: 237 (1975).

7. T.J. Dougherty, G.B. Grindey, R. Fiel, K.R. Weishaupt, and
    D.G. Boyle, Photoradiation therapy 2. Cure of animal tumours
    with haematoporphyrin and light, J. Natl. Cancer Inst. 55: 115
    (1975).
8. R. Bonnett, R.J. Ridge, P.A. Scourides, and M.C. Berenbaum, On
    the nature of haematoporphyrin derivative, J. Chem. Soc.,
    Perkin Trans. 1, 3139 (1981).
9. P.S. Clezy, T.T. Hai, R.W. Henderson, and L. van Thue, The
    chemistry of pyrrolic compounds 45. Haematoporphyrin
    derivative, Austral. J. Chem. 33: 585 (1980).
10. M.C. Berenbaum, R. Bonnett, and P.A. Scourides, In vivo
    biological activity of the components of haematoporphyrin
    derivative, Br. J. Cancer, 45: 571 (1982).
11. R. Bonnett, R.J. Ridge, P.A. Scourides, and M.C. Berenbaum,
    Haematoporphyrin derivative, J. Chem. Soc., Chem. Comm. 1198
    (1980).
12. R. Bonnett and M.C. Berenbaum, HpD − A study of its components
    and their properties, Adv. Exp. Biol. Med. 160: 241 (1983).
13. R. Hayward, In vitro demonstration of the photodynamic effect
    on human brain tumours, Ann. Roy. Coll. Surg. 54: 272 (1974).
14. B.L. Wise and D.R. Toxdal, Studies of the blood-brain barrier
    utilising haematoporphyrin, Brain Research, 387 (1967).
15. I. Klatzo, Cerebral oedema and ischaemia, Recent Adv. Neuro-
    pathol. 1: 27 (1979).
16. C.J. Gomer, N. Rucker, C. Mark, W.F. Benedict, and A.L. Murphee,
    Tissue distribution of ^{3}H-haematoporphyrin derivative in athymic
    'nude' mice heterotransplanted with human retinoblastoma,
    Invest. Ophthalm. Vis. Sci. 22: 118 (1982).
17. A. Weindl, Neuroendocrine aspects of circumventricular organs,
    in: "Frontiers in Neuroendocrinology", W.F. Ganong and
    L. Martini, eds., p.3, Oxford Univ. Press, London (1973).
18. R.D. Broadwell and M.W. Brightman, Entry of peroxidase into
    nervous systems from extracerebral and cerebral blood, J.
    Compar. Neurol. 166: 257.
19. R. Bonnett, Oxygen activation and tetrapyrroles, Essays in
    Biochemistry 17: 1 (1981), and there p.39.
20. H. von Tappeiner, Action of fluorescent substances on red
    corpuscles, Biochem. Z. 13: 1 (1908).
21. W. Hausmann, The photodynamic action of plant extracts
    containing chlorophyll, Biochem. Z. 12: 331 (1907).
22. A.A. Lamola, T. Yamane, and A.M. Trozzole, Cholesterol hydro-
    peroxide formation in red cell membranes and photohaemolysis
    in erythropoietic protoporphyria, Science, 179: 1131 (1973).
23. A. de Paolis, S. Chandra, A.A. Charalambides, I.A. Magnus, and
    R. Bonnett, Photohaemolysis: the effect of porphyrin structure,
    to be published.

A CHROMATOGRAPHIC STUDY OF HEMATOPORPHYRIN DERIVATIVES

Stein Sommer, Johan Moan, Terje Christensen
and Jan F. Evensen

Norsk Hydro's Institute for Cancer Research
Montebello, Oslo 3
Norway

INTRODUCTION

Hematoporphyrin derivative (Hpd), a porphyrin mixture first introduced as a tumorlocalizer by Lipson et al.[1] is the most widely used drug in clinical trials for photoradiation therapy (PRT) of cancer. Furthermore, due to its fluorescence and tumorlocalizing properties, it may be used in cancer diagnosis[1-5]. The components in Hpd have different tumorlocalizing and photosensitizing properties which should be characterized in order to select the component with the best properties for clinical use and for further investgations.

Since the main constituents of the chemical precursor of Hpd are porphyrin acetates, it has been proposed that hematoporphyrin diacetate should be used in the clinical experiments instead of the mixture Hpd[6,7]. However, the porphyrin acetates hydrolyze readily in aqueous solutions[8,9] and as shown in the present work, upon hydrolysis give rise to a porphyrin mixture not much different from Hpd. When hematoporphyrin diacetate is dissolved in dimetylsulfoxide and injected immediately in tumorbearing mice it does not sensitize tumors to photoinactivation[8]. Sensitizing properties develop gradually with time after dissolving the diacetate[8]. This led us to study the time course of the reactions taking place upon dissolving hematoporphyrin diacetate.

Many porphyrins are rapidly degraded by exposure to light[20]. Such degradation may also take place in tumors during PRT. Therefore, Hpd and its major components were studied with respect to light sensitivity and generation of photoproducts.

Finally, the problem of selecting the best tumorlocalizer of the Hpd components was approached by injecting Hpd in tumorbearing mice, extracting the porphyrins from the tumors and analyzing the extracts by HPLC.

MATERIALS AND METHODS

Chemicals

Hpd was prepared from hematoporphyrin dihydrochloride (Koch-Light) as described by Lipson et al.[1]

Hematoporphyrin diacetate was synthesized as described elsewhere[10]. Protoporphyrin, hematoporphyrin and photoprotoporphyrin were purchased from Porphyrin Products, Logan, Utah.

Chromatography

High pressure liquid chromatography (HPLC) was carried out with a LDC chromatograph equipped with a gradient elution system, a variable wavelength absorption detector (LDC spectromonitor III, model 1204) and a fluorescence detector (LDC fluoromonitor III). Absorption and fluorescence intensity were recorded simultaneously. The absorption detector was usually operated at 392 nm where most of the porphyrins studied in the present work have their absorption maximum under the conditions described below. The excitation light in the fluorescence detector was filtered by a broad band interference filter with maximum transmission at 360 nm and bandwidth 60 nm. Stray light was eliminated from the fluorescence by means of a cut-off filter transmitting only light with wavelengths longer than 410 nm.

A Supelcosil LC 18 column (250 x 4.6 mm) was used and the mobile phase was a variable mixture of methanol and water, buffered with 1.5 mM sodium phosphate. Usually a linear, gradient elution was applied. Solvent A: methanol/water (60/40), pH 7.0, 1.5 mM phosphate. Solvent B: methanol/water (90/10), pH 7.5, 1.5 mM phosphate. Gradient time: 30 min. More than 90% of the injected amount of Hpd was eluted from the column in a typical run.

Gel permeation chromatography was carried out by means of a Bio-gel P10 column (Bio-Rad, 260 x 10 mm) with Dulbecco's phosphate-buffered saline (PBS) as the mobile phase.

Spectroscopy

Absorption and fluorescence spectra were recorded by means of

a Cary 118 spectrophotometer and a Hitachi Perkin-Elmer MPF - 2A
spectrofluorimeter, respectively.

Biological experiments

Lewis lung carcinomas were inoculated subcutaneously into the
back of B6D2 mice weighing 16 - 20 g. Tumors were allowed to grow
until 5 - 10 mm in diameter. Three hours before the animals were
sacrificed 3.7 mg Hpd was injected intraperitoneally. After sacri-
ficing the mice,livers and tumors were isolated and weighed. The
porphyrins in tumor and liver tissue were extracted according to
the method described in (11), with a few modifications.

The composition of crude Hpd was unchanged when brought through
the entire extraction procedure.

Light exposure

The light source used for photodegradation of Hpd consisted
of four fluorescent tubes (Phillips TL 20W/09) emitting light
mainly in the wavelength region 330 - 420 nm. The light fluence
was 17 W/m^2 as measured with a calibrated thermopile (YSI, 65A,
Yellow Springs, OH).

RESULTS AND DISCUSSION

Hematoporphyrin dihydrochloride treated with sulfuric and
acetic acid according to the method described by Lipson et al.[1]
gives rise to a mixture of porphyrins which is rich in porphyrin
acetates. This mixture is called Hpa. According to our earlier
work[8], Hpa gives rise to another porphyrin mixture when hydrolysed
in 0.1 N NaOH: The clinically used hematoporphyrin derivative,
Hpd. Many of the components of Hpa and Hpd have been identified[9,10,12,13]. Referring to the assignment shown in the chromatograms in the present work (figure 1a + b) the following identi-
fications have been performed: 2 as hematoporphyrin, 3A and 3B as
the isomers of O-acetylhematoporphyrin, 4A and 4B as the isomers
2(4)-1-hydroxyethyl-4(2)vinyl-deutero-porphyrin, 5 as 0,0'-
diacetyl-hematoporphyrin, 6A and 6B as the isomers 2(4)-0-acetyl-
4(2)-vinyl-deutero-porphyrin and pp as protoporphyrin. Components
4B and 5 may be hard to separate with methanol/water-based
chromatographic system[13]. However, figure 1a shows that the use
of an exponential gradient makes separation possible. A satisfactory separation is obtained without the use of ion-pairing
reagents which may cause problems if the separated components are
to be used in biologic experiments.

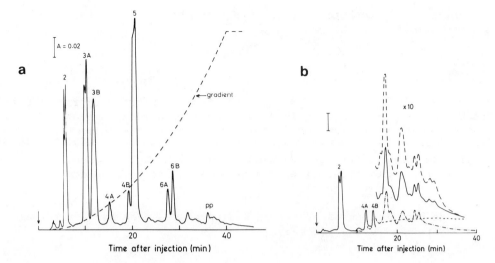

Fig. 1a.   HPLC of Hpa giving separation of component 4B and 5.
           Identifications of the components are given on page 3.
           Solvent A: Methanol/water (60/40); 1.5 mM sodium phos-
           phate buffer, pH 7.0. Solvent B: methanol/water (90/10);
           1.5 mM sodium phosphate buffer, pH 7.5. Gradient time
           100% A ➔ 100% B 40 min.
Fig. 1b.   HPLC of Hpd. ——— absorbance at 390 nm, —————— absor-
           bance at 365 nm, ... absorbance baseline, .—.—.—.-
           fluorescence. All curves are normalized to give the same
           peak height of component 2, 4A and 4B. The bar corres-
           ponds to A = 0.05 at 390 nm and A = 0.02 at 365 nm.
           Gradient time: 30 min. Linear gradient.

           Systems with a linear gradient may be used for the separation
of Hpd. By comparing figure 1a and 1b it turns out that Hpd contains no acetates.

           A large fraction of the components with retention times
exceeding 16 min (Fig. 1b) are aggregated. This is clearly demonstrated by their low fluorescence yield and their strong absorbance
at 365 nm (Fig. 1b). One small peak appearing just ahead of 4A may
also be attributed to aggregates for the same reason.

           With the exception of protoporphyrin, the chemical identity of
these components have not been determined. It has been suggested
that covalent bonds may play a role in keeping the porphyrin molecules in dimers, oligomers and aggregates[8]. In accordance with
this, the aggregates do not dissociate even when dissolved in
methanol which is known to favour a monomer configuration of protoporphyrin, one of the most hydrophobic components of Hpd[14].

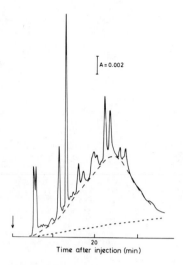

Fig. 2.   HPLC of the aggregated fraction of Hpd. Aggregates were
          isolated from Hpd by means of gel permeation chromato-
          graphy on a P10 column with PBS as the mobile phase.

As one could expect, a large fraction of the aggregates in Hpd are
not well resolved in our chromatograms, but appears as an unstruc-
tured broad band. Thus, when aggregates are isolated on a P10
column and analyzed by HPLC a similar broad band is obtained (Fig. 2).

    We propose that the sharp peaks with low fluorescence in
component 7 are due to dimers or oligomers.   A dimer of Hp and
hydroxyethylvinyl-deuteroporphyrin (Hvd), for instance, will probably give a number of peaks in a chromatogram, due to positional
isomers and stereoisomers. Our finding that all major fractions of
component 7 are converted mainly to protoporphyrin when heated to
160° C (results not shown), may indicate that they are isomers of
Hp/Hvd. (Heating results in conversion of Hp and Hvd to protoporphyrin.) Thus, component 7 may be less complex than the chromatogram indicates.

    It has been proposed that aggregates are formed during hydro-
lysis of the hematoporphyrin acetates in alkali[8]. Our results
confirm this suggestion. Aggregation is clairly indicated by the
change in the absorption spectra shown in figure 3b. A further
analysis of this change and of the chromatograms recorded during
hydrolysis of hematoporphyrin diacetate (Fig. 3a) give a reaction
kinetics as shown in figure 4. Similar reactions take place in
aqueous solutions at pH 7.3 (PBS) as in 0.1 M NaOH although somewhat slower in the former case (Fig. 4). There is one difference:
much smaller amounts of component 4 is formed in PBS than in 0.1 M
NaOH. It can be seen from figure 1b and figure 3a that hydrolysis

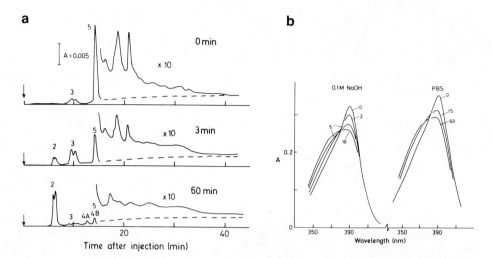

Fig. 3a. Absorption spectra of hematoporphyrin diacetate (component 5) during hydrolysis in 0.1 M NaOH and in PBS
(pH 7.3). The time of hydrolysis in minutes are given on
each curve. The hydrolysis was stopped by diluting the
samples 20 times in Methanol/H_2O (60/40). The pH was
stabilized at 7.0 by 1.5 mM phosphate buffer and by
addition of 0.1 M HCl when necessary. The spectra were
recorded within a few minutes after dilution.

Fig. 3b. HPLC chromatograms of hematoporphyrin diacetate during
hydrolysis in 0.1 M NaOH.

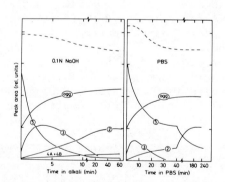

Fig. 4. Peak areas of the main components seen in the chromatograms of hematoporphyrin diacetate during hydrolysis in
0.1 M NaOH and PBS. The peak area of the aggregates is
estimated by assuming that its shape is the same as that
of the aggregates shown in Fig. 3. The dotted curves
correspond to the sum of the peak areas.

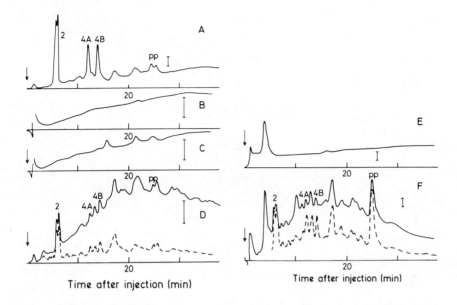

Fig. 5.   HPLC of Hpd and extracts from livers and tumors of mice.
          A: Hpd, B: blind extract, C: extract from liver without
          Hpd, D: extract from the liver of a mouse which was
          injected with Hpd, E: extract from tumor, F: extract from
          the tumor of a mouse which was injected with Hpd. The
          bars correspond to an absorbance of 0.005.
          ——————— absorbance, —————— fluorescence.

of hematoporphyrin diacetate gives rise to a porphyrin mixture not
much different from Hpd. Thus, it is not surprising that these two
porphyrin mixtures have been shown to have similar efficiencies
in sensitizing animal tumors to photodestruction[8]. This sensitizing efficiency is not predominantly due to the monomers of hematoporphyrin[8,15,6]. The most active material was found to be strongly
retained on a reversed phase RP-18 column, and it was supposed that
is was composed of dimers or aggregates[8]. Largely, these findings
and suggestions are in agreement with those of Dougherty et al.[15].
Our results (Fig. 5) also indicate that a large amount of aggregated porphyrins is found in tumors and livers of mice 3 hours
after an intraperitoneal injection of Hpd. Monomers seem to play
a less significant role. Results in agreement with this conclusion
were obtained when the components of Hpd were injected in tumor-
bearing mice[17]. The present results should be interpreted with some
care, since we have injected large quantities of Hpd in the animals
and analysed the tissues only 3 hours after the injections. This
was done in order to extract enough material for HPLC analysis.
Furthermore, the extraction procedure may change the porphyrins at

low concentrations (< 5 µg/ml). At these concentrations modifications of component 2, 4A and 4B may occur if too large amounts of
salts are present in the ether phase before evaporation. These
modifications gave low fluorescence and longer HPLC retention
times. Some chromophores from the extracted tissues may also appear
in the chromatograms, as seen in that of the tumor in figure 5.
Therefore, it is always necessary to chromatograph control samples
of tissue from animals not injected with Hpd.

The accumulation of aggregated material in tumors should be
considered in light of the histologic distribution of Hpd. Aggregates are likely to be taken up by pinocytosis and, in fact, Kupffer
cells in the liver and macrophages in the tumor have been shown to
contain high levels of Hpd (18). Experiments in progress in our
laboratory also indicate that accumulation of Hpd correlates with
high phago/pino-cytiotic activity in several tissues. (J. Evensen,
manuscript under preparation). We have also shown that the photosensitizing effect of Hpd on cells in vitro is mainly due to its
least polar and aggregated components (19).

It is well known that porphyrins are degraded by light.
A product of such a degradation of protoporphyrin is photoprotoporphyrin (20). However, this compound is not formed in detectable amounts when Hpd is exposed to light (figure 6a). From Hpd
one (or more) polar compound (marked as component 1 in figure
6a) is formed. The optical absorption- and fluorescence properties of the corresponding HPLC fraction are illustrated in figure
6b. For comparison spectra of photoprotoporphyrin and hematoporphyrin are also shown. The high absorbance of component 1 and
photoprotoporphyrin in the red part of the spectrum are of interest from a photoradiation therapeutic point of view, since light
of these wavelengths penetrates relatively deeply into tissues.
The tumorlocalizing and photosensitizing capacity of these two
components is not known yet. Notably, if component 1 is formed
inside cells during light exposure, it may play some role in
photoradiaton therapy, as it probably will be strongly retained
in cells because of its high polarity. These observations show
that porphyrins with strong absorbance above 600 nm and with
widely different polarity are easily generated. This should be
taken advantage of in the future search for new sensitizers for
photoradiation therapy. As shown in figure 7, component 4A and
4B are the most sensitive ones to light exposure. This was
verified by exposing the separated components to light. We
observed that the rate of photodegradation was reduced when nitrogen was bubbled through the solution during irradiation, suggesting
that oxydation processes are involved.

The present work was supported by The Norwegian Cancer
Society (Landsforeningen mot Kreft) and NAVF (The Norwegian Research Council for Science and the Humanities).

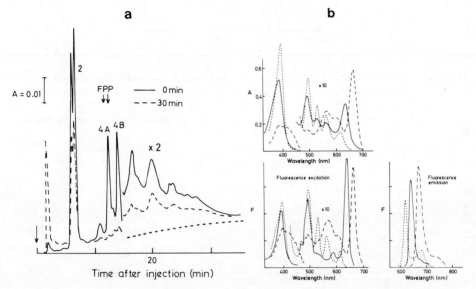

Fig. 6a.   HPLC of Hpd exposed to light for 0 min (————) and 30 min
           (- - - - -) in the presence of 1% serum. The Hpd concentra-
           tion was 62 µg/ml and the optical path-length of the
           exposed sample was 1.4 mm. The arrows marked FPP indi-
           cated where the isomers of photoprotoporohyrin are eluted.

Fig. 6b.   Absorption-, fluorescence-excitation- and fluorescence
           emission spectra of component 1 (————), photoprotopor-
           phyrin (- - - - -) and hematoporphyrin (·····). The fluor-
           escence spectra were recorded with a resolution of 5 nm.
           The excitation spectra were recorded at the following
           emission wavelengths: component 1: 643 nm, photoprotopor-
           phyrin: 672 nm and hematoporphyrin: 618 nm. The emission
           spectra were recorded with the excitation monochromator set
           at 638, 660 and 395 nm, for component 1, photoprotoporphy-
           rin and hematoporphyrin, respectively.

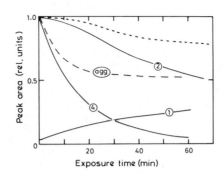

Fig. 7.   Normalized peak areas of the main components of Hpd as
           functions of the exposure time. Conditions as described
           in the legend of fig. 8. The dotted line corresponds to
           the optical absorption of the samples at 390 nm before
           injection.

REFERENCES

1. R. L. Lipson, E. J. Baldes, and A. M. Olsen, The use of a de-
    rivative of hematoporphyrin in tumor detection. J. Natl.
    Cancer Inst. 26:1 (1961).
2. R. L. Lipson, E. J. Baldes, and M. J. Gray, Hematoporphyrin
    derivative of detection and management of cancer. Cancer
    20:2255 (1967).
3. G. A. Kyriazis, H. Bolin, and R. L. Lipson, Hematoporphyrin
    derivative-fluorescence test colposcopy and colphotography
    in the diagnosis of atypical mataplasia, dysplasia and car-
    cinoma in situ of the cervix uteri. Am. J. Obstet Gynecol.
    117:375 (1967).
4. A. E. Profio, and D. R. Doiron, A feasibility study of the
    use of fluorescence bronchoscopy for localization of small
    lung tumors. Phys. Med. Biol. 22:949 (1977).
5. R. C. Benson, G. M. Farrow, J. H. Kinsey, D. A. Cortese,
    H. Zincke, and D. C. Utz, Detection and localization of
    in situ carcinoma of the bladder with hematoporphyrin de-
    rivative. Mayo Clin. Proc. 57:548 (1982).
6. R. W. Henderson, G. S. Christie, P. S. Clezy, and J. Lineham,
    Haematoporphyrin diacetate: A probe to distinguish malign-
    ant from normal tissue by selective fluorescence. Br. J.
    exp. path. 61:345 (1980).
7. M. C. Berenbaum, R. Bonnett, and P. A. Scourides, In vivo
    biological activity of the components of haematoporphyrin
    derivative. Br. J. Cancer 45:571 (1982).
8. R. Bonnett and M. C. Berenbaum, HPD - A study of its com-
    ponents and their properties. In: Porphyrin Photosensiti-

zation", D. Kessel and T. J. Dougherty, ed., Plenum Press, New York, London (1983).

9. J. Moan, S. Sandberg, T. Christensen, and S. Elander, Hemato-porphyrin derivative: Chemical composition, photochemical and photosensitizing properties. In: "Porphyrin Photo-sensitization", D. Kessel and T. J. Dougherty, ed., Plenum Press, New York, London (1983).

10. R. Bonnett, R. J. Ridge, P. A. Scourides, and M. C. Berenbaum, On the nature of haematoporphyrin derivative. J. Chem. Soc. Perkin I : 3135 (1981).

11. M. Salmi, and R. Tehunen, New method for liquid-chromatogra-phic measurement of erythrocyte protoporphyrin and copro-porphyrin. Clin. Chem. 26:1832 (1980).

12. P. S. Clezy, T. T. Hai, R. W. Henderson, and L. Thuc, The chemistry of pyrrolic compounds. VLV * Haematoporphyrin derivative: Haematoporphyrin diacetate as the main pro-duct of the reaction of haematoporphyrin with a mixture of acetic and sulfuric acids. Aus. J. Chem. 33:585 (1980).

13. P. A. Cadby, E. Dimitriades, H. G. Grant, and D. Ward, Se-paration and analysis of haematoporphyrin derivative com-ponents by high-performance liquid chromatography. J. Chromatography 231:273 (1982).

14. D. Kessel and E. Rossi, Determinants of porphyrin-sensitized photooxidation characterized by fluorescence and absorp-tion characterized by fluorescence and absorption spectra. Photochem. Photobiol. 35:37 (1982).

15. T. J. Dougherty, D. G. Boyle, K. R. Weishaupt, B. A. Hender-son, W. R. Potter, D. A. Bellnier, and K. E. Wityk, Photo-radiation therapy - Clinical and drug advances. In: !"Por-phyrin Photosensitization", D. Kessel and T. J. Dougherty, ed., Plenum Press, New York, London (1983).

16. D. Kessel, Components of hematoporphyrin derivative and their tumor-localizing capacity. Cancer Res. 42:1703 (1982).

    J. Moan, J. F. Evensen, T. Christensen, A. Hindar, S. Sommer and J. B. McGhie, Chemical composition of hematoporphyrin derivative, tumorlocalizing and photsensitizing properties of its main components. Abstr. from the 10th ann. meeting of the American Society for Photobiology, Vancouver 1982 (pp. 173-174).

    P. J. Bugelski, C. W. Porter, and T. J. Dougherty, Autoradio-graphic distribution of hematoporphyrin derivative in normal and tumor tissue of the mouse. Cancer Res. 41:4608 (1981).

    J. Moan, T. Christensen, and S. Sommer, The main photosensi-tizing components of hematoporphyrin derivative. Cancer Lett. 15:161 (1982).

    D. Dolphin (ed.) The porphyrins. Vol. 1 pp. 303-308, Acad. Press, New York, San Francisco, London (1978).

PROTECTION BY CAROTENOIDS FROM SINGLET OXYGEN PHOTOPRODUCED BY PORPHYRINS

R.V. Bensasson*, T.A. Moore§, D. Gust§, A.L. Moore§,
A. Joy§, T. Tom§, G. Nemeth§ and E.J. Land†
*Laboratoire de Biophysique, Muséum National d'Histoire
Naturelle 61, Rue Buffon 75005 Paris, France ; § Dept.
of Chemistry, Arizona State University, Tempe AZ 85287
USA ; † Paterson Laboratories, Christie Hospital and
Holt Radium Institute, Manchester M20 9BX, UK

The plant photosynthetic agent β carotene, a successful
oral photoprotective agent in erythropoietic protoporphyria[1]
might also decrease the discomfort of patients after treatment by
hematoporphyrin phototherapy.

Carotenoids prevent the porphyrin-photosensitized formation of highly destructive singlet oxygen by quenching the
porphyrin triplet states and may also scavenge additional singlet
oxygen present. Synthetic carotenoporphyrins consisting of a
carotenoid of variable length covalently linked to a porphyrin by
different linkages help to define the structural requisites for
the photoprotection function of carotenoids [2-5].

Singlet oxygen was detected by spectroscopically monitoring its reaction with a chemical probe, diphenylisobenzofuran,
whose bleaching was followed at 390 nm. Filtered light (630 nm
long pass cut off and a water filter) from a 150 W tungsten-halogen
lamp was used to illuminate the carotenoporphyrins in toluene solutions or in polystyrene or cellulose triacetate matrices at room
temperature. Intramolecular triplet energy transfer between the
porphyrin and the carotenoid was studied by nanosecond laser
flash photolysis.

It was observed that photoprotection was related both
to the triplet energy level of the carotenoid polyene and to the
rate of triplet energy tranfer. The energy transfer rate was in
turn determined by both static and dynamic aspects of the
carotenoporphyrin structure.

REFERENCES

1. M.M. Mathews-Roth in the Science of Photomedicine, Ed. by Regan
   and Parrish (Plenum Publishing Corporation, 1982).
2. G. Dirks, A.L. Moore, T.A. Moore, D. Gust, Photochem. Photobiol.
   32. 277 (1980).
3. A.M. Moore, G. Dirks, D. Gust, T.A. Moore, Photochem. Photobiol.
   32, 691 (1980).
4. R.V. Bensasson, E.J. Land, A.L. Moore, R.L. Crouch, G. Dirks,
   T.A. Moore, D. Gust, Nature 290, 329 (1981).
5. A.L. Moore, A. Joy, R. Tom, D. Gust, T.A. Moore, R.V. Bensasson
   and E.J. Land, Science 216, 982 (1982).

EFFECT OF He-Ne LASER ON HUMAN ERYTHROCYTES INCUBATED WITH HEMATO-PORPHYRIN DERIVATIVE AND BONELLIN: COMPARATIVE STUDY

G. Monfrecola,[*] D. Martellotta,[*] R. Galli,[*] G. Bruno,[*]
L. Cariello,[°] L. Zanetti[°] and P. Santoianni[*]
[*]Department of Dermatology, II Faculty of Medicine
University of Naples
[°]Biochemistry laboratory, Stazione Zoologica, Naples
[*]Via S. Pansini 5 - 80131 - Naples - Italy

INTRODUCTION

Bonellin is a green pigment extracted from Bonellia viridis (Echiurida).

This sea worm aroused great interest in biologists. for its peculiar behaviour and morphological characteristics. The male is 1-2 mm long; the female consists of a large body of about 8 cm with a proboscis more than 1 m long. The worm lives permanently in the

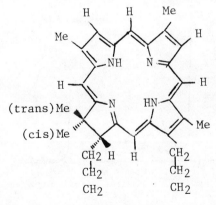

Fig. 1 Structural formula of bonellin

95

dark under sand or rocks on the sea bed: sunlight kills it. The
larvae which settle on the female proboscis change into males, while
those taken out of sea, differentiate into female subjects, several
orders of magnitude bigger.

Baltzer (1931) showed that the aqueous extract of the proboscis
masculinized the larvae. Lederer (1939) isolated from the proboscis
bonellin whose structure was identified by Pelter et al. (1976),
who showed that bonellin is a peculiar chlorin (fig. 1).

In 1979 Agius et al. showed the photodynamic activity of bonellin and, three years later, Cariello et al. demonstrated that this
substance and porphyrins act in a similar way. The absorption spectrum of bonellin (fig. 2) has a peak at 630 nm.

In the present study we have compared the irradiative effect
of He-Ne laser (λ = 632.8 nm) on human erythrocytes incubated
respectively with hematoporphyrin derivative (HpD) and bonellin,

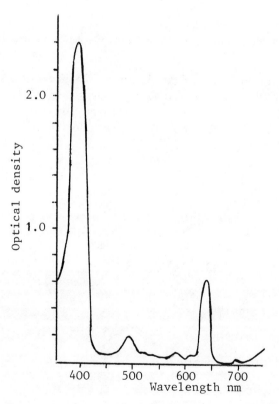

Fig. 2 Absorption spectrum of Bonellin

in order to establish the photodynamic propriety of bonellin.

MATERIALS AND METHODS

Bonellin and HpD Solutions

Bonellin was extracted according to the method previously described (Cariello et al. 1978). Bonellin stock solution (0.4 mg/ml in Na_2CO_3 0.1 M) and HpD stock solution (5 mg/ml in 0.9% NaCl) were dissolved in 5 mM sodium phosphate buffer PH 7.4 - 0.15 M NaCl.

Erythrocyte suspensions

Human blood (5 ml) was collected into tubes containing 0.4 ml of 0.2 M EDTA, diluited with an equal volume of cold 5 mM sodium phosphate buffer PH 7.4 - 0.15 M NaCl and centrifuged. The pellet was washed three times in the same saline buffer and resuspended in the buffer to obtain $4-5 \cdot 10^5$ cells mm^3. 1 ml of saline buffer containing bonellin or HpD was added to 1 ml of erythrocyte suspension to obtain final concentration of 0.5-1-2.5-4-5-10 µg/ml and 1-2.5-5-10-20 µg/ml respectively. The mixture was incubated in the dark, in plates 3 cm in diameter, for 1 h at $4°C$.

Irradiation

A He-Ne laser (λ=632.8 nm; 25mW output) was employed. The laser was equiped with a beam expander to irradiate the whole surface of the plate containing the erythrocyte suspension. The samples were irradiated up to find the minimal dose ($J \cdot cm^{-2}$) to obtain total haemolysis. Haemolysis was extimated from the amount of hemoglobin released into the supernatant (absorption at 579 nm).

RESULTS

The results are reported in fig. 3. For the same concentration, bonellin needs irradiative doses ten times smaller than HpD to determine total haemolysis.

Experiments with HpD at the concentration of 0.5 µg/ml were not performed because of exceedingly long times of irradiation required.

DISCUSSION

Using sea urchin gametes as test system, Cariello et al. (1978, 1980, 1982) and De Nicola Giudici et al. (1979) demonstrated that bonellin: i) acts on the plasma and nuclear membranes; ii) increases the incorporation rate of amino-acids into proteins; iii) pre-

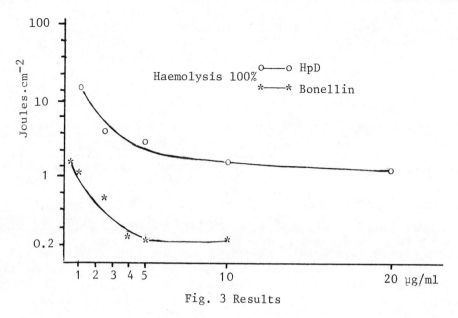

Fig. 3 Results

vents the cleavage in fertilized eggs; iv)does not damage the mitochondria; v)acts in the same way as porphyrins.

The photodynamic activity of the bonellin was carefully studied
by Agius et al. (1979) on erythrocytes and on echiuroid sperm and
developing eggs. Their results showed that: i)bonellin induce erythrocytes haemolysis only in presence of light; ii)the photoreaction
depends on the bonellin concentration; iii)the rate of haemolysis
was retarded in absence of oxigen and by addition of quenchers of
$^1O_2^*$ (ß-carotene and α-tocopherol) or benzoquinone

According to Cariello et al. (1982) who used a 150 W tungsten
lamp, our results show that bonellin is much more active than HpD,
at least with monochromatic source at 632.8 nm. This may be due in
part to the greater absorption of bonellin between 620 and 640 nm.

Control experiments showed no haemolysis if erythrocyte suspensions were irradiated (20 J· cm^{-2}) in absence of bonellin or incubated for 15 hs with bonellin in the dark. Moreover haemolysis was
not produced when bonellin was laser irradiated in the absence of
erythrocytes and this solution added to a red blood cell suspension.
The above data confirm that, as reported by Agius et al. (1978),
the activity of bonellin is not due to a stable photoproduct active
in the dark.

In agreement with Nigrelli et al. (1967), we have not eviden-
tiated toxic effects of bonellin into albino rats, at the dose of
4 mg/kg body weight (intraperitoneally injected).

In conclusion: the potent photodynamic activity by us eviden-
tiated for bonellin suggests that this substance presents an exceedingly high interest for future studies of photodynamic inactivation
of cancer cells, as a substitute for hematoporphyrin. We also pre-
conize a clinical use more favourable than hematoporphyrin in cancer
photochemiotherapy. Urgent studies are needed in this direction.

REFERENCES

Agius L., Jaccarini V., Ballantine J.A., Ferrito V., Pelter A.,
    Psaila A.F. and Zammit V.A., 1979, Photodynamic action of
    bonellin, an integumentary chlorin of Bonellia viridis,
    Rolando (Echiura, Bonelliidae), Comp. Biochem. Physiol.,
    63b: 109.
Baltzer F., 1931, Echiurida, Handb. Zool., 2: 62.
Cariello L., De Nicola Giudici M., Zanetti L., Prota G., 1978, Neo-
    bonellin, a new biologically active pigment from Bonellia
    viridis, Experientia, 34: 1427.
Cariello L., De Nicola Giudici M., Zanetti L., 1980, Partial activa-
    tion of sea-urchin eggs by bonellin, Gamete Res., 3: 309.
Cariello L., De Nicola Giudici M., Tosti E., Zanetti L., 1982, On
    the mechanism of action of bonellin on the sea urchin egg,
    Gamete Res., 5: 161.
De Nicola Giudici M., Cariello L., Zanetti L., 1979, Effects of bo-
    nellin on fertilization and cleavage of the eggs of the
    sea urchin, Sphaerechinus granularis, Gamete Res., 2: 247.
Lederer E., 1939, Sur l'isolament et la costitution chimique de la
    bonelline pigment vert de Bonellia viridis, Cir. Acad.
    Sci. Paris, 209: 528.
Nigrelli R.F., Stempien M.F., Ruggieri G.D., Liguori V.R., Cecil
    J.T., 1967, Substances of potential biomedical importance
    from marine organisms, Fed. Proc., 26: 1197.
Pelter A., Ballantine J.A., Ferrito B., Jaccarini V., Psaila A.F.,
    Schembri P.J., 1976, Bonellin, a most unusual chlorin,
    J. Chem. Soc. Chem. Commun., 23: 999.

SURVEY OF POTENTIAL PRT DYES

AND THEIR SPECTROSCOPIC PROPERTIES

Fred M. Johnson and Joseph F. Becker

Department of Physics
California State University
Fullerton, California 92634

INTRODUCTION

There exists a growing literature [1, 2, 3, 4, 5, 6,] describing the use of HPD in the treatment of malignant tumors, as well as extensive studies relating to the various possible aspects of the photodynamic processes in vitro and in vivo. The more recent topical conferences on the subject, in particular, have shown how the field is growing and how specialists in various disciplines bring their collective research talents to bear on the highly promising modality of cancer treatment. There is little doubt now that PRT will become one of the major weapons in the arsenal against solid tumors, largely as a result of Dr. T. J. Dougherty and the efforts of his disciples.

In this paper, we report the results of spectroscopic studies of a number of compounds potentially useful for use in PRT. In addition to the usual absorption and fluorescence measurements, we have extended our studies to include measurements of fluorescence lifetimes.

EXPERIMENTAL RESULTS

An extended list[7] compiled about twenty years ago was re-examined and analyzed. The results are shown in Table I, which includes additional potential dyes. We also measured the lifetimes of HPD, protoporphyrin IX and uroporphyrin (see Tables 2, 3, and 4).

101

TABLE I

Substance	Absorption	Excitation	Fluorescence Emission
B$_{12}$ Vitamin	broad UV 630	501 404	631w 679st 631
Protop. IX	400, 500, 537, 572, 628	572	632
Uroporphyrin	497, 530, 570 626	421, 499, 531, 570	626
Tetracyclene	400	423	630
Disodium Fluorescein	499	400	525
Brilliant Sulfoflavine		441	518
Nile Blue Perchlorate	630	536, 600, 630	670
Oxazine Perchlorate 750	663	675	690
Methylene Blue	660	550	700
Acriflavin	458	468	491
Riboflavin	350 450	366 468	570 517
Rose Bengal	550	556	571
Crystal violet	592	515	637
Neutral red	457	468	585
Stilbene 420	400	426	850
Eosin B	521	583	586
Kiton Red	558	457	591

TABLE 2

HPD LIFETIMES

Concentration μl/ml	Lifetime ns
10	15.56
3.3	15.54
1.1	15.58
0.11	15.88 *

* N_2 bubbling - no change
Room temp. ph 7.0

Fluorescence measurements were taken on a Perkin-Elmer MPF-44 spectrofluorimeter and the absorption measurements were taken on a Cary 15. The fluorescence lifetime apparatus is essentially as shown in Fig. 1. The ns flash lamp was a Model 510 B lamp (Photo Chemical Research, Inc.). The single photon detection consisted of a Model 270 PMT base and Model 403 A Time-Pick-Off Control (EGG). The Time to amplitude converter is Model 437 A (EGG).

The data acquisition system consisted of a ND-66 with a A/D converter (Nuclear Data Corp.) The data was analyzed on CYBER 170/730 computer (Control Data Corp.) using the non-linear regression program contained in the Biomedical Data Program, Series P (University of California Press).

TABLE 3

HPD Lifetime ns	Temperature Deg. C
15.54	23
15.32	37
15.10	50

* Concentration 3.3 μl/ml
ph 7.0

TABLE 4

LIFETIMES

Protoporphyrin IX	16.03 ns	
Uroporphyrin	(a) 16.92 ns	ph 7
	(b) 10-12 ns	
+BSA	(c) 16.92 ns	
	only	

DISCUSSION AND CONCLUSIONS

In comparing the uroporphyrin and protoporphyrin lifetimes with HPD (Tables 2, 3, 4), we note that uroporphyrin and proto-porphyrin individually have a longer lifetime than HPD. The HPD sample is a conglomerate which may contain trace compounds, which may be responsible for the quenching of the fluorescence lifetime of uroporphyrin and protoporphyrins in the HPD "mix".

Our experiment showed no change in lifetime of HPD subse-quent to N_2 bubbling, which is believed to displace dissolved oxygen. This suggests that either O_2 does not quench HPD fluor-escence or that the O_2 is so tightly bound to the fluorescent compounds in HPD that it is not removed by N_2 bubbling.

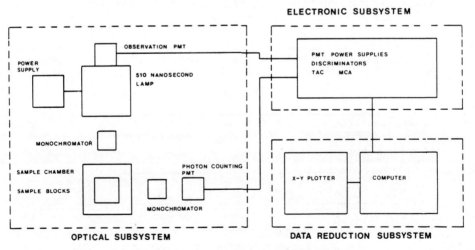

Fig. 1.   Block diagram of the integrated PRA fluorescence lifetime system.

Referring to Table 2, since there were no marked changes in lifetime as a function of concentration, we believe that concentration quenching effects are essentially not present.

Next, we wish to discuss our lifetime results as a function of temperature (Table 3). It should be pointed out that our measurements were taken at low intensity light levels. However, during normal PRT treatments using high intensity laser radiation, substantial local heating does occur. Based on our results, this would suggest an additional possible enhancement effect, since shorter lifetimes indicate higher fluorescence intensities. These higher intensities will produce more effective photodynamic activity.

In conclusion, studies as these of the spectroscopic properties of photodynamic dyes may enhance our understanding of the fundamental processes. In addition, these studies may suggest methods by which screening for other PRT dye candidates becomes possible without the use of complicated biological systems.

REFERENCES

1. D. Kessel and T.J. Dougherty, ed., "Porphyrin Photosensitization", Plenum Press, New York-London (1983).
2. Proceedings of the Clayton Foundation Symposium on Porphyrin Localization and Treatment of Tumors, April 24-28, 1983, Santa Barbara (Ca, USA), to be published.
3. A. Dahlman, A.G. Wile, R.G. Burns, G.R. Mason, F.M. Johnson, and M.W. Berns, Laser photoradiation therapy of cancer, Cancer Res. 43:430 (1983).
4. M.W. Berns, A. Dahlman, F.M. Johnson, R.G. Burns, D. Sperling, M. Guiltinam, A. Siemens, R. Walter, W. Wright, M. Hammer-Wilson, and A. Wile, In vitro cellular effects of Hematoporphyrin Derivative, Cancer Res. 42:2325 (1982).
5. J.D. Spikes, Photodynamic reactions in photomedicine, in: "The Science of Photomedicine", J.D. Regan and J.A. Parrish, ed., Plenum Press, New York-London (1982).
6. J.D. Spikes, Photosensitization in mammalian cells, in: "Photoimmunology", J.A. Parrish, M. Kripke, and W.L. Morison, eds., Plenum Press, New York (1983).
7. H.H. Seliger and W.D. McElroy, "Light: Physical and Biological Action", Academic Press, New York (1965).

Chapter 2

Interactions of Porphyrins with Model Systems and Cells

FLUORESCENCE OF PORPHYRINS IN CELLS

Johan Moan

Norsk Hydro's Institute for Cancer Research
Montebello, Oslo 3
Norway

INTRODUCTION

Two fields of research in biology and medicine are concerned
with the study of cellular uptake of porphyrins: research on porphyria and research on diagnosis and photoradiation therapy of
cancer. Porphyrins have a characteristic pattern of fluorescence.
Thus, cellular uptake and retention of porphyrins are often
studied by means of fluorescence measurements.

The fluorescence emission and excitation maxima of porphyrin
molecules as well as their fluorescence quantum yields vary with
their microenvironments. Characteristic changes take place when
the porphyrin concentration, the solvent dielectric constant or
the solvent viscosity are varied [1,2]. Binding to macromolecules
such as hemopexin and albumin is also accompanied by significant
and specific variations[3,4]. Thus, the fluorescence pattern of
porphyrins in cells may give valuable information about the
binding sites and the localization of the chromophores.

MATERIALS AND METHODS

Chemicals

Hematoporphyrin derivative (HPD) was prepared according to
the method described by Lipson et al.[5], dissolved in 0.1 M NaOH,
neutralized with 0.1 M HCl and supplied with NaCl to a total concentration of 0.15 M. The HPD stock solution (5 mg/ml) was kept
frozen until used.

All other chemicals used were of the highest purity commercially available.

Cultivation of cells

Cells from the NHIK 3025 line were cultured and kept in exponential growth as previously described[6]. About 7×10^5 cells were inoculated in 6 cm Petri dishes (Falcon) and incubated with HPD as described in the figure legends. In most experiments HPD from the stock solution (5 mg/ml in a 0.15 M aqueous solution of NaCl) was diluted to 12.5 µg/ml in E2a medium containing 1% human serum and 2% horse serum, in the following abbreviated to "medium with 3% serum". After incubation with HPD the cells were washed three times with icecold Dulbecco's phosphate buffered saline (PBS) and brought into a small volume (1 to 3 ml) of PBS by means of a cell scraper (Falcon).

Spectroscopy

Absorption spectra and fluorescence spectra were recorded by means of a Cary 118 spectrophotometer and a Hitachi Perkin Elmer MPF-2A spectrofluorimeter, respectively. The spectrofluorimeter was equipped with a red-sensitive Hammamatsu R 928 photomultiplier tube. In most cases the cells were brought into suspension before the analysis. Fluorescence spectra of cells growing on 12 mm cover glasses could also be recorded. The cover glasses were kept immersed in PBS and placed at an angle of 40° with the excitation light beam.

Chromatography

Extracts of cells were analyzed by high pressure liquid chromatography (HPLC). The equipment and the procedure have been described by Sommer et al. in the present volume. The porphyrins were extracted from about 1.5×10^7 HPD-labelled cells directly into a small volume of the mobile chromatographic phase (methanol/water 60/40, pH 7.0). Less than 15% of the initial porphyrin absorbance and fluorescence was left in the cell debris after an extraction.

Photoinactivation of cells

The cells were inoculated in 25 cm^2 tissue culture flasks (500 cells/flask) and allowed to attach to the flasks (2 h, 37° C). Then the cells were incubated with HPD for a given time and exposed to the light from four fluorescent tubes (Philips TL 20W/09), emitting light mainly in the wavelength region 330 - 440 nm.

The fluence rate at the position of the cells was 17 W/m^2 as measured
with a calibrated thermopile (YSI, 65A, Yellow Springs, OH). This
light source was also used to study the photodegradation of HPD.
After irradiation the HPD solution was removed from the cells
which were then incubated for 1 week in E2a medium with 30% serum
for colony formation.

RESULTS

Cells labelled with HPD show a relatively intense red fluorescence (Fig. 1). By comparing the transmission and the fluorescence
microscopic pattern of a cell population one may occasionally
observe cells with a high porphyrin content and a surprisingly weak
fluorescence (Fig. 1). However, this is not the general rule, and
we will assume that the amount of cell-bound porphyrins can be
determined by fluorescence measurements.

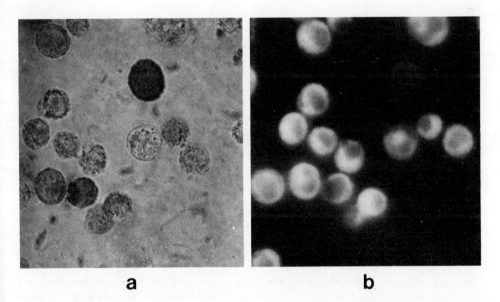

a   **b**

Fig. 1. NHIK 3025 cells exposed in suspension to 0.5 mg/ml HPD in
PBS for 30 min. The cells were then washed with cold PBS
and mounted in the microscope (Leitz diavert with a 40/1.3
fluorescence objective. a) is a Polaroid picture taken in
light field with monochromatic light (λ = 400 nm ± 20 nm)
to visualize the porphyrin absorption in the cel·ls. b) is
a similar picture taken of the fluorescence of the same
cells (filter block B).

The fluorescence excitation- and emission spectra of HPD in cells show some characteristic features: 1) The fluorescence excitation spectrum has two peaks (398, 410 nm) in the Soret region and a shoulder on each side of the Soret band (Figs 2 and 3). 2) The fluorescence excitation spectrum closely resembles the absorption spectrum (Fig. 2). It should be taken into account that for experimental reasons the latter spectrum is recorded with lower resolution than the former. In the visible region the fluorescence excitation spectrum has a peak at 610 nm which has no counterpart in the absorption spectrum (Fig. 4). However, this peak is also found in cells without HPD and has an emission spectrum different from that of porphyrins (Fig. 4 lower right). 3) The fluorescence emission spectrum is red-shifted compared with the emission spectrum of HPD in buffer solution (Fig. 2). 4) The shape and position of the fluorescence emission spectrum is dependent on the wavelength of the excitation light (Fig. 2). A change of the excitation wavelength from 398 to 410 nm gives a 2 nm red shift and a decrease in the line width of the emission spectrum. As a consequence of this, the shape of the fluorescence excitation spectrum is dependent of the bandwidth and the wavelength at which the emission monochromator is set.

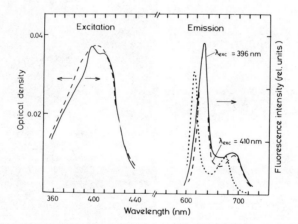

Fig. 2.   Optical absorption spectrum (--), fluorescence excitation spectrum (—) and fluorescence emission spectra of HPD in cells. The emission spectra were recorded for two excitation wavelengths: 396 nm and 410 nm. The dotted emission spectrum is that of HPD in PBS (λ_{exc} = 392 nm). The cells were incubated for 18 h with 12.5 µg/ml HPD in E2a medium with 3% serum.

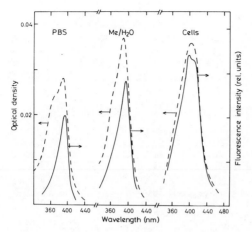

Fig. 3.   Absorption spectra (---) and fluorescence excitation
          spectra (——) of HPD (Soret region) in PBS, methanol/water
          (volume ratio 60/40, pH 7.0) and in cells after 18 h
          incubation with HPD (12.5 µg/ml, E2a with 3% serum).

The absorption spectrum of HPD in an aqueous solution has a
shoulder at about 360 - 370 nm (Fig. 3).   This shoulder decreases
when the concentration of HPD is reduced and when methanol is
added to the aqueous solution.   However, in no case is it completely absent.   The fluorescence quantum yield is lower in the region
of this shoulder than at and above 390 nm.

In the concentration range from 1 to 6 µg/ml, the absorption
spectrum of HPD in PBS changes drastically (Fig. 5).   This drastic
change is not associated with any abrupt change in the cellular
uptake of HPD although a certain decrease is observed (Fig. 5).
In medium with 3% serum the cellular uptake of HPD is lower than
in PBS by a factor of about 15 at similar incubation times and the
cellular uptake was found to be nearly proportional to the concentration (data not shown).

The shape of the fluorescence excitation spectrum of HPD in
cells is dependent on the incubation time with HPD (Fig. 6).   The
peak at 398 nm is more pronounced for short than for long incubation times.   Furthermore, when the cells were washed for half an
hour with medium without HPD, their fluorescence was reduced,   the
peak at 398 nm in the excitation spectrum more than the peak at
410 nm (Fig. 6).   In the case of 18 h incubation with HPD such a

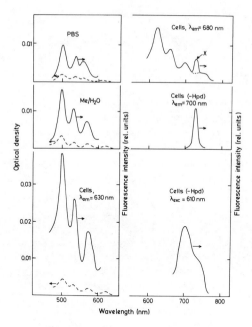

Fig. 4.   Absorption spectra and fluorescence excitation spectra of
          HPD in the visible region.   Conditions as for Fig. 3.

a washing removed about 30% of the HPD bound to the cells but did
not reduce their photosensitivity (Table 1).   In the case of 1 h
incubation with HPD the amount of cell-bound dye and the photosensitivity were both reduced by 60% during a similar washing.

Protoporphyrin and hematoporphyrin (HP) bound to cells have
fluorescence excitation spectra as shown in Fig. 6.   These dyes
are relatively efficiently removed from the cells by washing, even
after an incubation time of 18 h.

In our HPLC system HPD has a chromatogram as shown in Fig. 7A.
The components, which have been given numbers according to an
earlier publication (7), may be divided into three groups:
1) Components with relatively high quantum yields of fluorescence
(Table 2) and sharp peaks in the chromatogram (comp. 2, 4A, 4B and
7C).   2) Components with somewhat lower quantum yields of
fluorescence (Table 2) and sharp peaks in the chromatogram (comp.
3, 7A, 7B, 7D - 7F) and 3) one or more components with a low
quantum yield of fluorescence and a broad, structureless peak in the
chromatogram stretching from about 10 to about 35 min in elution
time (Fig. 7).

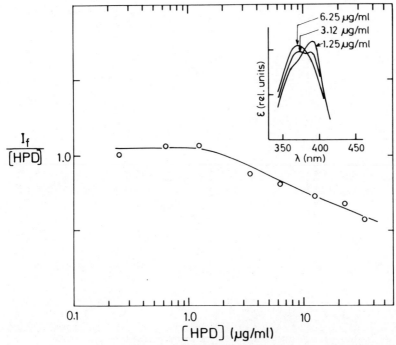

Fig. 5.   Cellular uptake of HPD during 30 minutes incubation in PBS.
The ordinate gives the ratio of the HPD fluorescence of the
cells (λ_{exc} = 410 nm ± 12 nm, λ_{em} = 632 nm, $\Delta\lambda_{em}$ = 5 nm)
to the HPD concentration, and the abscissa gives the HPD
concenctration.   In the upper right of the figures is shown
the wavelength dependence of the extinction coefficient of
HPD at three concentrations in PBS.

        The cells accumulate some of the components selectively,
notably those with elution times longer than 15 minutes (Fig. 7B).
When the cells were washed with medium for half an hour, component 2,
4A, 4B and 7C (i.e. those with a high quantum yield of fluorescence)
were almost completely removed (Fig. 7C).

        HPD in cells is degraded (bleached) by light (Fig. 8) while HPD
in PBS is much more stable (data not shown).   The fluorescence
excitation spectrum does not change significantly during light
exposure.

        Cells exposed to light after a short time incubation with HPD
accelerate their uptake of HPD, and the shape of the fluorescence
excitation spectrum changes as shown in Fig. 9.

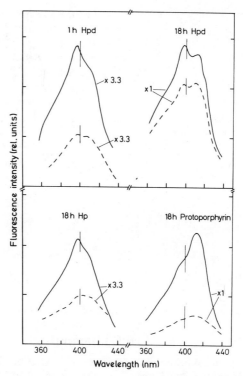

Fig. 6.   Fluorescence excitation spectra of HPD, hematoporphyrin
          and protoporphyrin in cells after incubation times as given
          on the figure. The medium was E2a with 3% serum. The
          stippled lines are the spectra of the porphyrins in the
          cells after a similar HPD labelling followed by 30 minutes
          washing in E2a medium without HPD (3% serum, 37°C). The
          emission monochromator was in each case set at the maximum
          of the emission spectrum (Δλ = 12 nm).

DISCUSSION

     An aqueous solution of HPD is extremely complex. It contains
several porphyrins which may be present as monomers, dimers,
oligomers and aggregates. Some of the dimers, oligomers and aggregates may even be tied together with covalent bonds[8-10] and
therefore not subjected to the normal monomerization process upon
dilution, addition of alcohols or binding to proteins. In aqueous
solutions monomers and dimers have their absorption maximum at
about 390 nm while the absorption maximum of aggregates is located
at about 360 - 370 nm[11]. Furthermore, monomers probably have the
highest fluorescence quantum yields of the species present in
HPD[7,10]. The absorption spectrum of HPD has a shoulder at

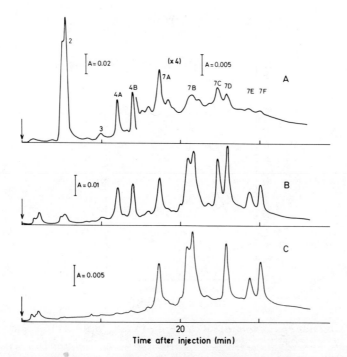

Fig. 7.   High pressure liquid chromatography of HPD.   A) HPD directly
          diluted in the mobile chromatographic phase.   B) HPD
          extracted into the mobile chromatographic phase from cells
          after 1 h incubation with 100 µg/ml HPD in E2a medium with
          3% serum.   C) Similar to B) except that the cells were
          washed with pure E2a medium (3% serum) for 30 minutes
          before the porphyrins were extracted.

360 - 370 nm even at low concentrations in a water/methanol solution (Fig. 3).   This solvent is known to favor monomer formation[2].
Thus, our data support the assumption that stable oligomers and/or
aggregates exist in HPD.

      The complexity of HPD is demonstrated by its chromatogram
(Fig. 7).   The following components have been identified (see 7 and
references cited there):   2 is hematoporphyrin, 4A and 4B are the
isomers of hydroxyethyl-vinyl-deuteroporphyrin and 7C is protoporphyrin.   The high fluorescence quantum yields (Table 2) indicate
that these components are in a monomeric form in the mobile chromatographic phase.   A number of other relatively sharp peaks are seen
in the chromatogram.   The corresponding HPD components have significantly lower fluorescence quantum yields than that of monomers
(Table 2).   We propose that these components are dimers or oligo-

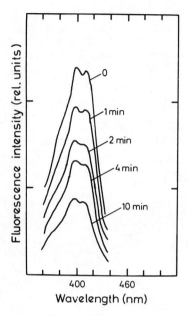

Fig. 8. Photodegradation of HPD in cells. The cells were incubated for 18 h with 12.5 µg/ml HPD in E2a medium with 3%
serum and then exposed to light as given on the figure.
The excitation spectra were recorded with λ_{em} = 630 nm
± 12 nm.

Table 1.

Incubation time with HPD	Washing time	Relative cellular content of HPD	t_{10}^{-1} (rel. units)
1 h	0	1.0	1.0
1 h	0.5 h	0.4	0.4
18 h	0	3.8	7.8
18 h	0.5 h	2.9	7.8

Relative amount of HPD bound to cells and t_{10}^{-1} values for cells incubated with 12.5 µg/ml HPD in E2a medium with 3% serum for 1 and
18 h at 37° C respectively. Washing was performed with the same
medium without HPD. t_{10} is the exposure time to light needed to
reduce the cellular survival by a factor 10. (t_{10} (1 h) = 5.6 min,
t_{10} (18 h) = 44 s). Data from three independent experiments.
Standard error about 15%.

Table 2.

	2	3	4A	4B	7A	7B	7C	7D	7E	7F
Φ_{rel}	0.7	0.2	0.65	0.65	0.3	0.3	0.65	0.4	0.2	0.2

Relative fluorescence quantum yields (Φ_{rel}) of HPD components in the mobile chromatographic phase (methanol/water).

mers, since higher aggregates will probably be of variable composition and give rise to broad peaks in the chromatogram. Such a broad peak is also present in the chromatogram of HPD. This is convincingly demonstrated by the HPLC chromatogram of the fast-running fraction of HPD separated on a P10 column (Sommer et al. in present volume). Dimers of components 2 and 4 will give a number of peaks in the chromatogram due to isomerization.

A comparison of the chromatograms A, B and C in Fig. 7 leads to the following conclusions:

1) HPD components with long retention times on a reversed phase column (i.e. components of low polarity) and sharp peaks in the chromatogram are selectively bound to the cells. This is in agreement with earlier findings[12,13].

2) Under the present conditions (1 h incubation with HPD in medium containing 3% serum) the larger aggregates (i.e. the component(s) corresponding to the broad peak in the chromatogram) are less concentrated by the cells than the better resolved components mentioned under 1).

3) Monomers (HP, 4A, 4B and protoporphyrin) are almost completely removed from the cells by washing with medium containing serum. This indicates that the monomers are predominantly bound in the plasma membrane. A certain fraction of the non-monomer components is also removed by washing the cells and therefore probably bound in the plasma membrane. This fraction decreases with increasing incubation time with HPD.

When we take the fluorescence excitation spectra (Fig. 6), the effect of washing on these spectra, the chromatogram and the data for photoinactivation of cells (Table 1) into account, the following further suggestions can be made:

4) The peak in the fluorescence excitation spectrum at 398 nm mainly corresponds to component 2, 4A and 4B while that at 410 nm corresponds to the components 7A - 7F.

5) Under conditions where most of the HPD in a solution is aggregated (i.e. in PBS at concentrations higher than 3 µg/ml) the cells seem to accumulate slightly less porphyrins than under conditions where aggregation is less dominating (Fig. 5). Thus, aggregated porphyrins are not generally more efficiently taken up than mono- and dimers.

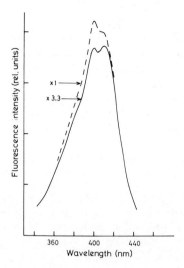

Fig. 9. Fluorescence excitation spectra of cells after incubation
with 25 µg/ml HPD in E2a medium with 3% serum. Full line:
1.5 h incubation with HPD. Stippled line: 1 h incubation
with HPD, 3 minutes irradiation, corresponding to about
90% cellular inactivation, and 0.5 h further incubation
with HPD.

6) The relative mean sensitizing efficiency of a porphyrin
molecule is about a factor 2 higher after an incubation time of 18 h
than after an incubation time of 1 h (Table 1).

7) The fraction of the cell-bound HPD that may be removed by
washing has some sensitizing effect on cells incubated for 1 h with
HPD while it has no influence on the photosensitivity of the cells
after 18 h incubation with HPD (Table 1), even though it constitutes
about 25% of the amount of HPD bound to the cells prior to washing.

If, as suggested above, we assume that this HPD fraction is
located mainly in the plasma membrane, we may conclude that membrane
damage plays a significant role in photosensitizing cells incubated
for a short time (about 1 h) with HPD. Such damage seems to be much
less important in the case of long-term incubation (about 18 h) with
HPD[14]. These findings closely correspond with those of Henderson et
al. . They suggested that long-term uptake resulted in the migra-
tion of HPD or some of its components to sites within the cell where
photodamage is more critical for cell survival.

Microscopic observation of irradiated HPD-labelled cells also
supports the above reasoning. A D_{10} fluence (i.e. a fluence inacti-

vating 90% of the cells) generates blebs on the membrane of cells
after short-term labelling with HPD[6,15], while practically no such
membrane damage can be observed in cells which are photoinactivated
after long-term incubation with HPD[16].Photodamage to the membrane of
cells after short-term incubation with HPD is also demonstrated by
Fig. 9. A D_{10} fluence generates a membrane damage that results in
an accelerated accumulation of HPD, components corresponding to the
398 nm peak in the fluorescence excitation spectrum being slightly
favoured. A similar photoinduced accumulation of HP has been reported earlier[17].

     The binding and transport studies of Kessel and Kohn[1] are in
agreement with the present work. They observed a rapid accumulation
of mesoporphyrin at a relatively hydrophilic cellular environment,
supposedly the outer cell membrane. Photodamage caused by light
absorption of porphyrins in this pool, which could be readily
removed by washing the cells, manifested itself as a reduced membrane transport of the nonmetabolized amino acid cycloleucine.
Another, more slowly accumulating, and more firmly bound pool, was
not efficient in sensitizing membrane photodamage. The maximum of
the fluorescence excitation spectrum and the fluorescence emission
spectrum of the latter pool was red-shifted compared with the
corresponding spectra of the former pool.

     It is well known that porphyrins are sensitive to photodegrada-
tion. However, this phenomenon has been paid little attention to in
the research aimed at improving photoradiation therapy. From data
like those shown in Fig. 8 one may estimate the significance of
photodegradation for a therapeutic situation. If a tumor is exposed
to a parallel beam of light, the fluence at a depth x below the
surface is approximately given by:

$$D = D_o \exp\left[-\frac{x-\delta}{\delta}\right]$$ (L. Svaasand, personal communication)

where D_o is the fluence delivered at the surface and δ is defined
as the penetration depth, typically of the order of 1 - 2 mm for
human tumors[18]. Assume that the concentration of unbleached dye
when a fluence D is delivered is $C = C_o \exp(-kD)$, where C_o is the
initial concentration and k is a wavelength-dependent constant.
(From Fig. 8 one can estimate k at 360 - 370 nm to be about
2×10^{-4} m^2/J). Further assume that the quantum yield of bleaching
is the same, and that the extinction coefficient of HPD is about a
factor 30 larger in the Soret band than at 630 nm. Accordingly,
the value of k at 630 nm is about 1.2×10^{-5} m^2/J. The concentration of unbleached dye as a function of position and incident
fluence is

$$C = C_o \exp\left[-k\,D_o \exp\left(-\frac{x-\delta}{\delta}\right)\right]$$

Relevant fluences in photoradiation therapy are of the order of

$D_0 = 500/kJ/m^2$ at 620 - 640 nm^9. According to the present considerations and calculations, such a fluence will degrade more than 50%
of the HPD at a depth of x = 3 δ.

Bleaching of HPD is obviously more important the lower the dye
concentration in the tumor is, since a low dye concentration calls
for a high fluence. The crucial point is whether a tumor contains
enough dye to be inactivated before the dye is bleached.

There are a number of uncertain points in the above estimation.
In addition to those stated as assumptions, one may mention the fact
that the oxygen concentration in a tumor is usually low. A low
oxygen concentration may reduce the yields of tumor inactivation and
dye bleaching to different degrees. Furthermore, the photoproducts
of HPD may themselves be photosensitizers. In view of recent experiments with protoporphyrin[19] this may well be the case. Nevertheless,
some of the reports of failure of HPD sensitized photoradiation
therapy may be due to dye bleaching in the tumor. Such problems
call for further elucidation of the effects of bleaching.

Our main conclusions are that:

1) Cells selectively bind HPD components of low polarity.
2) The HPD components that are selectively bound and retained
in cells have lower fluorescence quantum yields than porphyrin monomers and are probably dimers and/or oligomers of the type HP...HVD.
3) NHIK 3025 cells seem to have a lower affinity for higher
porphyrin aggregates than for the components mentioned under 2).
4) Porphyrin monomers (HP, hydroxyethyl-vinyl-deuteroporphyrin
and protoporphyrin) are removed from cells by washing with media
containing serum. These porphyrins are assumed to be bound in the
plasma membrane.
5) The loosely bound fraction of HPD in cells (i.e. the fraction that is removed by 30 minutes washing with media containing
serum) decreases with increasing incubation time of the cells with
HPD.
6) The quantum yield of photoinactivation of cells increases
with increasing incubation time with HPD.
7) Membrane damage seems to play a significant role in the
photoinactivation of cells after short-term incubation with HPD but
no role in the case of long-term incubation.
8) Photobleaching of HPD in cells is significant and may
reduce the efficiency of photoradiation therapy of cancer when the
HPD concentration in the tumor is low.

The present work was supported by The Norwegian Cancer
Society (Landsforeningen mot Kreft).

REFERENCES

1. D. Kessel and K.I. Kohn, Transport and binding of mesoporphyrin IX by leukemia L 1210 cells, Cancer Res. 40:303 (1980).
2. D. Kessel and E. Rossi, Determinants of porphyrin-sensitized photooxidation characterized by fluorescence and absorption spectra, Photochem. Photobiol. 35:37 (1982).
3. A.A. Lamola, I. Asher, U. Muller-Eberhard and M. Pole-Fitzpatrick, Fluorometric study of the binding of photoporphyrin to haemopexin and albumin. Biochem. J. 196:693 (1981).
4. W.T. Morgan, A. Smith and P. Koskelo, The interaction of human serum albumin and hemopexin with porphyrins. Biochem. Biophys. Acta 624:271 (1980).
5. R.L. Lipson, E.J. Baldes and A.M. Olsen, The use of a derivative of hematoporphyrin in tumor detection. J. Natl. Cancer Inst. 26:1 (1961).
6. J. Moan, E.O. Pettersen and T. Christensen, The mechanism of photodynamic inactivation of human cells in vitro in the presence of haematoporphyrin. Br. J. Cancer 39:398 (1979).
7. J. Moan, S. Sandberg, T. Christensen and S. Elander, Hematoporphyrin derivative: Chemical composition and photosensitizing proporties, in: "Porphyrin Photosensitization", D. Kessel and T.J. Dougherty, Plenum Press, New York, London (1983).
8. R. Bonnett and R. Berenbaum, HPD - a study of its components and their properties, in: "Porphyrin Photosensitization", D. Kessel and T.F. Dougherty, Plenum Press, New York and London (1983).
9. T.J. Dougherty, D.G. Boyle, K.R. Weishaupt, B.A. Henderson, W.R. Potter, D.A. Bellnier and K.E. Wityk, Photoradiation therapy - clinical and drug advances, in: "Porphyrin Photosensitization", Plenum Press, New York and London (1983)
10. A. Andreoni, R. Cubeddu, S. de Silvestri, P. Laport, G. Jori and E. Reddi, Hematoporphyrin derivative: Experimental evidence for aggregated species. Chem. Phys. Lett. 88:33 (1982).
11. S.B. Brown, M. Shillcock and P. Jones, Equilibrium and kinetic studies of the aggregation of porphyrins in aqueous solutions. Biochem. J. 153:279 (1976).
12. J. Moan, J.B. McGhie and T. Christensen, Hematoporphyrin derivative: Photosensitizing efficiency and cellular uptake of its components. Photobiochem. Photobiophys. 4:337 (1982).
13. D. Kessel, Effects of photoactivated porphyrins at the cell surface of leukemia L 1210 cells. Biochem. 16:3443 (1977).
14. B.W. Henderson, D.A. Bellnier, B. Ziring and T.J. Dougherty, Aspects of the cellular uptake and retention of hematoporphyrin derivative and their correlation with the biologic responses to PRT in vitro, in: "Porphyrin Photosensitization", D. Kessel and T.J. Dougherty, Plenum Press, New York and London (1983).

15. J. Moan, J.V. Johannessen, T. Christensen, T. Espevik and J.B. McGhie, Porphyrin-sensitized photoinactivation of human cells in vitro, Am. J. Pathol. 109:184 (1982).

16. T. Christensen, T. Sandquist, K. Feren, H. Waksvik and J. Moan, Retention and photodynamic effects of haematoporphyrin derivative in cells after prolonged cultivation in the presence of porphyrin. Br. J. Cancer, in press.

17. J. Moan and T. Christensen, Cellular uptake and photodynamic effect of hematoporphyrin. Photobiochem. Photobiophys. 2:291 (1981).

18. D.R. Doiron, L.O. Svaasand and A.E. Profio, Light dosimetry in tissue: Application to photoradiation therapy, in: "Porphyrin Photosensitization", Plenum Press, New York and London (1983).

19. G.S. Cox, C. Bobillier and D. Whitten, Photooxidation and singlet oxygen sensitization by protoporphyrin IX and its photooxidation products. Photochem. Photobiol. 36:401 (1982).

HEMATOPORPHYRIN DERIVATIVE: FLUOROMETRIC STUDIES IN SOLUTION AND CELLS

Giovanni Bottiroli, Franco Doccio*, Isabel Freitas,
Roberta Ramponi* and Carlo Alberto Sacchi*

Centro di studio per l'Istrocimica del CNR, Istituto di
Anatomia Comparata dell'Università, Pavia, Italy
* Centro di Elettronica Quantistica e Strumentazione
Elettronica del CNR, Istituto di Fisica del Politecnico
Milano, Italy

INTRODUCTION

Hematoporphyrin Derivative (HpD) is a mixture of porphyrins, widely used in detection and therapy of cancer[1,2]. HpD was introduced in 1961 by Lipson et al.[3] as a better tumor-locating drug than Hematoporphyrin (Hp). They proposed that the crude Hp be treated with a mixture of acetic acid and sulfuric acid, followed by adjustment of the final pH to neutrality. The derivative obtained in such a way is a complex mixture whose chemical composition has yet to be completely clarified. In particular the active components in HpD solution have not been determined. Moreover, many questions about the interaction of this drug with the cellular structures have not been solved.

Therefore, the mechanisms leading to tumor specificity of HpD are not known. Many studies have been done in order to clarify the chemical and biological basis of the mechanism of selective retention of HpD by tumor tissue and to define the precise workings of the cytotoxic effect[4,5,6].

Here we give some data on the dependence of HpD fluorescence on the cell functional state. To this end, time-resolved fluorescence microscopy has been employed. Analysis of the fluorescence waveforms obtained in single cells can provide information both on the quantitative distribution of the fluorescent molecules (which is proportional to fluorescence peak-intensity) and on the way the

125

drug interacts with the microenvironment (through the decay times). The biological model chosen were normal human lymphocytes, both in the quiescent state (G_0 phase) and in the pre-replicative (G_1) phase, after stimulation with Phytohemagglutinin (PHA).

A spectral band in the 570-590 nm region was found, in which the differences between quiescent and stimulated lymphocytes are more evident. The definition of this emission band, corresponding to a new porphyrin species (NPS), seems to be very important, since it was also found in material extracted from tumor cells. Therefore the absorption, excitation and emission spectra of HpD in saline were measured in different environmental conditions, and also time-resolved fluorescence measurements were performed on the same solutions.

MATERIALS AND METHODS

Chemicals

HpD was purchased from Oncology Research and Development Inc. (Cheetowaya, N.Y., USA) under the trade name of Photofrin (5mg/ml in normal saline, corresponding to 6.623×10^{-3} M, if we assign to HpD the molecular weight of Hp diacetate, 755). HpD solutions, in the 10^{-5} to 10^{-7} M range, were obtained by diluting Photofrin in saline. Whenever de-aerated HpD solutions were required, the saline was bubbled with Nitrogen (chromatografic grade) for one hour before use. After the addition of Photofrin, the solution was bubbled again with Nitrogen for one minute, and then sealed with parafilm. Care was taken to protect all solutions from light and to minimize their exposure during the recording of the spectra. Unless otherwise stated, temperature during storage and measurements was 22°C.

Lymphocyte Preparation

Lymphocytes were separated by density gradient with Ficoll (d = 1.077) from normal sterile human blood, diluted 1:1 (v/v) in 5% glucose solution. Chromosome Medium B with PHA and Chromosome Medium A without PHA from Seromed (W. Germany) were used as the culture media. Aliquots with the same cell concentration ($5 \cdot 10^6$ cells/ /0.1 ml) were added to the culture medium with and witout PHA, after which the cells were incubated for 12 h, and for 45 min, respectively. HpD was then added, in order to obtain a final drug concentration of $5 \cdot 10^{-5}$ M. After 1 h of incubation, the supensions were centrifuged, and the cells were separated and smeared on slides.

Emission decay time measurements

Fluorescence decay-time measurements were performed, using a pulsed-laser microfluorometer developed in our laboratories and already extensively described in[7]. Fig. 1 shows the block diagram of

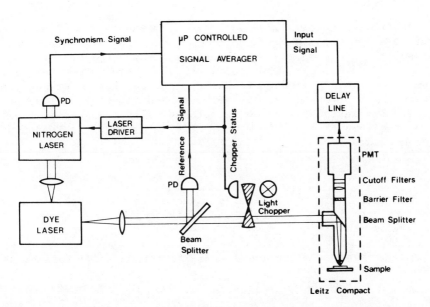

Fig. 1. Block-diagram of the pulsed-laser microfluorometer.

the apparatus. The excitation source was a nitrogen-laser-pumped dye-laser (10^{-3} M solution of α-NPO in ethanol), which generates pulses of $\sim$ 200 ps duration, 50 Hz repetition rate, and tuned at $\sim$ 400 nm. Suitable optics and a microscope were used to focus the laser light on the sample and to collect the fluorescence, barrier, and/or interference filters to select the spectral region of observation and to cut off unwanted laser reflections. The microscope was also used in the measurements on HpD solution, in such a way as to be in the same experimental conditions as those used for measuring HpD fluorescence in cells, thus making immediate comparisons significant. A fast photomultiplier tube (XP 1210, $\sim$ 0.5 ns rise--time) was used to detect the fluorescence signal, and a microprocessor-controlled signal-averager to acquire and process the data. The measurement apparatus makes use of a sampling oscilloscope as a fast acquisition unit.

The fluorescence curves, each obtained by averaging over 200 sweeps, were considered for statistical analysis by the non-linear, least-square method, in order to fit them with a sum of exponential curves. The accuracy of the fit obtained by computer was evaluated through analysis of the residuals and of their autocorrelation function.

Spectroscopy

Absorption spectra were recorded by means of a Beckman DU$^{(R)}$8 UV-visible computing spectrophotometer, equipped with a λ-scanning compuset$^{(TM)}$ and sample holder under electronic temperature control (accuracy: T $\pm$ 0.1°C). The fluorescence spectra were obtained by means of an SP-2 Applied Photophysics spectrofluorometer equipped with an EMI 9558/Q photomultiplier tube and an Ortec Photon Counter System. Excitation spectra were automatically adjusted to the output of the lamp (Thorn, 250 W D.C. XE/D) by means of a Rhodamine quantum counter.

Analytical procedure

The equilibria among chemical species in the porphyrin solutions are usually studied by means of indices derived from spectroscopic measurements[8].

In our case, we introduced a NPS formation index refined as

$$R_1 = E_{obs405}/E_{obs395}$$

where E_{obs405} and E_{obs395} are the extinction coefficient observed at wavelength corresponding to the NPS and the monomer absorption peaks, respectively. The influence of the NPS formation process on the monomer-dimer equilibrium was evaluated by means of the dimerization index

$$R = E_{obs365}/E_{obs395}$$

where E_{obs365} is the extinction coefficient observed at the wavelength corresponding to the dimer.

RESULTS AND DISCUSSION

Fluorescence analysis in human lymphocytes was performed in the 520-650 nm region.

First of all, the primary fluorescence of both stimulated and unstimulated lymphocytes was studied. In both cases, primary fluorescence was pratically absent in the freshly-prepared smears of cells in the red part of the spectrum. On the other hand, primary fluorescence was present in the yellow region. We observed, however, that repeated measurements in different lymphocytes systematically gave a peak intensity smaller than that given by HpD in lymphocytes. It is worth remembering that, as already reported in [9], primary fluorescence is substantially stabilized in cells treated with HpD. This effect had also already been observed in human lymphocytes[10].

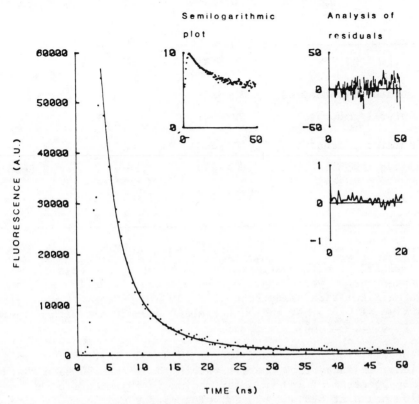

Fig. 2.   Fluorescence waveform of an HpD-treated stimulated human
          lymphocyte.   Spectral region: 521-581 nm.

The fluorescence of HpD-treated lymphocytes was then analyzed.
Fig. 2 shows an example of a fluorescence waveform of HpD in a stimulated lymphocyte. Both the experimental points and the fitting
curve are given. The method of analysis is also shown.

Table 1 summarizes the results obtained with a set of measurements on several samples once the primary fluorescence contribution
has been subtracted. The measurements were performed in different
spectral regions. The fluorescence curve of both stimulated and
unstimulated lymphocytes, in the red region, is well fitted by the
sum of two exponential decays with similar decay times in the two
samples ($\sim$ 3.5 and $\sim$ 16 ns). Going from the red to the yellow region of the spectrum the 16 ns component disappears and only the
3.5 ns one remains. Moreover, the absolute peak amplitude is higher

Table 1.   HpD Fluorescence in Unstimulated and Stimulated Lympho-
           cytes.

	spectral range (nm)	peak intensity	decay times (ns)
Unstimulated lymphocytes	521–581	I_1	3.5
Stimulated lymphocytes	521–581	3.9 I_1	3.5
Unstimulated lymphocytes	604–649	I_2	3.5–16
Stimulated lymphocytes	604–649	1.6 I_2	3.5–16

$$(I_2 = 2.5 \ I_1)$$

in stimulated than in unstimulated lymphocytes, and this difference
is greater in the yellow part of the spectrum. Thus, we may consider two main emission bands, one at about 570–580 nm with a typical
decay time of $\sim$ 3.5 ns, and one at about 610–620 nm, with a typical
decay time of $\sim$ 16 ns.

The emission band around 580 nm is absent in fresh HpD or Hp
solution. In fact, from the literature[4,8], it can be seen that the
emission spectrum of HpD in polar medium is characterized by two
emission peaks at 610 and 670 nm. The corresponding excitation
spectrum shows, in the Soret region, a narrow band at about 395 nm,
ascribed to monomeric forms, which exhibit a fluorescence decay
time of about 16 ns. The absorption spectrum, however, shows a
second, larger band at about 365 nm, ascribed to non-fluorescent
dimeric forms. The spectral characteristics of fresh HpD solution
are shown in Fig. 3 (dashed curves).

Nevertheless, the yellow emission region is particularly interesting, since it has been observed in the "in vivo" spectra of
HpD in mice with mamma tumor[11], and in the spectra of HpD components extracted with SDS micelles from tumors (MBL-2 Lymphoma and
Yoshida Hepatoma), but not from normal tissue[12]. Finally, it has
been observed in the spectra of suspension of HpD-treated mouse
3T3 cells[13]. In the latter case, the band is centered at 590 nm,
and its relative importance, in the fluorescence spectrum, increases with time after HpD treatment. A similar emission band in cells
had already been observed in some of our previous works[14,15].

Thus, definition of the conditions responsible for the appearance of this fluorescence peak may be useful for a better understanding of the interaction of HpD with cellular structures and,

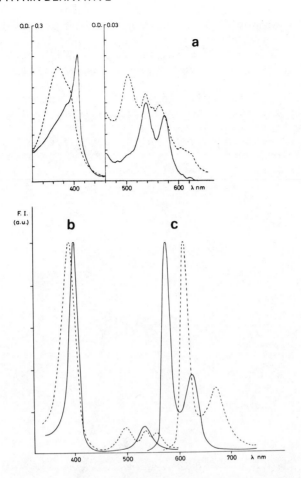

Fig. 3.   Absorption (a), excitation (b), and emission (c) spectra
          of HpD solution in saline. Dashed curves refer to air-
          -equilibrated solution immediately after preparation.
          Unbroken curves refer to N_2-equilibrated solution 24 h
          after preparation (HpD concentration: $3 \cdot 10^{-6}$ M).

therefore, for clarifying its tumor specificity.

A porphyrin species emitting in the yellow region may by observed in HpD in saline, after aging of the solution. In the Soret region, it is characterized by a narrow absorption peak centered at
$\sim$ 405 nm, and two emission peaks around 575 and 630 nm (Fig. 3, un-
broken curves), and a typical fluorescence decay time of about 3.5 ns.

The environmental parameters that influence the appearance of this porphyrin species were investigated. In particular, the dependence of the NPS formation kinetics on gases diluted in the solution, on pH, on concentration, and on temperature was studied.

The process of formation of the species emitting around 580 nm was studied by recording the absorption spectra in the Soret region, at fixed time intervals, using fresh solutions as a reference. The Soret region was chosen, since, in it, the differences in the component absorption features are more evident. The study was carried out in different solution aeration conditions. It was found that

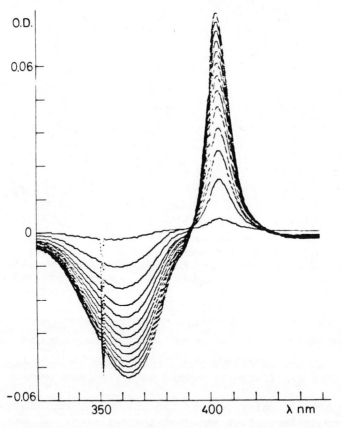

Fig. 4. Kinetics of the formation of the porphyrin species absorbing at 405 nm in N_2-equilibrated solution. Time interval between consecutive curves: 15 min.

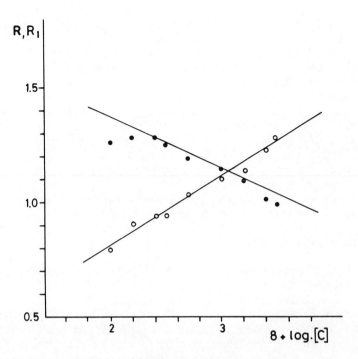

Fig. 5.   R (o) and R_1 (●) values vs concentration of 24 h-old de-
          -aerated solutions.

the presence of Oxygen is an inhibiting or, at least, a strongly
delaying, factor for the formation of the species absorbing at 405 nm.
In fact, the rate of formation in air-equilibrated solution is much
lower than in de-aerated solutions. Fig. 4 shows an example of
formation kinetics in N_2-equilibrated solution. In air-equilibrated solution the formation rate was 8-10 times slower.

        From Fig. 4 it can be seen that the dimer is more influenced
by the formation of the NPS than is the monomer. However, the rate
of formation of the species absorbing at 405 nm decreases as the
HpD concentration increases, in agreement with Pasqua et al.[16].
This can be seen from Fig. 5, where the R and R_1 values are shown
for 24 h-old solutions. On the other hand, the degree of dimerization increases as the HpD concentration increases; thus, this process is probably competitive with the formation of the NPS. Therefore, it is reasonable to assume that the NPS forms directly from
the monomer. The whole equilibrium may be explained by assuming
that NPS formation induces a dissociation of the dimer to compensate

for the transformation of the monomers into the new porphyrin species. As to the effect of hydrogenionic concentration on the formation of the NPS, it can be seen that acid pH's inhibit the appearance of the 405 nm absorption peak. In a basic environment, inhibition occurs only for pH values greater than 8. At higher pH's, with
aging, a non-fluorescent species with an absorption peak at 408 nm
appears. It is worth noting that all measurements were performed
in N_2-equilibrated solutions. It should also be stressed that measurements at different pH's were not performed in buffered solutions,
since the NPS formation kinetics, in such a case, seems to be influ-
enced in a different way by the ionic species in the solution.

The effect of pH on the spectral characteristics of the NPS
was evaluated, starting from an aged N_2-equilibrated solution of
HpD, containing only NPS. The solution pH was adjusted by adding
concentrated NaOH or HCl.

In basic environment, up to pH 12, the spectral characteristics of the NPS do not change. In the case of acidification, however, the absorption peak at 405 nm initially decreases, but without
any evident spectral shift. At a pH value of about 3, the absorption peak shifts to 400 nm. A similar absorption peak can be found
in fresh solution at the same pH value, and is attributed to a di-
cationic form[17]. The corresponding emission peak is centered at
595 nm.

The NPS formation kinetics is temperature-dependent. In particular, the temperature-increase is a factor favouring the appearance of NPS up to about 80°C. At higher temperatures, a gradual
decrease of the absorption at 405 nm can be seen.

We have thus pinpointed the environmental factors influencing
the appearance and formation rate of the NPS. Let us now see how
the presence of this new species may be explained in lymphocytes.
Two hypotheses may be advanced: 1) lymphocytes in a different functional state exhibit a different uptake capability; 2) lymphocytes
in a different functional state favour, to a different extent, the
formation of NPS, due to their microenvironmental conditions.

As to the first hypothesis, the different membrane conditions
surely justify a higher HpD uptake in stimulated lymphocytes. Indeed, considering the whole HpD emission spectrum, the fluorescence
peak intensity resulting from time-resolved measurements is higher
in stimulated lymphocytes, which indicates a greater overall HpD
content. However, the content differences are much more evident in
the yellow emission band, as if there were a preferential uptake
for the NPS. To see if this was reasonable, we studied the behaviour of HpD in the culture media used in lymphocyte preparation.
Only 48 h after adding HpD to the culture media, it was possible to

observe the appearance of a small peak corresponding to the NPS
(data not given). It is worth noting that both the absorption/ex-
citation and the emission spectra are red-shifted by about 10 nm
in culture media, as compared with the saline solution. Since the
incubation time in our experiments was no longer than 1 h, we may
assume that the HpD absorbed by cells had no 585 nm fluorescence
component in it; thus, the new species should form directly inside
the cells, as stated by the second hypothesis. Indeed, in the light
of the results obtained in solution, the greater oxygen consumption
in stimulated lymphocytes, due to their higher metabolic activity,
may be assumed to favour NPS formation in these cells.

In conclusion, the finding of the aforementioned fluorescence
differences in the yellow spectral region, related to a specific
fluorescent compound, if widely confirmed in tumor cells, should be
useful for two main purposes: (i) to clarify the interaction of
HpD with tumors, the main aspects of which are not yet understood,
and (ii) to increase sensitivity in the location of early-stage
tumors through the detection of fluorescence, a promising technique
that is increasingly used.

REFERENCES

1. A. E. Profio, D. R. Doiron, and E. G. King, Laser fluorescence
    bronchoscope for localization of occult lung tumor, Med.
    Phys. 6:523 (1979).
2. T. J. Dougherty, J. E. Kaufman, A. Goldfarb, K. R. Weishaupt,
    D. Boyle, and A. Mittleman, Photoradiation therapy for the
    treatment of malignant tumors, Cancer Res. 38:2628 (1978).
3. R. L. Lipson, E. J. Baldes, and A. M. Olsen, The use of a de-
    rivative of Hematoporphyrin in tumor detection, J. Natl.
    Cancer Inst. 26:1 (1961).
4. J. Moan, and S. Sommer, Fluorescence and absorption properties
    of the components of Hematoporphyrin Derivative, Photobio-
    chem. Photobiophys. 3:93 (1981).
5. R. Bonnett, R. J. Ridge, P. A. Scourides, and M. C. Rosenbaum,
    On the nature of Hematoporphyrin Derivative, J. Chem. Soc.
    Perkin T. 12:3135 (1981).
6. D. Kessel, and T. Chow, Tumor-localizing components of the
    porphyrin preparation Hematoporphyrin Derivative, Can. Res.
    43:1994 (1983).
7. F. Docchio, R. Ramponi, C. A. Sacchi, G. Bottiroli, and I.
    Freitas, An automatic pulsed laser microfluorometer with
    high spatial and temporal resolution, to be published.
8. S. B. Brown, H. Hatzikonstantinov, and D. G. Herries. The
    structure of porphyrins and haems in aqueous solution, Int.
    J. Biochem. 12:701 (1981).

9. F. Docchio, R. Ramponi, C. A. Sacchi, G. Bottiroli, and I. Freitas, Time-resolved fluorescence microscopy of Hemato-porphyrin-Derivative in cells, Lasers in Surgery and Medicine 2:21 (1982).

10. F. Docchio, R. Ramponi, C. A. Sacchi, G. Bottiroli, and I. Freitas, Time-resolved fluorescence microscopy of Hemato-porphyrin-Derivative in tissue- and culture-cells, in: "Laser Tokyo '81", K. Atsumi and N. Nimsakul, eds., Inter Group Corp., Tokyo (1981).

11. W. J. M. Van der Putten, and M. J. C. Van Gemert, Hematopor-phyrin Derivative fluorescence spectra in vitro and an animal tumor, in: "Proc. Laser '81 Opto-Elektronik , München, West Germany" (1981).

12. G. Jori - Personal communication.

13. M. W. Berns, A. Dahlam, F. M. Johnson, R. Burns, D. Sperling, M. Guiltinan, A. Siemens, R. Walter, W. Wright, M. Hammer--Wilson, and A. Wile, In vitro cellular effects of Hemato-porphyrin Derivative, Cancer Res. 42:2325 (1982).

14. F. Docchio, R. Ramponi, C. A. Sacchi, G. Bottiroli, and I. Freitas, Fluorescence studies of biological molecules by laser irradiation, in: "New Frontiers in Laser Medicine and Surgery", K. Atsumi, ed., Excerpta Medica, Amsterdam (1983).

15. G. Bottiroli, I. Freitas, F. Docchio, R. Ramponi, and C. A. Sacchi, Towards a better understanding of the mechanism of action of Hematoporphyrin Derivative at the cellular level, in: "Proc. 13th Cancer Congress, Seattle U.S.A." (1982).

16. A. Pasqua, A. Poletti, and S. M. Murgia, Ultrafiltration techniques as a tool for the investigation of Hematoporphy-rin aggregates in aqueous solution, Med. Biol. Environ. 10:287 (1982).

17. K. M. Smith, General features of the structure and chemistry of porphyrin compounds, in: "Porphyrins and Metalloporphy-rin Compounds", K. M. Smith, ed., Elsevier Sci. Publishing Co., Amsterdam (1975).

TIME-RESOLVED LASER FLUORESCENCE AND PHOTOBLEACHING OF SINGLE CELLS

AFTER PHOTOSENSITIZATION WITH HEMATOPORPHYRIN DERIVATIVE (HpD)

H. Schneckenburger, E. Unsöld, W. Weinsheimer[*], and
D. Jocham

Abteilung f. Angewandte Optik
Gesellschaft f. Strahlen- und Umweltforschung mbH München
Ingolstädter Landstr. 1, D-8042 Neuherberg, F.R. Germany

*) Urologische Klinik und Poliklinik, Klinikum Großhadern
   Marchioninistr. 15, D-8000 München 70, F.R.Germany

INTRODUCTION

Because of its preferential retention in tumor cells hematoporphyrin derivative (HpD) is used for diagnosis[1,2] and phototherapy [3]
of tumors. The cytotoxic effect has been attributed to the formation
of singlet oxygen after intermolecular energy transfer $HpD \rightarrow O_2$ [4] or
to the production of HpD radicals [5].

Quantitative fluorometric detection of HpD is limited by cell
autofluorescence which cannot be completely suppressed by spectral
filtering. However previous results obtained using mouse tissue cells
and human lymphocytes [6] indicate that HpD fluorescence and autofluorescence can probably be separated according to their different decay times. These different decay patterns have been investigated further in this paper using human bladder cells and rabbit Brown-Pearce
tumor cells.

EXPERIMENTAL

Cultures of human cells (normal urothelial and bladder cancer
cells) or Brown-Pearce carcinoma cells [7], were incubated with an
aqueous HpD solution (5 µg/ml) for 12 or 36 hours, respectively.

Single cells were irradiated in a fluorescence microscope
(Fig. 1) with UV pulses of 364 nm and 100 psec duration from a mode-
locked argon ion (Ar^+) laser. Laser pulses with a repetition rate

137

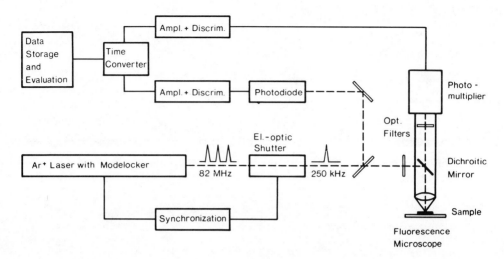

Fig. 1. Experimental setup for time-resolved fluorescence
         microscopy

of 250 kHz were selected from the 82 MHz pulse train by means of an
electro-optic shutter.

     The laser beam, focused to a diameter of 100 µm, illuminated
the cells homogeneously with a pulse energy of $2 \cdot 10^{-11}$ Joule. The
fluorescence decay curve was obtained using a single photon counting
system, as well as optical long pass and interference filters appropriate for HpD emission (600–700 nm)[2]. The time-resolution of the
entire detecting system was about 0.5 nsec.

RESULTS AND DISCUSSION

     Fig. 2 shows the fluorescence decay curves for a single human
bladder cell incubated with HpD and for a reference cell not exposed
to HpD. Both curves show fast decay times of about 1 nsec which are
attributed to autofluorescence. The cell treated with HpD also shows
a long-lived fluorescence component which decays with a time constant
of (6.5 ± 2) nsec. The same decay time was measured for all normal
and tumor cells incubated with HpD, in agreement with results recently obtained by Docchio et al.[6] using mouse tissue cells.

     A decrease of fluorescence intensity due to photobleaching was
observed within a few minutes of irradiation. Fig. 3 shows the
bleaching behaviour of an HpD treated Brown-Pearce tumor cell at an
average irradiance of 300 mW/mm^2. The fading of short-lived autofluorescence is relatively weak, but the fluorescence photon rate of HpD
is reduced by more than a factor of 3. Even at a power density of
only 3 mW/mm^2, the value commonly used for time-resolved fluorescence

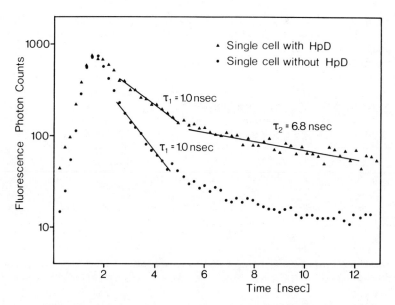

Fig. 2.   Fluorescence decay curves for single human urinary
          bladder cells. The semilogarithmic plot reveals two ex-
          ponential components for the cell treated with HpD.

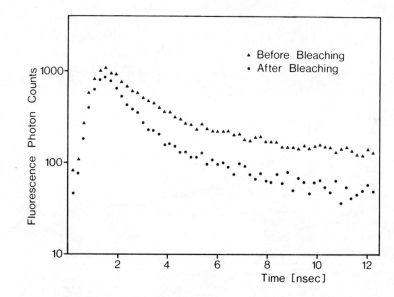

Fig. 3.   Fluorescence decay curves for a single HpD treated
          Brown-Pearce tumor cell before and after 8 min of
          photobleaching (power density 300 mW/mm^2).

measurements, significant photobleaching of HpD emission was detected. Similar results were obtained with both normal and tumor cells from human urinary bladder.

The different bleaching behaviour was verified by measuring the integral fluorescence intensity as a function of the time of irradiation. The results are shown in Fig. 4. Whereas the fluorescence of all cells incubated with HpD decreased by a factor of 2-4 within 8 minutes of laser exposure (300 mW/mm^2), that of cells not treated with HpD decreased by a factor of only 1.15-1.5. At a laser power of only 3 mW/mm^2 (s. above), the fluorescence intensity remained constant for cells without HpD, but still decreased by about 20% within 8 minutes for cells incubated with HpD.

The results show that the fluorescence due to HpD can easily be differentiated from autofluorescence on the basis of the different decay times. However, quantitative determination of HpD content within normal and tumor cells is complicated by the effect of photobleaching that occurs during laser irradiation. Since the fluorescence decay time of HpD is the same for normal and tumor cells within the experimental limits of error, no differences in fluorescence quantum efficiency or in energy transfer HpD $\rightarrow O_2$ can be deduced from these experimentes.

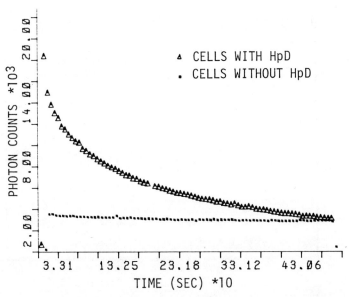

Fig. 4.   Photobleaching of Brown-Pearce tumor cells as a function of irradiation time (power density 300 mW/mm^2). Integral fluorescence detection after spectral filtering at (650 $\pm$ 40) nm.

REFERENCES

1. A. E. Profio, D. R. Doiron, and E. G. King, Laser fluorescence
    bronchoscope for localization of occult lung tumors, Med.
    Phys. 6:523 (1979).
2. J. H. Kinsey, D. A. Cortese, and D. R. Sanderson: Mayo Clin.
    Proc. 53:593 (1978).
3. T. J. Dougherty, J. E. Kaufman, A. Goldfbar, K. R. Weishaupt,
    D. Boyle, and A. Mittleman, Photoradiation therapy for the
    treatment of malignant tumors, Cancer Res. 38:2628 (1978).
4. K. R. Weishaupt, Ch. J. Gomer, and T. J. Dougherty, Identifica-
    tion of singlet oxygen as cytotoxic agent photoinactivation
    of murine tumor, Cancer Res. 36:2326 (1979).
5. A. Andreoni, R. Cubeddu, S. De Silvestri, P. Laporta, and O.
    Svelto, Two step laser activation of Hematoporphyrin Deri-
    vative, Chem. Phys. Lett. 88:37 (1982).
6. F. Docchio, R. Ramponi, C. A. Sacchi, G. Bottiroli, and I.
    Freitas, Fluorescence studies of biological molecules by
    laser irradiation, in: "New Frontiers in Laser Medicine and
    Surgery", K. Atsumi, ed., Excerpta Medica, Amsterdam-Oxford-
    -Princeton (1983).
7. D. Jocham, E. Unsöld, G. Staehler, and Ch. Chaussy, Proc. Symp.
    Porphyrin Localizatin and Treatment of Tumors (St. Barbara,
    USA) (1983).

EFFECTS OF HpD AND LASER ON TRANSFORMED AND CORRESPONDING NORMAL CULTURED CELLS: DIFFERENTIAL CYTOTOXICITY AS AN IN VITRO MODEL FOR TUMOR PHOTOCHEMOTHERAPY

Francesco Saverio Ambesi-Impiombato, Alessandra Andreoni[*], Rinaldo Cubeddu[*], Mario Esposito, Michele Mastrocinque, and Donatella Tramontano

Centro di Endocrinologia ed Oncologia Sperimentale del CNR, c/o Istituto di Patologia Generale, Università di Napoli, Italy

[*]Centro di Elettronica Quantistica e Strumentazione elettronica del CNR, c/o Istituto di Fisica del Politecnico, Milano, Italy

INTRODUCTION

In vivo studies on tumor-bearing animals have demonstrated a preferential uptake of several exogenous dyes - and particularly of the Hematoporphyrin-Derivative (HpD) - within the tumor mass [1-4] (reviewed in Ref. 5). Consequently, photoactivation of the dye resulted in selective destruction of the tumor tissue. Such photodynamic effects have been utilized in experimental photochemotherapy of induced or spontaneous tumors in animals [3,6-8]. After HpD administration, tumor tissues have been irradiated by laser light either directly or through optic fibres. Success reported with this strategy lead recently to the application of similar protocols to human tumors [9,10].

The basis of the photodynamic effect are however still unclear. In a recent report the generation of triplet oxigens (after 1 photon absorption) and of ionization products (after 2 photon absorption) have been demonstrated following respectively continuous wave or pulsed (10 nsec duration) laser irradiation of HpD [11]. Presently, despite the widespread and growing interest in the potentially of tumor photochemotherapy by HpD and laser several questions are still under debate, such as: a) the existence of tissue or cellular basis of tumor selectivity, and b) the cellular or subcellular localization and site(s) of interaction of HpD.

143

To provide a definitive answer to the first question, a difference in sensitivity to HpD treatment followed by laser irradiation have been demonstrated on "in vitro" cultured strains of differentiated normal and "in vitro" virally transformed cells from rat thyroid [12]. The transformed, tumorigenic cells resulted 2-3 times more sensitive when compared to the corresponding normal cells under various but strictly parallel treatments.

The aim of the present report is to demonstrate: a) that the selective cytocidal effect of HpD and laser treatment occurs on different in vitro cell lines, rather than being a peculiar characteristic of the differentiated epithelial cells already described; and b) that the greater sensitivity is an intrinsic property of the tumor cells resulting from specific and different cell-dye interactions.

MATERIALS AND METHODS

Cells

a) Epithelial Cells. FRT Cl 1 is a strain epithelial, non-tumorigenic and undifferentiated cells derived from adult normal rat thyroids and established as a permanently-growing strain [13].

FRT Cl 1 KiKi transformed strain has been obtained from the previous by infection with an RNA tumor virus (Ki-MSV(Ki-MuLV)) [14]. Viral tranformation of the epithelial cells has been thus achieved using the sarcoma virus, and transformation has been demonstrated, as already reported, by morphological changes in individual cells and colonies, by the presence of reverse transcriptase in the culture medium of infected cells, by the acquired ability to clone in semi-solid media and by growth in syngenic animals forming solid, carcinoma-like tumors.

b) Mesenchimal Cells. FRT FIB: is a fibroblastic (as defined by morphological appearance of single cells and colonies) strain derived from adult rat thyroids. They are capable of apparently indefinite growth "in vitro". This appears to occur very easily in rat cells and - unlike human fibroblasts - without any sign of crisis or spontaneous transformation. FRT FIB are unable to grow in semisolid media or to form tumors in syngeneic animals.

FRT FIB KiKi: obtained from the previous normal cells by infection with the same RNA virus (Ki-MSV(Ki-MuLV)). True transformation has been obtained, as demonstrated by the same criteria already mentioned for the FRT Cl 1 KiKi cells.

Cell Culture Conditions

Cells were maintained in modified Ham F-12 medium [13] supple-

mented with 5% calf serum (Gibco), in Falcon plastic 100 mm. diam.
dishes, in 95% air-5% CO_2 humid incubators at 37°C, and split by
trypsinization when confluent or when needed. All cell manipulations
were performed in sterile conditions.

Hematoporphyrin

Commercially available HpD (Photofrin, Oncolory Research &
Development, Inc., Cheektowaga, N.Y., USA) has been used.

Laser

A continuous-wave dye laser (Rhodamine B) at 631 nm, pumped by
an argon laser has been used. The wavelength was measured by a
Jarrel-Ash Model 82-410 monochromator. The irradiation average power measured by a calibrate thermopile, was adjusted to 100 mW/cm^2.

Incubation and Irradiation Experiments

These were performed as previously described [12]. Briefly, suspensions of 10^7 trypsinized cells in 10 ml of medium lacking serum
were treated with 0 (controls) or 20 µg/ml HpD for 2 hours in a CO_2
incubators at 37°C with occasional mixing.

After incubation, if laser irradiation was to follow, 200 ul
aliquots of washed cell suspensions were put in 5 mm optical path
quartz cuvettes and uniformly irradiated (mixing every min.).

At the end of experiments, cell viability was evaluated counting cells in a haemocytometer before and after irradiation using
trypan blue (1%) in isotonic (0.9% NaCl) solution. All experimental
points represent the average of several experiments.

RESULTS

Two different strains of cultured cell have been studied, one
epithelial (undifferentiated) and one of mesenchimal origins (fibro-
blast) from rat thyroid, each studied in parallel with their corresponding malignant counter part previously produced "in vitro" by
retrovirus transformation.

Treatments with HpD Alone

Preliminary control experiments in which normal and tumor cells
were incubated with HpD but not exposed to laser light thereafter,
gave results superimposable to those already reported for the FRTL5/
/FRTL KiKi system (differentiated, normal and transformed thyroid
cells) [18]: in essence, HpD treatment did not effect significantly
cell viability (more than 90% survival) and never had long-term effects on cells as demonstrated by plating efficiency and growth

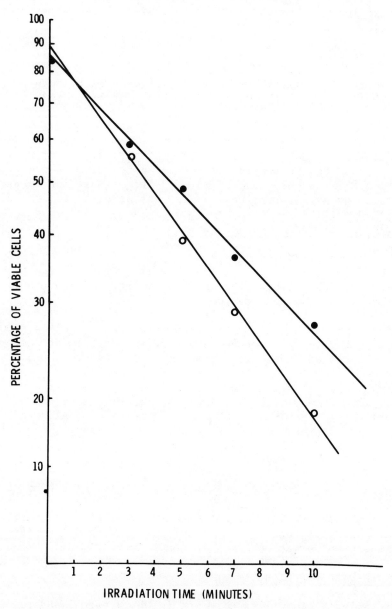

Fig. 1. Percentage of viable FRT Cl 1 (●) and FRT Cl 1 Kiki (o) cells versus irradiation time after HpD incubation and laser irradiation.

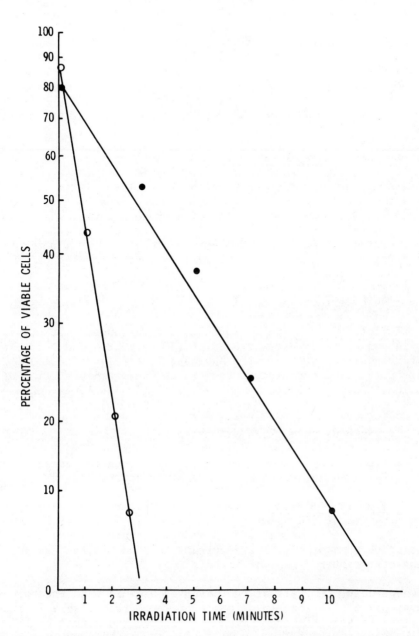

Fig. 2.   Percentage of viable FRT FIB (●) and FRT FIB KiKi (o)
          cells versus irradiation time after HpD incubation and
          laser irradiation.

curves experiments. Furthermore, laser irradiation <u>per se</u>, not pre-
ceded by HpD treatment was also without effect on these cells.

With another set of preliminary experiments, the dosage of HpD
to be used has been determined for the different cells. This was
necessary because of the different sensitivity found among various
cell types with respect to HpD. A concentration of 20 μg/ml, the
maximum HpD dosage accounting for less than 10% of cell death (in
the absence of irradiation) has been used for irradiation experiments.

Absorbance and Fluorescence Spectra

After incubation with HpD, cells (10 per sample) were washed
and pelletted. The pellet was then dissolved in a mixture of H_2O
(0.5 ml) and Protosol (NEN, 2 ml). The whole material was transferred in a quartz cuvette (1 cm light path) and spectra were obtained
in a recording Beckman UV 5230 spectrophotometer (O.D.: 350-700 nm)
or in a Perkin-Elmer 650-40 fluorometer (Fluorescence: 550-700 nm,
excitation wavelength: 405/395 nm).

Irradiation Experiments

FRT Cl 1/FRT Cl 1 KiKi. Normal and transformed epithelial
cells responded to complete treatment (20 μg/ml HpD and laser) with
a pattern qualitatively similar but quantitatively different. Treatment resulted in a cytocidal effect which increased with time of irradiation (Fig. 1). Decrease in cell viability is linear when plotted on a semi-logarithmic scale from 0 to 10 min. Percentages of
cell survival following treatment were determined by dye exclusion
tests (trypan blue straining: see methods).

The selectivity of the effect (i.e. preferential damage of the
tumor cells) also increased with time of irradiation.

FRT FIB/FRT FIB KiKi. Fibroblastic cells responded to the same
treatment protocol (20 μg/ml HpD and laser) in a similar fashion
(Fig. 2) but both cytocidal effect and selectivity were greater, to
the point that no significant survival was found in the case of malignant cells after 3 min. of irradiation.

Comparative analysis of the results obtained with the two cell
systems, epithelial and fibroblastic, reveals that (Table 1) the
difference in sensitivity between transformed and normal cells, measured as % of cells killed per unit time of irradiation is significantly greater in the case of the fibroblastic cells (Ratio: 4.46)
than in the case of the epithelial cells (Ratio: 1.25).

Table 1. Photosensitivity of Normal and Transformed Cells.

Cell Type	% of Cells Killed x min.$^{-1}$	Ratio Transf./Norm.
FRT Cl 1	5.85	
FRT Cl 1 KiKi	7.3	1.25
FRT FIB	7.4	
FRT FIB KiKi	33.0	4.46

HpD Uptake

Selective cytocital effect could be due to different HpD up-take, or to other mechanisms, such as different interactions or lo-calization inside the tumor cells. To discriminate between these several possibilities, HpD uptake in normal and tumor cells have been measured.

After incubation with the dye, cells were washed and pelleted as usual. Cell pellets were dissolved in H_2O/Protosal mixture. Typical HpD absorption (Fig. 3) and fluorescence (Fig. 4) spectra were obtained from undiluted pellets of treated FRT FIB KiKi cells, where untreated blank cells were lacking of any interfering optical activity in the same conditions. It was clear, from those determi-nations, that cell-bound HpD can be specifically quantitized by op-tical methods in the cell pellet.

O.D. determinations at 400 nm, gave higher values for tumor cells, indicating a higher HpD uptake, with an increase over normal cells of 144% and 251% respectively in the case of the epithelial and fibroblastic cells (see Table 2).

Confluent vs.log Phase Growing Cells

The higher HpD uptake inside tumor cells and consequently the greater sensitivity to photochemiotherapy could be due to a variety of reasons, from specific differences between normal and tumor cells which could be interesting to pursue, to unspecific differences such as higher division or metabolic rates. To discriminate between these possibilities, non-confluent (log phase growing) and conflu-ent (growth arrested) cells were treated with HpD and laser. FRT FIB normal cells were chosen for these experiments for their ability to remain almost indefinitly in a confluent, completely growth ar-rested state without any apparent cell death and consequent repla-

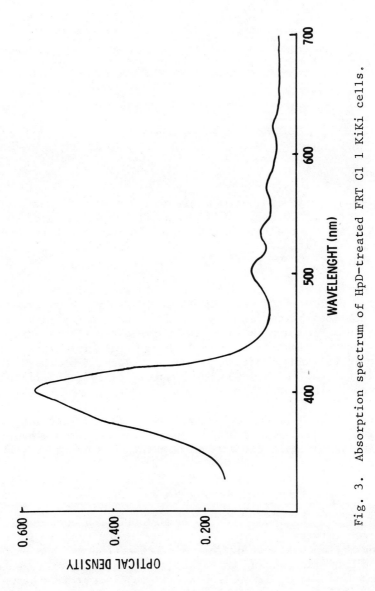

Fig. 3.   Absorption spectrum of HpD-treated FRT Cl 1 KiKi cells.

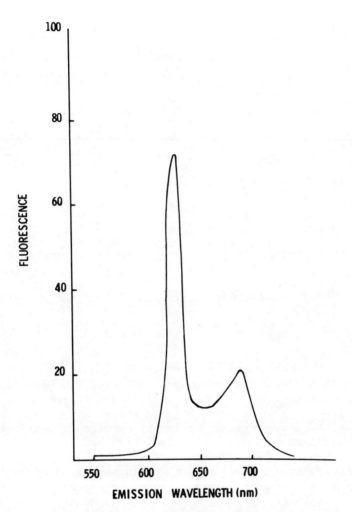

Fig. 4. Fluorescence spectrum of HpD-treated FRT Cl 1 KiKi cells.
Fluorescence intensity (y axis) is expressed in arbitrary
units.

ment by cell duplication. Cells from confluent dishes were treated
in parallel with log phase cells following the usual protocol. As
illustrated in Table 2, HpD uptake was practically the same and,
correspondingly, no differences in % of viable cells were observed

Table 2. Uptake of HpD Determined by Optical Density of 10^6 Pel-
          letted Cells

Cell Type	HpD uptake (O.D. at 400 nm)	Variations % (Transf./Norm.)
FRT Cl 1	.500	–
FRT Cl 1 KiKi	.720	144
FRT FIB	.152	–
FRT FIB KiKi	.383	251
FRT FIB LOG PHASE	.145	
FRT FIB CONFLUENT	.135	

at any time of laser irradiations (Fig. 5), the two curves being
clearly superimposable.

DISCUSSION

In addition to the results recently obtained on differentiated
cells [12] the existence of a tumor-specific, selective cytocidal effect has been now proven on both epithelial and fibroblastic cells
of thyroid origins. The normal cells have been directly compared
"in vitro" to the corresponding malignant cells obtained by retro-
viral transformation of the same cells "in vitro".

Preliminary experiments in which cells were treated with HpD
or laser irradiation alone demonstrated minor unspecific cell damage,
and served to evaluate the best experimental conditions and HpD concentrations which were used thereafter.

Complete HpD and laser treatment gave higher tumor cells mor-
tality rates in all conditions tested. Selectivity was already significant in the epithelial cells system (FRT Cl 1/FRT Cl 1 KiKi)
but was sensibly greater (almost 4 times, see Table 1) in the fibroblastic cell system (FRT FIB/FRT FIB KiKi).

Cell-bound HpD has been directly measured in the pellet with
both fluorescence and O.D. measurements, and such quantitative determinations showed a good correlation between higher uptake of the
dye and selective cytocidal effect. Tumor cells have a significantly higher uptake than corresponding normal cells. Furthermore, a
higher difference in uptake was found in the fibroblastic cell sys-

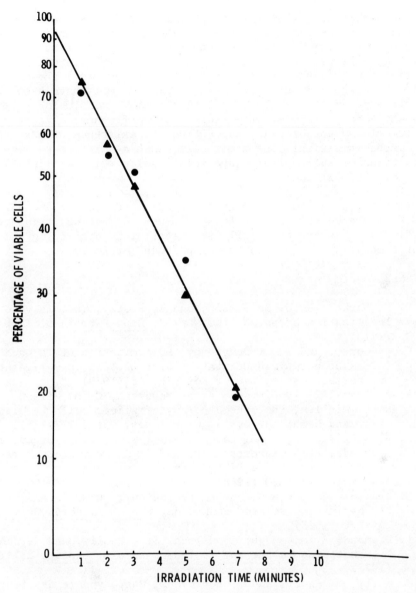

Fig. 5. Percentage of viable cells in log phase growing (•) and
confluent (▲) FRT FIB cells, versus irradiation time after
HpD incubation and laser irradiation.

tem (FRT FIB/FRT FIB KiKi) where also the selectivity (therapeutic margin) was greater.

The possibility that higher HpD uptake and consequently lower survival after treatment were due to faster duplication or metabolic rate of the tumor cell has been ruled out by the last experiment described. The same kind of cells in completely different metabolic conditions (confluence arrested and log phase growing) showed identical HpD uptake and survival rates. FRT FIB cells have been chosen for this experiment for their ability to remain viable for several weeks while completely growth-arrested at confluency. This results is particularly encouraging, suggesting the existence of more specific mechanisms within the tumor cell, such as different cell-dye interactions or intracellular dye localization which will be the object of further studies.

Investigations now in progress in our laboratories are also aimed to increase our ability to selectively damage the tumor cells. Such "in vitro" experiments will be essential in optimizing the therapeutic margins of "in vivo" tumor photochemotherapy.

REFERENCES

1. D. S. Barker, R. W. Henderson, and E. Storey, The "in vivo" localization of porphyrins, Br. J. Exp. Pathol. 51:628 (1970).
2. C. J. Gomer, and T. J. Dougherty, Determination of ^{3}H- and ^{14}C-Hematoporphyrin Derivative distribution in malignant and normal tissue, Cancer Res. 39:146 (1979).
3. S. G. Granelli, I. Diamond, A. F. McDonagh, C. B. Wilson, and S. L. Nielsen, Photochemotherapy of glioma cells by visible light and Hematoporphyrin, Cancer Res. 35:2567 (1975).
4. H. B. Gregorie Jr, E. O. Horger, J. L. Ward, J. F. Green, T. Richards, H. C. Robertson Jr, and T. B. Stevenson, Hematoporphyrin-Derivative fluorescence in malignant neoplasms, Ann. Surg. 167:820 (1968).
5. M. Tsutsui, C. Carrano, and E. A. Tsutsui, Tumor localizers: Porphyrins and related compounds, Ann. N.Y. Acad. Sci. 244:674 (1975).
6. I. Diamond, A. McDonagh, C. Wilson, S. Granelli, and R. Jaenicke, Photodynamic therapy malignant tumors, Lancet. 2:1175 (1972).
7. J. Kelly, M. Snell, and M. Berenbaum, Photodynamic destruction of human bladder carcinoma, Br. J. Cancer. 31:237 (1975).
8. S. H. Tomson, E. A. Emmett, and S. H. Fox, Photodestruction of mouse epithelial tumors after oral acridine orange and argon laser, Cancer Res. 34:3124 (1974).
9. T. J. Dougherty, J. E. Kaufman, A. Goldfarb, K. R. Weishaupt, D. Boyle, and A. Mittleman, Photoradiation therapy for the treatment of malignant tumors, Cancer Res. 38:2628 (1978).

10. T. J. Dougherty, T. J. G. Lawrence, J. H. Kaufman, D. Boyle, K. R. Weishaupt, and A. Goldfarb, J. Natl. Cancer Inst. 62:231 (1979).

11. A. Andreoni, R. Cubeddu, S. De Silvestri, P. Laporta, and O. Svelto, Two-step laser activation of Hematoporphyrin Derivative, Chem. Phys. Lett. 88:37 (1982).

12. A. Andreoni, R. Cubeddu, S. De Silvestri, P. Laporta, F. S. Ambesi-Impiombato, M. Esposito, M. Mastrocinque, and D. Tramontano, Effects of laser irradiation on Hematoporphyrin-treated normal and transformed thyroid cells in culture, Cancer Res. 43:2076 (1983).

13. F. S. Ambesi-Impiombato, L. A. M. Parks, and H. G. Coon, Culture of hormone-dependent functional epithelial cells from rat thyroids, Proc. Natl. Acad. Sci. U.S.A. 77:3455 (1980).

INTERACTION OF FREE AND LIPOSOME-BOUND PORPHYRINS WITH NORMAL AND MALIGNANT CELLS: BIOCHEMICAL AND PHOTOSENSITIZATION STUDIES IN VITRO AND IN VIVO

I. Cozzani, G. Jori[*] E. Reddi[*] L. Tomio[§] P.L. Zorat[§]
T. Sicuro and G. Malvaldi

Istituto di Biochimica e Istituto di Patologia Generale
Università di Pisa; *Istituto di Biologia Animale e
§ Divisione di Radioterapia,Università di Padova,Italy

The porphyrins used in combination with visible light for the early diagnosis and phototherapy of neoplasias are so far limited to hematoporphyrin (Hp) alone or associated with some derivatives obtained by acid treatment (HpD). Several evidences indicate that the cytoplasmic membrane represents a hydrophobic barrier limiting the uptake of HpD and, to a greater extent, of Hp by cells; in most cases, a significant aliquot of cell-bound porphyrin is rapidly cleared from both isolated cells[1] and animal tissues[2]. The release is markedly slower for malignant cells and tissues[3] thus providing favourable tumor-to-normal tissue ratios of porphyrin concentrations, which are exploited in diagnostic and therapeutic oncology. Clearly, further enhancements of these ratios would be of paramount clinical importance. In this paper, we report some experimental indications that liposome-bound hematoporphyrin (Hp_{lip}) and its water-insoluble dimethylester (HpDME) are taken up by cells and tissues at a higher rate and in greater amounts as compared with aqueous Hp solutions (Hp_{aq}) of corresponding concentrations. Moreover, the release from the cells of porphyrins vehiculated via liposomes is slower. Although normal cells take up and retain considerably higher levels of porphyrin when incorporated into liposomes, the phenomena are enhanced in neoplastic cells and tissues, both in vitro and in vivo. As a consequence, when neoplastic systems are treated with Hp_{lip} or HpDME, remarkably enhanced and long-lasting sensitivity to photodynamic effects has been observed in preliminary experiments.

MATERIALS AND METHODS

Dipalmitoylphosphatidylcholine (DPPC, Sigma) and Hp or HpDME (Porphyrin Products) (70:1, molar ratio) were dissolved in chloroform:methanol, 9:1 (v/v) and dried in a rotary evaporator. The

lipid film was resuspended in 0.01 M phosphate buffer pH 7.4, containing 150 mM NaCl, and the liposome suspension was sonicated at
50°C for 30 min.

Normal and neoplastic hepatocytes were isolated by liver perfusion with collagenase[4] of either normal rats or rats bearing a
chemically induced solid hepatoma. Ascites hepatoma cells (Yoshida
AH-130) were obtained on the seventh day from intraperitoneal transplantation into Wistar rats. All isolated cells were washed with
isotonic phosphate-buffered solution (PBS) and tested for trypan
blue exclusion; preparations containing at least 80 % cells exclu-
ding the dye were used for in vivo incubations.

Hp_{aq}, Hp_{lip} or $HpDME_{lip}$ were injected either intraperitoneally
or intravenously at a dose of 5 mg/kg body weight to Wistar albino
rats either normal or affected by a subcutaneously implanted solid
Yoshida hepatoma. The rats were 20 ± 1 days old and the porphyrin was
administered at 10 days after tumor implantation. At predetermined
intervals, rats were sacrificed. The porphyrin content was estimated
spectrophotofluorimetrically both in selected whole tissues and in
subcellular fractions isolated as previously detailed[5].

RESULTS

Uptake of Aqueous and Liposomal Hematoporphyrin by Normal and
Neoplastic Cells of Liver Origin

Normal and malignant cells of rat liver origin (isolated normal
hepatocytes, neoplastic hepatocytes isolated from solid hepatomas
and cells of AH-130 Yoshida ascites hepatoma) were incubated with
various Hp concentrations either in buffer solution at pH 7.4 (Hp_{aq})
or bound to unilamellar DPPC liposomes (Hp_{lip}). The net Hp uptake
(in the Hp concentration range 0.5-20 µg/ml) was linear during the
initial 5 min. of incubation, a plateau concentration of cell-bound
Hp being approached. These features were reproduced when liposome-
bound porphyrins were used or serum albumin was added to Hp_{aq} solutions (Fig. 1 and Fig. 2). Apparently, the kinetics and amount of
Hp accumulation by neoplastic cell is faster in comparison with
normal hepatocytes (it should be taken into account that the size
of normal hepatocytes is about 15-fold and 5-fold greater than that
of ascites and, respectively, solid malignant hepatocytes).

On incubation with liposomal Hp (Fig. 2.) or HpDME, rapid porphyrin uptake leading to a steady state was observed for both normal
and malignant liver cells. Considerable differences in cell-bound
Hp concentrations were observed by comparing normal and neoplastic
cells: the plateau values of porphyrin uptake, expressed as molar
Hp concentration/wet cell volume, were 60, 825 and 570 µM for
normal hepatocytes isolated from solid hepatomas and Yoshida asci-
tes-hepatoma cells, respectively.

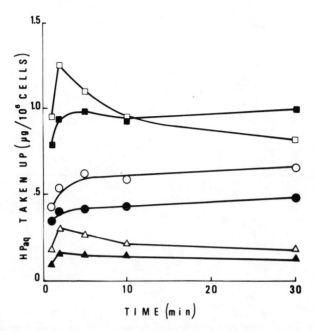

Fig. 1.   Kinetics of uptake of Hp_{aq} by normal hepatocytes (circles),
by malignant hepatocytes (squares) and by ascites hepatoma
cells (triangles), in the absence (open symbols) and in the
presence (closed symbols) of 1 % BSA. The cells were incu=
bated with 10 μg/ml Hp_{aq} at 37° in the dark.

Effects of Serum Albumin on the Uptake and Release of Hp_{aq} by
Normal and Neoplastic Cells

      Distinct features of BSA addition were observed, according to
the cell type. In the case of normal hepatocytes the uptake of Hp_{aq}
was reduced in the presence of 1 % BSA, although this effect was
lower than that observed for normal and neoplastic cells of non-liver
origin. In the case of malignant cells of liver origin a biphasic
effect of BSA on the time-course of Hp_{aq} uptake was observed (Fig. 1):
for short incubation times, the Hp_{aq} uptake was reduced, a larger
effect being observed with ascites hepatoma cells than with malignant hepatocytes from solid tumors; for longer incubations, the
presence of BSA produced an increased net uptake of Hp_{aq}. These
effects may be explained by assuming that neoplastic cells have a
higher affinity for porphyrins than normal cells, and normal hepatocytes have a higher affinity for BSA than malignant cells of liver
origin and cells of origins other than liver. Likely, albumin protects cell permeability at extents that are proportional to its
affinity for the given cell type. These assumptions appear to be

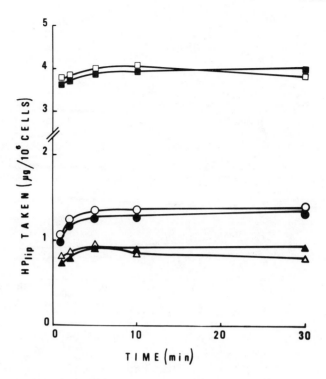

Fig. 2. Kinetics of uptake of Hp_{lip} by normal neoplastic hepatocytes
and by ascites hepatoma cells, in the absence and in the
presence of BSA. The symbols and the experimental conditions
are the same as in Fig. 1.

supported by the experiments of Hp_{aq} release from isolated cells
(Fig. 3) and by photodynamic experiments in vitro and in vivo (to be
published elsewhere). In striking contrast with the complex action
of BSA on Hp_{aq} uptake, no appreciable effect of BSA was observed on
the uptake and release of Hp_{lip} (Fig. 2 and Fig. 4).

Release of Aqueous and Liposomal Hematoporphyrin from Normal and Malignant Cells

Both normal and neoplastic hepatocytes release an important
fraction of the porphyrin taken up from Hp_{aq} solutions, when the
cells are washed free of excess porphyrin and incubated in PBS
(Fig. 3 and Fig. 4). However, the neoplastic cells retain considerably higher levels (especially in terms of molar concentrations) than
the normal cells incubated with Hp_{lip}. The presence of BSA affects
the release of Hp_{aq} from normal cells (presumably by protecting the
permeability of the cell membrane, Fig. 3), but has no detectable
effect on the kinetics of Hp_{aq} release from neoplastic cells, or the

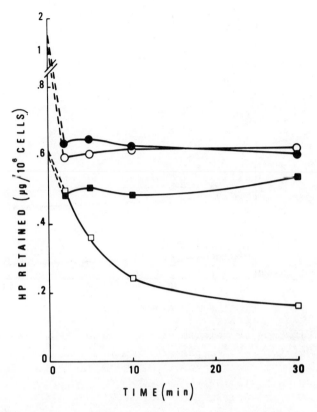

Fig. 3. Kinetics of release of Hp_{aq} by normal (squares) and mali-
        gnant (circles) hepatocytes, in the presence (closed symbols)
        and in the absence (open symbols) of 1% BSA. The porphyrin
        bound to the cells was measured, after incubation with
        10 μg/ml Hp_{aq} for 10 min. at 37°C in the dark, cell washing
        and incubation with PBS for the times indicated.

release of Hp_{lip} from normal and neoplastic cells.

Time-dependence of Porphyrin Distribution in Normal and Tumor-bearing
Rats

        The time-dependence of Hp_{aq} or Hp_{lip} recovery from liver, kidneys
and eventually tumor of normal rats an rats affected by Yoshida
hepatoma is shown in table 1 and, respectively, table 2. Clearly,
the liposomal porphyrins accumulate in the liver in greater amounts
but at a lower rate as compared with Hp_{aq}. The affinity of liposo-
me-incorporated drugs for organs of the reticuloendothelial system
has been observed by other authors[6]. Surprisingly, a significant
fraction of Hp_{lip} and $HpDME_{lip}$ is eliminated via kidneys indicating

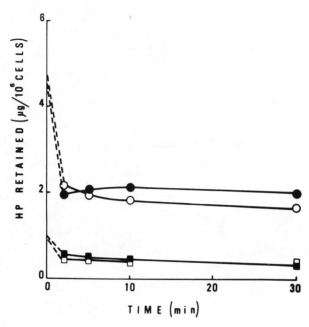

Fig. 4. Kinetics of release of Hp_{lip} from normal and malignant
         hepatocytes, in the presence and in the absence of BSA.
         The symbols and the experimental conditions are the same
         as in Fig. 3.

that the mechanisms controlling the transport and elimination of
liposome-bound porphyrins differ from those typical of Hp_{aq}. The
largest difference between normal and aqueous Hp is observed at relatively long times after injection. Actually, Hp_{lip} is cleared from
the liver with a kinetic similar to that found for Hp_{aq}; on the
other hand, elimination of Hp_{lip} from the tumor is remarkably slower
than that of Hp_{aq}. The phenomenon is even more evident for HpDME.As
a consequence, tumor-to-liver ratios of porphyrin concentration as
high as 6.25, 18.39 and 11.58 are estimated at 72 h after injection
of Hp_{aq}, Hp_{lip} and $HpDME_{lip}$, respectively.

     The high affinity of liposomal porphyrins for neoplastic cells
is probably due to a tight binding with membrane receptors. Subcellular fractionation studies indicate that about 80-90 % of endocel-
lular porphyrins is associated with the cytoplasmic membrane at 48 h
after injection.

DISCUSSION

     The liposomal system for delivery of porphyrins to tumor cells

Table 1. Recovery of Hp_{aq} (ng/g) from tissues of normal and tumor-bearing rats

Time	Normal rats		Tumor-bearing rats		
(h)	L	K	L	K	T
1	18.1	4.3	10.2	3.6	12.5
6	6.3	3.5	5.7	3.9	12.9
12	3.7	2.1	3.0	1.5	10.9
24	2.8	1.8	3.0	1.7	9.7
72	2.7	1.4	2.7	0.7	7.8

L = liver   K = kidneys   T = tumor

Table 2. Recovery of Hp_{lip} (ng/g) from tissues of normal and tumor-bearing rats

Time	Normal rats		Tumor-bearing rats		
(h)	L	K	L	K	T
1	34.0	12.4	9.5	11.4	27.9
6	9.6	7.5	3.6	10.3	45.9
12	7.3	4.9	2.5	8.9	49.7
24	4.2	6.3	2.0	8.7	55.8
72	2.0	2.3	2.3	2.4	79.1

L = liver   K = kidneys   T = tumor

described in this paper is characterized by some important features.

i) Water-insoluble and -soluble porphyrins are readily incorporated in a pure monomeric form into the liposomal structure. Preliminary spectroscopic studies indicate that both Hp and HpDME are located in the lipid bilayer of DPPC unilamellar vesicles. In this way, aggregation of Hp and HpD or other porphyrins are possibly overcome.

ii) Both in vitro and in vivo studies reported above demonstrate that liposome-bound porphyrins are accumulated in higher amounts and eliminated at a lower rate by neoplastic than by normal cells and tissues. Evidently, the liposome carrier favours the binding of porphyrins across the hydrophobic barrier created by the cytoplasmic membrane. Studies are in progress to elucidate the detailed molecular mechanisms involved in the interaction of liposomal porphyrins with cells.

iii) The preferential uptake of Hp_{lip} and HpDME by neoplastic cells is due, at least in part, to the exclusion of BSA from the binding process of liposomal porphyrins with the cell components. This fact is likely to play a major role in the photodynamic process leading to cell necrosis in vivo, since albumin-bound Hp is known[7] to be ineffective as a cell photosensitizer.

iv) Actually, preliminary experiments demonstrate that HeLa cells loaded with liposomal Hp or HpDME undergo a very fast photody= namically induced damage and lysis: e.g., for a given dose of light energy, we obtain complete cell death upon irradiation of HeLa cells incubated with 1 μg/ml HpDME, whereas the same effect is obtained with about 40-fold higher concentrations of Hp_{aq}. Moreover, both rats bearing a solid Yoshida hepatoma or mice affected by MBL-2 lymphoma exhibit significant tumor regression when exposed to 80 mW/cm^2 of red light for 60 min. at 48 h after injection of 5 mg/kg Hp_{lip} or HpDME.

ACKNOWLEDGMENT

This work was financially supported by C.N.R. (Italy) under the Progetto Finalizzato "Lasers in Biology and Medicine".

REFERENCES

1. I. Cozzani and J. D. Spikes, Photodamage and photokilling of malignant human cells in vitro by hematoporphyrin-visible light: molecular bases and possible mechanisms of phototoxicity, Med. Biol. Environ. 10:269 (1982).
2. G. Jori, E. Reddi, L. Tomio, B. Salvato, and F. Calzavara, Time-course of hematoporphyrin distribution in selected tissues of normal rats and in ascites hepatoma, Tumori 65:43(1979)
3. I. Cozzani, G. Jori, E. Reddi, A. Fortunato, L. Tomio, and P. L. Zorat, Distribution of endogenous and injected porphyrins at the subcellular level in rat hepatocytes and in ascites hepatoma, Chem. Biol. Interactions 37:67 (1981).
4. K. N. Jeejeeboy, J. Ho, G. R. Greenberg, M. J. Phillips, A. Bruce-Robertson, and U. Sodtke, Albumin, fibrinogen and transferrin synthesis in isolated rat hepatocyte suspensions, Biochem. J. 146:141 (1975).
5. G. Jori, I. Cozzani, E. Reddi, E. Rossi, L. Tomio, G. Mandoliti, and G. Malvaldi, In vitro and in vivo studies on the interaction of hematoporphyrin and its dimethylester with normal and malignant cells, in:"Porphyrin Localization and Treatment of Tumors," D. Doiron, ed., Alan R. Liss Inc., New York(1983).
6. B. E. Ryman and D. A. Tyrrell, Liposomes: bags of potential,

Essays Biochem. 16:49 (1980).

7.   T. Ito, Cellular and subcellular mechanisms of photodynamic action: the $^1O_2$ hypothesis as a driving force in recent research, Photochem. Photobiol. 28:493 (1978).

PHOTODYNAMIC INACTIVATION OF L929 CELLS AFTER TREATMENT WITH

HEMATOPORPHYRIN DERIVATIVE

T.M.A.R. Dubbelman, K. Leenhouts and J. van Steveninck

Department Medical Biochemistry
Sylvius Laboratories, Wassenaarseweg 72
2333 AL Leiden, The Netherlands

INTRODUCTION

Porphyrin photoradiation therapy for the treatment of various malignant tumors is a recent rapidly developing technique and progress has been fast and promising[1,2]. The principle of porphyrin photoradiation therapy is relatively simple. Following systematic administration, porphyrins, especially the so-called hematoporphyrin-derivative (HpD) are accumulated to higher concentrations in malignant than in normal cells [3]. During subsequent exposure of the cells to visible light the accumulated porphyrin acts as photodynamic sensitizer [4] and causes oxidation of cellular constituent presumably by formation of singlet oxygen and possibly hydroxyl radicals. These oxidations lead to disturbed functions and, ultimately, cell death. Three mechanisms may be responsible e.g. membrane deterioration, DNA-damage and photodynamic inactivation of crucial enzyme systems. Studies of Kessel et al. indicate that membrane damage may be the direct cause of photodynamic cell death in tumors [5-7]. Illumination of L1210 and SS-1 cells incubated with porphyrin leads to cross-linking of membrane proteins [6] as described before with red cell membranes [8,9]. Further, loss of cell viability was correlated with inhibition of transmembrane cycloleucine transport [5]. Studies of Moan et al. also indicate that membrane damage is presumably the most important determinant in photodynamic cell killing. These authors showed that the sensitizer has to be bound to the cells in order to be effective [10,11].

Also DNA damage has been observed both in model systems utilizing isolated DNA and intact cells [12-14]. Most obvious is the photodynamic degradation of the guanine moiety [14]. Secondary to

167

this process photo-induced single- and double strand breaks have
been observed. The ability of DNA to serve as a template for DNA
dependent RNA synthesis is impaired by photodynamic treatment [15].
Recent studies have shown that DNA-protein crosslinks can be formed
photodynamically [16].

Numerous publications describe photodynamic inactivation of
many enzymes with a variety of sensitizers. In general it seems unlikely that photosensitized cell killing would be correlated with
inactivation of cellular enzymes. Only in a few cases such a correlation should be considered. DNA-dependent RNA polymerase appears
to be very sensitive to photodynamic inactivation [15,17].

In this report some characteristics of the uptake of HpD by
L929 cells will be described as well as the photodynamic action of
HpD on some transport processes across the membrane of these cells
and on its DNA.

METHODS

L929 cells were grown in minimum essential medium (modified)
with Earle's salts supplemented with 10% heat-inactivated calf serum,
penicillin (50 U/ml), streptomycin (50 µg/ml) and fungizone
(0.5 µg/ml). Confluent cell layers (about 7×10^4 cells/cm^2) were incubated with different concentrations of HpD in Dulbecco's phosphate
buffered saline (PBS) for 1 h at 37°C in the dark. The cells were
washed with PBS and illuminated in the same buffer with a slide projector equipped with a 150 W quartz halogen light bulb. The light
beam was reflected through the bottom of the culture discs by a
mirror after having passed a filter with a sharp cut-off at 590 nm.
The K^+ content of the cells was determined as described by Bader et
al. [18]. Uptake of 2-deoxyglucose, 2-aminoisobutyric acid and Rb^+,
all at a conc. of 2.5 µM, was determined by incubating the cell-layer
for 2 min at room temp. on a shaker in the dark. Passive Rb^+ influx
was measured by inhibiting the active influx with 1 mM ouabain. Uptake was stopped by washing the cell-layer 3x with 5 ml ice-cold PBS.
The cells were scraped into 2% SDS/10 mM sodiumphosphate buffer pH 7
and dissolved by incubation at 100°C for 4 min. Aliquots of this were
analyzed for radioactivity and for protein. Hexokinase activity was
determined according to Bergmeyer in the presence of 1% Triton
X-100 [19]. DNA damage was assessed by the alkaline elution technique
of Kohn et al. [20]. Porphyrins were extracted from the cells by subsequent treatment with acetone/HCl at -30°C, methanol/H$_2$O (2:1 v/v),
methanol/tetrahydrofuran/H$_2$O (1 : 1 : 1, v/v/v) and Ethylacetate/HAc
(4 : 1, v/v). The porphyrins were analyzed by HPLC on a Supelcosil
LC-18 column using tetrahydrofuran/3 mM tetrabutylammoniumphosphate
pH 3.0 (45 : 55, v/v).

RESULTS

    Incubation of L929 cells for 1 hr at 37°C with 5,10,25 and
50 µg/ml of HpD results in intracellular concentrations of porphyrins
of resp. about 0.3, 0.6, 1.5 and 1.8 µg/10^6 cells. Intracellular
porphyrins can be extracted with the procedure described in the methods section. The resulting protein pellet, after dissolution into
2% SDS does not fluoresce anymore. These porphyrins have been separated by HPLC as shown in fig. 1. Protoporphyrin along with some
other porphyrins appears to be concentrated intracellularly. The
origin of peak 1 is unknown; metabolic conversion cannot be excluded.
For reasons of comparison also the HpD chromatogram is shown. The intracellular porphyrins are mainly located perinuclearly as shown in
fig. 2.

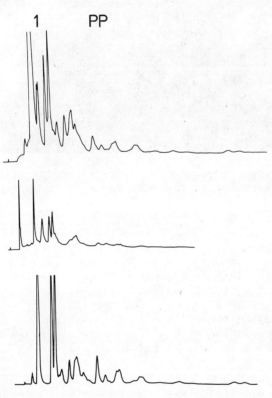

Fig. 1. HPLC profile of porphyrins after incubation of L929 cells for
        1 h at 37°C with 25 µg/ml. Top: porphyrins extracted from the
        supernatant, middle: intracellular porphyrins and bottom:
        HpD profile.

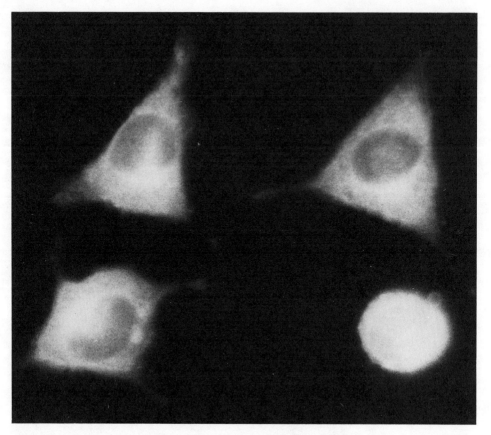

Fig. 2. Fluorescence microscopy of cells incubated with 10 µg/ml of
      HpD as described in the methods.

        Illumination of the cells, incubated with HpD results in K^+
leakage only after incubation with relatively high HpD concentrations
as shown in fig. 3. This is in agreement with the increased passive
Rb^+ uptake under the same conditions (fig. 4). 2-Deoxyglucose is
presumably taken up by a carrier mediated transport system and is
phosphorylated inside the cells [21]. This system is inhibited by illumination after incubation with all HpD concentrations used (fig. 5).
At both lower concentrations (5 and 10 µg/ml) the hexokinase activity
is still intact.

        Two active uptake systems have been studied: 2-aminoisobutyric
acid and Rb^+. The former is accumulated up to a ratio of about 15; it
is inhibited readily by the photodynamic action of HpD (fig. 6). The
same is true for the active Rb^+ uptake, but only at 10 and 25 µg
HpD/ml. The results of the uptake studies are summarized in fig. 7.

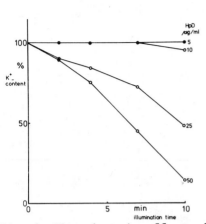

Fig. 3. Photodynamic effect of HpD on the K+ content of L929 cells.

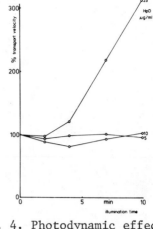

Fig. 4. Photodynamic effect of HpD on passive Rb+ uptake; the active Rb+ uptake was inhibited by incubation with 1 mM ouabain.

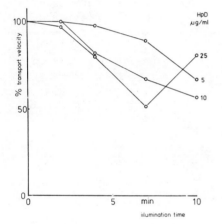

Fig. 5. Photosensitivity of the 2-DOG uptake system of L929 cells.

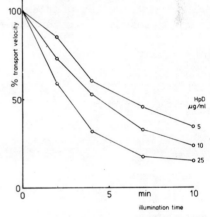

Fig. 6. Inhibition of 2-aminoiso-butyric acid uptake by photodynamic treatment of L929 cells with HpD.

DNA damage has been studied with the alkaline elution technique. Some of the results are shown in fig. 8. Fig. 9 is a summary of all results. Incubation with 10 µg HpD/ml, where already membrane damage has taken place at short illumination times only causes DNA damage at longer times.

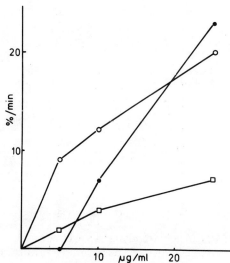

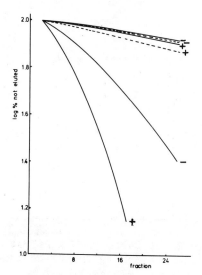

Fig. 7. Comparison of the inhibition of some transport
systems of the L929 cell
membrane by photodynamic
treatment with HpD. □-□:
2-DOG, ●-●: Rb+ and o-o:
AIB transport

Fig. 8. Alkaline elution of DNA
of L929 cells sorbed to
filters fter incubation
with 10 µg/ml of HpD and
illumination. —— (top)
controls with (+) and
without (-) proteinase
K treatment, --- after
30 min of illumination
and after 2 hr of illu-
mation (—— bottom)

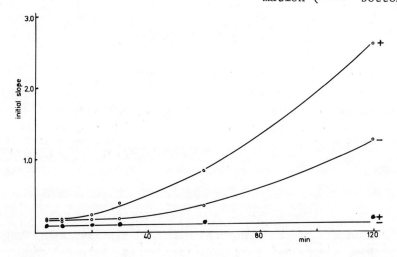

Fig. 9. Initial slopes of the alkaline elution profiles after illumination of L929 cells containing HpD.
●-● controls; +: with and -: without proteinase K treatment.

DISCUSSION

    Cell inactivation is often thought to be caused by membrane damage rather than by other possible mechanisms [5,10,11]. Key membrane functions include transport systems like the ones described here. These studies have been performed after incubation with three different HpD concentrations: 5, 10 and 25 μg/ml. At 5 and 10 μg/ml and subsequent illumination up to 10 min no K^+ leakage and no change in passive Rb^+ uptake could be observed. This means that the membrane barrier is still intact. Carrier mediated passive 2-DOG transport is already inhibited by the photodynamic action of HpD at these concentrations. 2-DOG is readily phosphorylated inside the cells; therefore hexokinase activity was determined. This activity is not inhibited at the lower concentrations, so the transport inhibition is a real effect on the transport system. The decrease of hexokinase activity, which is a cytoplasmic function, closely follows K^+ leakage, thus declines after the membrane barrier has been broken down. These observations are in agreement with previous studies of erythrocyte membrane transport. It was shown that carrier mediated transport of leucine, sulfate and glycerol was inhibited by photodynamic action, whereas passive permeability of glycerol and urea were increased [22] as it is the case with cation permeability [23].

    Two systems were included in this study that require energy: the active Rb^+ uptake, which is correlated with the Na-K ATPase and the 2-aminoisobutyric acid uptake. Both are readily inactivated by photodynamic action of HpD, although Rb^+ uptake inactivation requires a threshold concentration. It has been shown that mitochondria are easily damaged by photodynamic action [24]. This might explain the rather progressive damage of these transport systems, although of course damage of the protein carriers is also very likely. Together with some membrane functions, we have also studied the photodynamic effect on the DNA of these cells. In model experiments it was shown previously that covalent coupling of guanosine and derivatives to proteins takes place [16]. Alkaline elution of cell DNA sorbed to a filter proved to be a valuable technique to study cell DNA damage, whereby protein, eventually crosslinked to DNA is hydrolyzed by proteinase K. The results showed clearly strandbreak formation and protein-DNA crosslinking, because the elution profile with and without proteinase K treatment is different.

    It is clear from these studies that the energy dependent transport systems are most sensitive to photodynamic attack, followed by the carrier-mediated DOG transport, whereas in our experimental set-up DNA is least sensitive. This does not necessarily mean that cell inactivation is caused by the breakdown of the active permeability systems. Even one hit at a guanosine might be lethal and it is impossible to detect even a very limited guanosine oxidation with the kind of experiments described in this study.

REFERENCES

1. T.J. Dougherty, Photoradiation therapy for bronchogenic cancer, Chest 81:265 (1982).

2. I.J. Forbes, P.A. Cowled and A.S.Y Leong, Phototherapy of human tumours using haematoporphyrin derivative, Med.J.Austr. 2:489 (1980).

3. T. Dougherty, D. Boyle, K. Weishaupt, C. Gomer, D. Borcicky, J. Kaufman, A. ʰoldfarb and G. Grindey, Phototherapy of human tumors, in: "Research in Photobiology", A. Castellani, ed., Plenum Publishing Corp., New York (1977).

4. J.D. Spikes, Porphyrins and related compounds as photodynamic sensitizers, Ann.N.Y.Acad.Sci., 244:496 (1975).

5. D. Kessel, Effects of photoactivated porphyrins at the cell surface of leukemia L1210 cells, Biochemistry 16:3443 (1977).

6. K. Kohn and D. Kessel, On the mode of cytotoxic action of photoactivated porphyrins, Biochem.Pharmacol. 28:2465 (1979).

7. D. Kessel, Transport and binding of hematoporphyrin derivative and related porphyrins by murine leukemia L1210 cells, Cancer Res. 41:1318 (1981).

8. A.W. Girotti, Protoporphyrin-sensitized photodamage in isolated membranes of human erythrocytes, Biochemistry 18:4403 (1979).

9. T.M.A.R. Dubbelman, A.F.P.M. de Goeij and J. van Steveninck, Protoporphyrin sensitized photodynamic modification of proteins in isolated human red blood cell membranes, Photochem.Photobiol. 28:197 (1978).

10. J. Moan, E.O. Pettersen and T. Christensen, The mechanism of photodynamic inactivation of human cells in vitro in the presence of hematoporphyrin, Br.J.Cancer 39:398 (1979).

11. J. Moan and T. Christusen, Photodynamic effects on human cells exposed to light in the presence of hematoporphyrin. Localization of the active dye, Cancer letters 11:209 (1981).

12. R.J. Fiel, N. Datta-Gupta, E.H. Mark and J.C. Howard, Induction of DNA damage by porphyrin photosensitizers, Cancer Res. 41:3543 (1981).

13. C.J. Gomer, DNA damage and repair in CHO cells following hematoporphyrin photoradiation, Cancer letters 11:161 (1980).

14. B. Gutter, W.T. Speck and H.S. Rosenkranz, The photodynamic modification of DNA by hematoporphyrin, Biochim.Biophys.Acta 475:307 (1977).

15. D.A. Musser, N. Datta-Gupta and R.J. Fiel, Inhibition of DNA dependent RNA synthesis by porphyrin photosensitizers, Biochem. Biophys.Res.Commun. 97:918 (1980).

16. T.M.A.R. Dubbelman, A.L. van Steveninck and J. van Steveninck, Hematoporphyrin-induced photo-oxidation and photodynamic crosslinking of nucleic acids and their constituents, Biochim. Biophys.Acta 719:47 (1982).

17. B.R. Munson, Photodynamic inactivation of mammalian DNA dependent RNA polymerase by hematoporphyrin and visible light, Int. J.Biochem. 10:957 (1979).

18. J.P.Bader, T. Okazaki and N.R. Brown, Sodium and rubidium uptake in cells transformed by Rous sarcoma virus, J.Cell. Physiol. 106:235 (1981).
19. H.U. Bergmeyer, K. Gawehn and M. Grassl, Hexokinase, in: "Methods of enzymatic analysis", H.U. Bergmeyer, ed., Acad.Press Inc., New York (1974).
20. K.W. Kohn, L.C. Erickson, R.A.G. Ewig and C.A. Friedman, Fractionation of DNA from mammalian cells by alkaline elution, Biochemistry 21:4629 (1976).
21. P.G.W. Plagemann and D.P. Richey, Transport of nucleosides, nucleic acid bases, choline and glucose by animal cells in culture, Biochim.Biophys.Acta 344:263 (1974).
22. T.M.A.R. Dubbelman, A.F.P.M. de Goeij and J. van Steveninck, Protoporphyrin-induced photodynamic effects on transport processes across the membrane of human erythrocytes, Biochim. Biophys.Acta 595:133 (1980).
23. A.A. Schothorst, J. van Steveninck, L.N. Went and D. Suurmond, Protoporphyrin-induced photohemolysis in protoporphyria and in normal red blood cells. Clin.Chim.Acta 28:41 (1979).
24. S. Sandberg, Protoporphyrin-induced photodamage to mitochondria and lysosomes from rat liver, Clin.Chim.Acta 111:55 (1981).

BACTERIAL AND YEAST CELLS AS MODELS FOR STUDYING HEMATOPORPHYRIN PHOTOSENSITIZATION

G. Bertoloni, M. Dall'Acqua, M. Vazzoler, B. Salvato* and G. Jori*

Istituto di Microbiologia and *Istituto di Biologia Animale, Università di Padova, Italy

The photodynamic action of porphyrins has been mainly studied with eucaryotic cells or cells in a multicellular organism[1-3]. These cells represent a complex experimental model owing to the variety of potential binding sites for the sensitizing dyes; in the case of porphyrins, the precise subcellular location is still largely unknown, although it appears to depend on the porphyrin dose and the incubation time[4]. As a consequence, the main cellular targets involved in the photoprocess have not been identified as yet. For these reasons we are studying the photodynamic action of hematoporphyrin (HP) using bacteria and yeast cells[5]. Procaryotic cells were chosen for their simple structural organization and absence of endomembrane systems; moreover, they represent easily reproducible experimental models. Our investigations have been carried out on several strains for each species of microorganism (see table 1) in order to detect whether the effect of the photoprocess is typical of the strain or the species. Moreover, the use of cells with different organization and chemical composition of the cell wall allows one to investigate the interaction of porphyrins with various compounds (lipopolysac= carides, peptidoglycans, teichoic acids, etc.), thus hopefully increasing the present knowledge on the relationships between cell porphyrin binding sites and porphyrin-induced cell photodamage.

MATERIALS AND METHODS

The bacterial and yeast strains used in the present investigation (table 1) were grown in brain heart infusion broth and treated as described elsewhere[6]. The final cell suspensions in phosphate-buffered saline at pH 7.2 had A = 0.87 at 650 nm. The cell suspensions were air-equilibrated and maintained at either 18 °C or 37 °C by thermostated water. The irradiated systems were prepared by adding

Table 1. Bacterial and yeast strains investigated.

Type	Species	Strains
Gram-negative bacteria	Escherichia coli	PD O4 ATCC 23804 K12 CA265
	Klebsiella pneumoniae	NG2RI PD 4 PD 8
Gram-positive bacteria	Staphylococcus aureus	ATTCC 65389 PD 2 PD 4 6846/A
	Streptococcus faecalis	ATTCC 9790 PD 7 SS191 PD 9
Yeasts	Candïda albicans	PD 6 CDC O
	Candida guilliermondii	CDC O
	Candida krusei	CDC O
	Candida pseudotropicalis	CDC O
	Candida lipolytica	CDC O

ATTC - American Type Culture Collection
CDC - Center for Disease Control, Atlanta (Georgia)
PD - wild-type strain from the Istituto di Microbiologia, Padova
      (Italy)

a suitable volume of HP solution to the cell suspensions so that
the final dye concentration was in the 0.001-1 mg/ml range, as
estimated spectrophotometrically using an extirction coefficient
of $7.88 \cdot 10^3$ M^{-1} cm^{-1} at 400 nm^3. The irradiation apparatus[3] involved
four 250 W tungsten bulbs emitting white light: under these condi-
tions, cells were unaffected by 30 min.-illumination in the absence
of added HP. Typically, the strains were dark-incubated with HP at
20 °C, and then subjected to visible light-irradiation for variable
periods up to 30 min. The dark- and light-sensitivity of Streptococcus
faecalis to HP was investigated using the following lower and upper
limit values for the various parameters: HP dose 0.1-1 g/ml;
dark incubation time of cells and HP 6-30 min.; irradiation time
2-10 min.; irradiation temperature 18°-37 °C. At predetermined
times, aliquots of the dark-incubated or irradiated cell suspensions
were taken for analysis of the cell-bound HP concentration by a
spectrophotofluorimetric procedure[4] and/or cell viability by colony
counting at 24 h after incubation of plated samples at 37 °C[5].

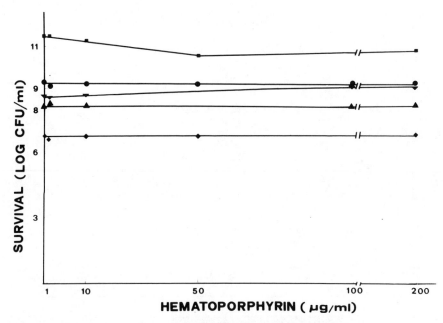

Fig. 1. Effect of various HP concentrations on the survival of typical bacterial and yeast strains in the dark. An identical behavior was observed for all other strains listed in table 1.

The determination of the specific accumulation of HP on the cytoplasmic membrane and the procedure for electron microscopy studies have been detailed previously[6].

RESULTS

All strains listed in table 1 are unaffected by dark incubation with HP doses up to 0.2 mg/ml (Fig. 1). The amount of cellbound HP is estimated to be in the order of 10^{-18} moles per cell by quantitative spectrophotofluorimetric analysis. Essentially all cell-bound HP is located in the cytoplasmic membrane, at least up to a dose of about 7 μg/ml. The Gram-negative bacteria examined by us, i.e. E. Coli and K. pneumoniae, are insensitive to visible light irradiation after dark-incubation for 30 min. with HP even if the cells have been pretreated with EDTA. On the contrary,Grampositive bacteria and yeasts are highly photosensitive to the treatment with HP and visible light (Fig. 2). The maximal photosensitivity is displayed by Str. faecalis in the logarithmic phase of growth: this bacterium undergoes 99.9 % killing when irradiated for 30 min.

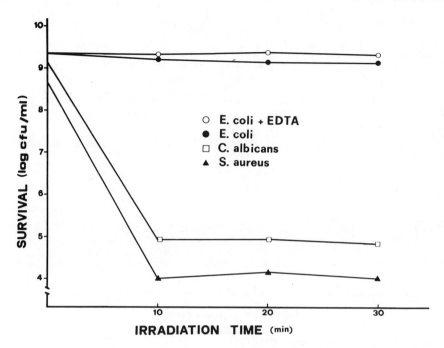

Fig. 2.   Time dependence of cell survival upon visible light-irra=
           diation of aqueous suspensions of S. aureus, C. albicans,
           E. coli, and E. coli + 5 mM EDTA, in the presence of 0.2 mg/ml
           HP. All irradiations were performed at 18°C after 60 min.-
           incubation of cells and HP in the dark at room temperature.

        Kinetic studies point out that, at 0.1 μg/ml HP, Str. faecalis
is photoinactivated by a monophasic process whereas, at 1 μg/ml
HP, cell death follows a biphasic trend (Fig. 3). The fluorescence
intensity of cell-bound HP decreases as a function of the irradiation time, owing to a change in the microenvironment of the porphyrin in the photodamaged cells.

        The cells of Str. faecalis exhibit no detectable ultrastructu-
ral modification when exposed to visible light in the absence of HP
(Fig. 4). On the other hand, some 5-10 % cells incubated with HP
(1 μg/ml) for 16 min. in the dark appear to be elongated with
either incomplete or complete septa. More drastic changes (70-80 %
cells) are obserwed after HP-light treatment for 10 min.: the formation of septa is inhibited, and mesosomes are visible at the level
of incomplete septa (Fig. 5).

DISCUSSION

        The results presented in this paper demonstrate that HP binds

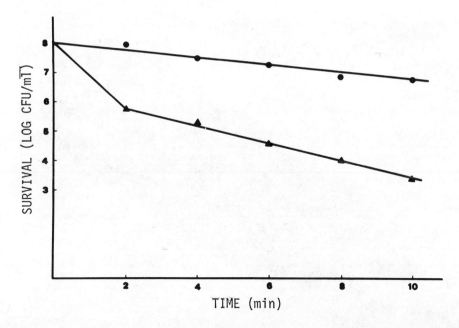

Fig. 3. Time dependence of cell survival upon visible light-irra-
         diation of aqueous suspensions of <u>Str. faecalis</u> in the pre-
         sence of 0.1 µg/ml ● and 1 µg/ml ▲ HP. The irradiations
         were performed at 18°C after 6 min.-incubation of cells and
         HP in the dark at room temperature.

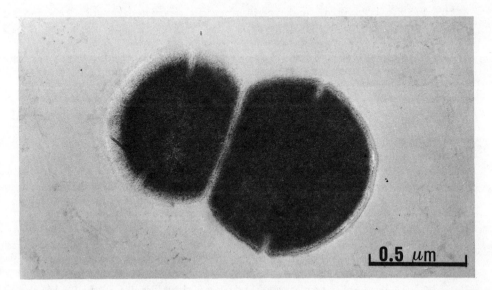

Fig. 4. Electron micrograph of <u>S. Faecalis</u> (10 min-irradiated, no HP)

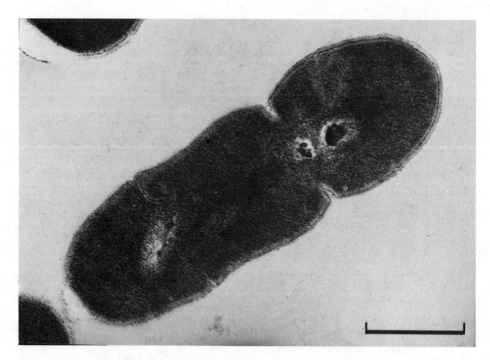

Fig. 5.   Electron micrograph of Str. faecalis cell treated with HP
          (1 µg/ml) and exposed to light (10 min.). Bar marker rep-
          resents 0.5 µm.

with all the bacterial and yeast strains examined by us. In general,
the porphyrin appears to interact with membrane sites, as suggested
by cell fractionation and electron microscopy studies. However,
this process causes no detectable cytotoxicity, at least within the
intervals of HP dose investigated. On the other hand, exposure to
visible light of the bacterial and yeast cells associated with HP
induces different types of responses, depending on the specie. The
largest photosensitivity is displayed by yeast and Gram-positive
bacterial strains, whereas Gram-negative bacteria appear to be
photochemically inert even EDTA if is added to the reaction medium
prior to irradiation.

     Therefore, the efficiency of the HP-photosensitized cell damage
appears to be critically related with the structure of the substrate.
The latter parameter may modulate the interaction of the photogenerated reactive intermediates with the potentially photolabile cell
targets, especially those present in the cytoplasmic membrane. This
hypothesis is further supported by the differences in photosensitivity observed for various Gram-positive bacteria. In conclusion,
the studies hitherto performed indicate that binding of HP to the
cell is not sufficient to ensure efficient photosensitized cell

killing. At present, we are pursuing our attempts to elucidate which factors further control the course of the photoprocess.

REFERENCES

1. T. J. Dougherty, E. Thoma, D. G. Boyle, and K. R. Weishaupt, Interstitial photoradiation therapy for primary solid tumors in pet cats and dogs, Cancer Res. 41:401 (1981)
2. T. Moan, E. O. Pettersen, and T. Christensen, The mechanism of photodynamic inactivation of human cells in vitro in the presence of hematoporphyrin, Br. J. Cancer 39:398 (1979)
3. E. Reddi, E. Rossi, and G. Jori, Factors controlling the efficiency of porphyrins as photosensitizers of biological systems to damage by visible light, Med. Biol. Environ. 9:357 (1981)
4. I. Cozzani, G. Jori, E. Reddi, A. Fortunato, L. Tomio, and P. L. Zorat, Distribution of endogenous and injected porphyrins at the subcellular level in rat hepatocytes and in ascites hepatoma, Chem. Biol. Interactions 37:67 (1981)
5. G. Bertoloni, M. Dall'Acqua, M. Vazzoler, B. Salvato, and G. Jori, Photosensitizing action of hematoporphyrin on some bacterial strains, Med. Biol. Environ. 10:238 (1982)
6. G. Bertoloni, B. Salvato, M. Dall'Acqua, M. Vazzoler, and G. Jori, Hematoporphyrin-sensitized photoinactivation of Streptococcus faecalis, Photochem. Photobiol., in press.

CHOLESTEROL IMPREGNATION INTO ERYTHROLEUKEMIA CELL MEMBRANE

INDUCES RESISTANCE TO HEMATOPORPHYRIN PHOTODYNAMIC EFFECT

Zvi Malik, Flavio Lejbkowicz, and Samuel Salzberg

Department of Life Sciences
Bar-Ilan University
Ramat-Gan, 52100 Israel

SUMMARY

Specific damage to the membrane of Friend erythroleukemic cells was the result of the hematoporphyrin derivative (HPD) photodynamic effect as analysed by scanning electron microscopy (SEM). Appearance of limited area of tiny holes in the outer membrane was followed by vesicular formation and complete decomposition of the membrane, while bare nucleus remained undamaged. In addition, a decrease in cell number as a function of HPD concentration used, as well as a reduction in protein synthesis, were detected in HPD-treated Friend cells. Furthermore, a parallel inhibition of virus release from these cells was also observed, as determined by the reverse transcriptase assay. Preincubation of the erythroleukemic cells with cholesterol hemisuccinate induced almost complete resistance to the HPD photodynamic damage and protein synthesis rate remained similar to control unsensitized cells.

INTRODUCTION

Cholesterol deficiency in the surface membrane of leukemic cells has been shown to be an important membranal feature in the development of leukemia.[1] Cholesterol deficiency stimulated a marked increase in the fluidity of the cell membrane.[2] On the other hand, human leukemic lymphocytes and other experimental leukemic cell lines were shown to bind protoporphyrin and by exposure to light were destroyed.[3] This photodynamic effect, expressed by cell lysis, was similar to that observed with red blood cells from erythropoietic protoporphyria patients.[4]

185

Normal reticulocytes treated with photoactivated protoporphyrin showed reduced (Na$^+$-K$^+$) ATPase activity, inhibition of ^{55}Fe incorporation by mitochondria, decreased globin synthesis,[5,6] and induced crosslinking of proteins[7] leading to a sponge-like appearance of the cell, with tiny holes and hemoglobin precipitates bound to the membrane.[5,6]

Friend leukemia cells (FLC) are of erythroid origin and are chronically infected with the Friend complex of murine leukemia virus (F-MLV).[8,9] It is clear now that at least two separate viruses are involved in these diseases. One is a replication defective spleen focus-forming virus, while the other is a replication competent helper virus.[10] It was, thus, important to study the photodynamic process of hematoporphyrin as expressed on both the growth-rate of FLC and the release of F-MLV from these cells. In addition, the effect of cholesterol incorporation into FLC on the same photodynamic process was also examined.

MATERIALS AND METHODS

Erythroleukemic cells: Friend erythroleukemic cells (FLC), line 745, of murine origin[11] were grown in Dulbecco's modified Eagle medium (DMEM, Gibco) supplemented with 10% fetal calf serum (FCS, Gibco). For determination of cell number, cells were harvested by low speed centrifugation (1500 rpm for 5 min), resuspended in DMEM and counted after staining with 0.3% trypan blue.

Photodynamic sensitization: Hematoporphyrin (Sigma) was esterified to hematoporphyrin derivate (HPD) by the method described by Dougherty.[12] Cells were washed from culture medium with phosphate buffered saline, containing 1% glucose (PBS). HPD (1mg/ml) was added to FLC suspended in PBS to the indicated final concentration. The cells were illuminated with a white tungsten light source (light intensity 4×10^{19} quanta/m^2/s) for the required times, as indicated in each experiment.

Determination of protein synthesizing capacity: FLC exposed to HPD and light for an indicated time, were washed in the dark with PBS, resuspended in PBS containing 10uCi ^{14}C-leucine (Amersham), then incubated for 10 min at 37°C. At the end of incubation time the cells were washed with PBS, precipitated with 10% TCA, filtered on glass fiber discs, samples were dried, toluene scintillation cocktail added and radioactivity was counted by a Kontron counter.

Reverse transcriptase (RT) assay: Friend cells were exposed to HPD and light for 10 min, sedimented, washed and resuspended in DMEM supplemented with 10% FCS for 24 hr. Viable cells were counted and removed by low speed centrifugation. The growth medium was collected, placed in ice and assayed for RT activity, as described by Aboud et al.[13]

Cholesterol enrichment medium: The FLC membrane was rigidified by incorporation of cholesterol hemisuccinate (CHS) into the lipid layer by the method of Shinitzky et al.[14] Briefly, cells were incubated for enrichment with CHS in medium containing 0.01mg/ml CHS 3.5% polyvinyl pyrrolidone (PVP), 1% bovine serum, and 0.5% glucose. Control cells were incubated in PVP medium without CHS. Chemicals were obtained from Sigma.

Electron microscopy: At the required period of time, the cells were collected and washed once with PBS and fixed in 1% glutaraldehyde in Na^+-K^+ phosphate buffer, pH 7.4. For SEM the fixed cells were sedimented on poly-L-lysine-coated glass coverslips and dehydrated with graded alcohol and Freon. After critical point drying, the cells were coated with gold and examined by a JSM-35 scanning electron microscope. Five hundred cells were examined and classified in each sample and the mean of each morphological phenomenon was calculated.

RESULTS

Ultrastructural Characterization of Cellular Damage Induced by HPD

Figs. 1-4 depict the time-dependent process of erythroleukemic cell destruction induced by photoactivated HPD. Figs. 1,2, show a

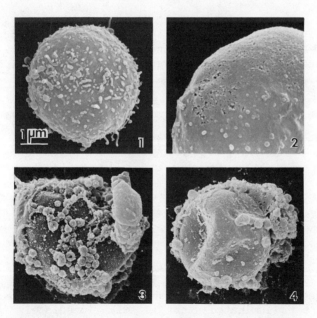

Figs. 1-4: The photodynamic damage to FLC analyzed by SEM. 1 - control cell. 2, 3, 4 - 5-, 15- and 30-min HPD-treated cells (20 µg/ml), respectively. Bar = 1µ.

control cell at time 0 of experiment in comparison to 5 min HPD sensitized cell demonstrating a limited area of tiny pits in the membrane. Fig. 3 shows formation of small vesicular blebs from outer membrane, whereas the inner nuclear envelope appears unaffected (15-min exposure). Fig. 4 demonstrates almost bare nucleus surrounded by remnant of cytoplasmic membrane after 30 min of HPD sensitization.

Effect of HPD on Cell Growth and F-MLV Release

In order to clarify whether HPD exerts a specific effect on F-MLV release from FLC, the cells were treated with different concentrations of HPD, followed by light activation for 10 min. After 24 hr, the number of viable cells was determined and RT activity was measured in the culture medium. As illustrated in Fig. 5, a parallel decrease was observed both in cell number and RT activity as a function of HPD concentration used. Fig. 6 presents the ratio between RT activity and cell number obtained at each concentration. It is obvious that this ratio remains constant indicating that there is no specific inhibitory effect of HPD on the release of F-MLV. A similar result was obtained when the amount of cells was determined by [3H] leucine incorporation in addition to cell number determinations (data not shown).

Induction of Resistance to the HPD Effect by Cholesterol Impregnation

Friend erythroleukemic cells were exposed to photoactivated HPD (20ug/ml), and at each time interval a sample of cells were tested for protein synthesizing capacity for additional 10 min of

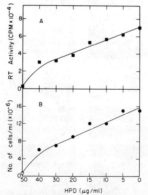

Fig. 5: Effect of HPD on FLC viability and virus release. The cultures were illuminated for 10 min immediately following addition of HPD to Friend cells and further incubated for 24 hr. Viable cell number and RT activity in the culture medium were then determined.

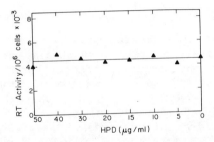

Fig. 6: Ratio between RT activity and cell number. This ratio was obtained from the results presented in Fig. 5.

incubation in the dark. After 30 min, the HPD-treated cells retained only 7.4% of their protein synthesizing capacity while control cells unsensitized by HPD retained 78.5% of their capacity (Table 1). Resistance to photodynamic damage of the leukemic cells was induced by 90 min preincubation in PVP medium containing cholestrol hemisuccinanate (CHS). The CHS pretreatment protected the cells from the HPD photodynamic effect and the cells retained 68% of their protein synthesizing capacity, while control cells preincubated only in PVP were markedly affected by HPD and remained with only 17% of their protein synthesis activity.

More than 80% of CHS pretreated cells were shown to be undamaged after the preincubation period and after exposure to HPD as determined by scanning electron microscopy.

TABLE 1. Protein synthesizing capacity of HPD- and CHS-treated cells

	^{14}C-leucine incorporation cpm/10^6 cells/10 min					% residual capacity
Illumination time:	0	5	10	20	30	
a. Control	7900	7900	7300	6500	6200	78.5
b. HPD	6800	4150	2400	1100	500	7.4
c. PVP-HPD	6400	5000	4100	1900	1100	17.2
d. PVP-HPD CHS	3600	3300	3050	2650	2450	68.1

Cells were preincubated for 90 min in PBS (a,b) or in polyvinyl pyrrolidone medium (c) or in PVP enriched with cholesterol (CHS, d). After cells were exposed to photoactivated HPD (20µg/ml), protein synthesis was measured for 10 min in the dark, with ^{14}C-leucine.

DISCUSSION

The present results indicate that the outer membrane of Friend erythroleukemic cells and protein synthesis activity was heavily damaged by the HPD photodynamic effect. Furthermore, a parallel inhibitory effect of HPD on the release of F-MLV from the cells was also observed. However, it appears that this effect was not due to a specific block of virus release, since, as clearly demonstrated in Fig. 6, the ratio between RT activity detected in the culture medium of HPD-treated cells and the number of cells at each HPD concentration used remained constant. It is, therefore, obvious that the inhibition of virus release is a direct result of the damage induced in FLC following HPD treatment. Cholesterol incorporation into the leukemic membrane reduced the basal protein synthesis rate as determined by ^{14}C-leucine incorporation, while ultrastructurally the cells preserved the undamaged morphology. By HPD treatment the CHS enriched cells retained their protein synthesizing capacity to the same rate as FLC untreated cells. Cholesterol deficiency of leukemic cells was described to be an accompanying phenomenon of malignant transformation.[1] On the basis of the present results, it is conceivable that cholesterol content may contribute to the tumor-localizing potential of porphyrins, while failure of porphyrins to bind specifically could be a consequence of cholesterol normal metabolism in the tumor-bearing animal.

The membrane and metabolic activity of FLC was affected by HPD similar to that observed previously in reticulocytes.[6] In both cases, membrane damage was produced, possibly as a result of a similar mechanism of cross-linking of membranal proteins[7] leading to hole-formation and decomposition of the membrane.[5] The resistance of nuclear envelope to HPD photosensitization examined by SEM is of particular interest; it is in good agreement with the lack of porphyrin fluorescence observed in the nucleus of FLC, whereas fluorescence was observed only as patches in the outer membrane.[3]

ACKNOWLEDGEMENT: We wish to thank Mrs. Bluma Lederhendler for assistance in editing and for typing this manuscript.

REFERENCES

1. M. Inbar and M. Shinitzky, Cholesterol as a bioregulator in the development and inhibition of leukemia. Proc. Natl. Acad. Sci. USA 71:4229 (1974).
2. H. Ben-Bassat, A. Poliak, S.M. Rosenbaum, E. Naparstek, D. Shouval and M. Inbar, Fluidity of membrane lipids and lateral mobility of Con A receptors in the cell surface of normal lymphocytes and lymphocytes from patients with malignant lymphomas and leukemias. Cancer Res. 37:1307 (1977).

3. Z. Malik and M. Djaldetti, Destruction of erythroleukemia, myelocytic leukemia and Burkitt lymphoma cells by photo-activated protoporphyrin. Int. J. Cancer 26:495 (1980).

4. A.A. Schothorst, J.V. Steveninck, L.N. Went and D. Suurmond, Metabolic aspects of the photodynamic effect of protopor-phyrin in protoporphyrin and in normal red blood cells. Clin. Chim. Acta 33:207 (1971).

5. Z. Malik and H. Breitbart, Cross-linking of hemoglobin and inhibition of globin synthesis in reticulocytes induced by photoactivated protoporphyrin. Acta Haemat. 64:304 (1980).

6. H. Breitbart and Z. Malik, The effects of photoactivated protoporphyrin on reticulocyte membranes into cellular activities and hemoglobin precipitation photochemistry and photobiology. Photochem. Photobiol. 35:365 (1982).

7. T.M.A.R. Dubbelman, A.F.P.M. de Goeig and J. Van Steveninck, Protoporphyrin induced photodynamic effects on transport processes across the membrane of human erythrocytes. Biochim. Biophys. Acta 595:133 (1980).

8. C. Friend, M.C. Patuleia and E. De Harven, Erythrocytic maturation in vitro of murine Friend virus-induced leukemic cells. Natl. Cancer Inst. Monog. 22:505 (1966).

9. C. Friend and G.B. Rosi, Transplantation immunity and the suppression of spleen colony formation by immunization with murine leukemia virus preparations. Internat. J. Cancer 3:523 (1968).

10. P.A. Marks and R.A. Rifkind, Erythroleukemic differentia-tion. Ann. Rev. Biochem. 47:419 (1978).

11. Z. Malik and Y. Langzam, Cell membrane maturation of Friend erythroleukemic cells and tocopherol-dependent erythro-poietin effect: A scanning electron microscopy study. Cell Differ. 11:161 (1982).

12. T.J. Dougherty, J.E. Kaufman, A. Goldfarb, K.R., Weishaupt, D. Boyle, D. and A. Mittelman, Photoradiation therapy for the treatment of malignant tumors. Cancer Res. 38:2628 (1978).

13. M. Aboud, O. Weiss and S. Salzberg, Rapid quantitation of interferon with chronically oncornavirus-producing cells. Infec. Immun. 13:1626 (1976).

14. M. Shinitzsky, Y. Skornik and N. Haram-Ghera, Effective tumor immunization induced by cells of elevated membrane-lipid microviscosity. Proc. Natl. Acad. Sci. USA 76: 5313 (1979).

PHOTODYNAMIC EFFECT OF THE HE-NE LASER WITH HpD ON THE ULTRASTRUCTURE OF RHABDOMYOSARCOMA CELL

Chen Ting-I   and Guo Zhong-he[*]

Institute of Radiation Medicine, Academy of Military
Medical Science, Beijing, China

[*]The Chinese PLA General Hospital, Beijing, China

INTRODUCTION

Photodynamic effect of Hematoporphyrin Derivative (HpD) on malignant cells has been widely studied; cells which have taken up HpD are killed "in vitro" or "in vivo", when the compound is activated by light. The light excitation of HpD produces singlet oxygen which, by its strong oxidizing power, breaks down the structure and alters the biological function of major biomolecules, including proteins, nucleic acids, cholesterol, fibrinogen, and various kind of enzymes etc. [1,2]. As all of these are the essential materials in the structure and function of the cell, photodynamic action of this kind may induce extensive damage or alteration in the ultrastructure of cells. It has been reported that photodynamic action dissolves the cell membrane, oxidizes phospholipid and cholesterol, causes damage of enzymes in membrane transferring system, inhibits Ca^{++} transportation of Chinese hamster ovarian cells [3], depresses oxidative phosphorylation in mitochondria as well as oxygen consumption [4], breaks down on DNA chain [5], and kills the tumor cells [6] especially those at G_1-S stage of the cell cycle [7]. The singlet oxygen action causes wide-spread damage of the cell which can be revealed easily by observing the ultrastructure under electron microscopy. Coppola [8] reported that mitocontria may be more sensitive to light and HpD, and therefore become the first organelles to be affected. We have observed the photodynamic action on tumor cells. The results are presented in the following.

193

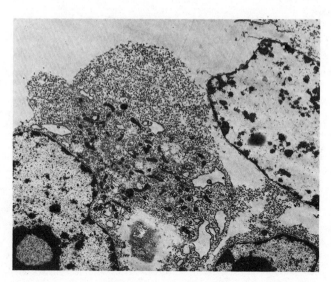

Fig. 1.   Cells in same field show various degree severity of lesion
          as shown by the different changes of the liable organelles
          in different cells.   x 4,000.

MATERIALS AND METHODS

The PLA-802[#] Rhabdomyosarcoma cells of human larynx (Alveolar
type) were cultured in $RPMI_{10}$ 1640 medium for 24 hours. HpD was
added to the medium at a concentration of 10^{-5} M and kept in the dark
for 20 minutes. The cells were irradiated inside the flask by an
He-Ne laser with the power density 10 mW/cm^2 for 20 minutes.

The cells were harvested from the flask, centrifuged, then fixed, embedded in EPON-812, and prepared for ultrathin section with
LKB microtome. After staining with lead and uranium, the preparations were observed under JEM-6c electron microscope[*].

RESULTS

Photodynamic action of the He-Ne laser and HpD induced various
and extensive changes in ultrastructure of PLA-802 cell. In the
electron-microscope observation field, one might disclose cells damaged at various degrees as shown by the structure changes in differ-

[#]Cells are provided by Department of Pathology of The Chinese PLA
General Hospital.

[*]The EM sections were prepared by Xiao Lou, and Zhan Si-min.

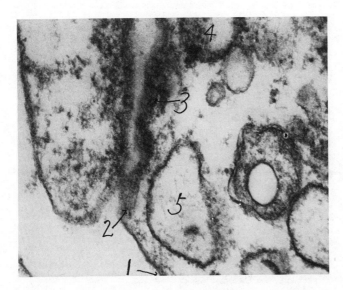

Fig. 2.   Membrane damage. 1. Plasma membrane with trilaminar ap-
          pearance blurred. 2. Desmosome membrane blurred. 3. Fila-
          ment fainted. 4. Mitochondrion with degradated materials.
          5. Dilated E R.   x 273,000.

ent cells (Fig. 1). As a result of receiving different quantities
of illumination from the light spot, a variety of cellular lesions
were produced. Such lesions were especially prominent in cells at
certain stages of the cell cycle. This is probably the reason why
the tumour cells react to light and HpD in different liability to
photodynamic treatment. The following stated facts are not proposed to describe the event of different sensitivities of cellular
organelles, but give a bird's eye view about the essential changes
in the ultrastructure of tumor cells.

Cell Membrane

     Plasma membrane lost its trilaminar appearance, became blurred.
The membrane material spread off and lost the characteristic structure of normal membrane. In desmosome, the microfilaments were
blurred and faint, no dense intercellular plate could be seen. In
the degenerated membrane the normal constituents were no more conspicuous (Fig. 2).

Nucleus

     Electron microscopy showed that in the majority of the treat-
ed tumour cells, chromatin appeared as coarse granules (Figs. 3,4)
as the dense heterochromatin with inactive DNA in normal cells[9]; in

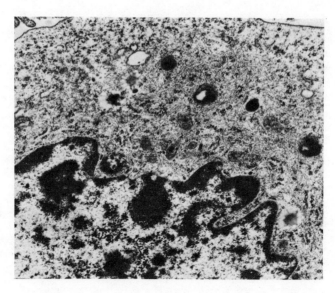

Fig. 3.   Tumor cell damage. 1. Nucleolus near N M, connected with
          heterochromatin. 2. Coarse granules of chromatin. 3. Chro-
          matin part fartly homogenus in appearance. 4. Secondary
          lysosome. 5. Brownish lipid droplets. 6. Microtubule zone.
          7. Mitochondrion. x 15,000.

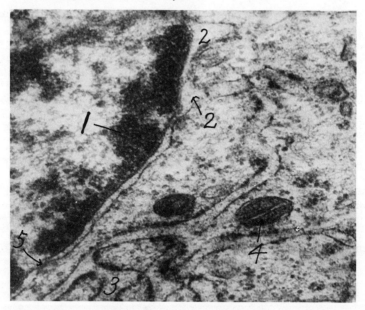

Fig. 4.   Tumor cell damage. 1. Coarse granular chromatin. 2. Sac
          formation of bulging N M, 3. Dilated R E R with rich ribo-
          some. 4. Mitochondrion. 5. Nuclear pore. x 255,000.

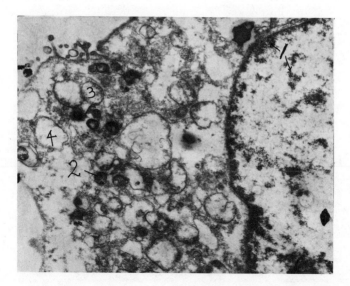

Fig. 5. Severely damaged cell. 1. Coarse granular chromatin. 2.
         Lysosome increased. 3. Degenerated mitochondrion. 4. Damag-
         ed cell membrane. 5. Dilated S E R. x 30,000.

some other nuclei, chromatin was aggregated as chromatin masses of
different sizes(Fig.s 1,3,4,5), while the heterochromatin became
scanty.

     Nuclear membrane looked apparently normal, but the membrane
pore were blurred. The severely damaged nuclear membrane had its
interspace widened, the out-layer might bulge out to form a sac of
about 0.1-0.3 μm in diameter, and communicated with dilated endoplasmic reticulum (Fig. 4).

Mitochondrion

     The early lesions of mitochondria manifested widening of cris-
tae, on which they appeared as opaque areas and circumscribed gra-
ular particles. The inter-cristae space was unevenly distended and
no cristae granules could be seen (Fig. 6).

     The majority of the treated tumor cells were severely damag-
ed; their mitochondria were swellen with very few autolysed or degenerated residues inside.

Other Organelles

     The smooth endoplasmic reticulum was markedly distended. Its
cross-section looked like a sac about 1 μm diameter. Many ribosome

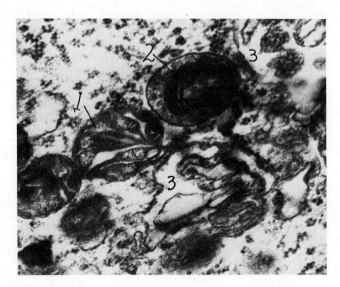

Fig. 6. Early damaged tumor cell. 1. Mitochondrion (see text).
         2. Secondary lysosome with myelin structure. 3. The dilat-
         ed S E R tends to engulf the degenerated structure.
         x 228,000.

granules attached on the surface of the distended rough endoplasmic
reticulum (Fig. 4).

    The amount of lysosome increased while the secondary lysosome
contained a lot of degraded materials. As presented in Fig. 3, a
lysosome contained the myelin structure. The damaged and degenerated organelles were engulfed by the extenting smoot endoplasmic reticulum in which the autophagosome formation was progressing. Area
of microfilament appeared in cytoplasm (Fig. 3).

    Electron lucent droplets and faint opaque droplets could be
seen in the same cell (Fig. 3).

    Finally the damaged cells lost their cytoplasmic and nuclear
contents, and disintegrated into cell debris left behind.

DISCUSSION

    Laser acts on the HpD treated cells generating singlet oxygen
that attacks the biomolecules of the cell leading to extensive
changes of the ultrastructure.

    Cell membrane loses its trilaminar appearance. This is un-
doubtedly favoured by the photodynamic action on phospholipid, protein

and other membrane materials, firstly dissolving the membrane, especially at the site near desmosome.

The chromatin of large number of cells treated with laser and HpD usually changes from homogeneous appearance to coarse granules. This indicates the lowering of the activity of DNA from active to the inert form at early stage of photodynamic action. This may be in accordance with the degree of damage of DNA and that of cells at G_1-S state in the cell cycle. Cell in G_0, or early G_1 stage showed some light change in chromatin in the early lesion. There are cells (Fig. 3) with one nucleolus located near the nuclear membrane, may be at the early stage of cell formation after completion of miotic division, that exhibit less degree of damage.

Variation of electron opacity in a single cristae of lightly damaged mitochondria may reflect the inhibition of oxidative phosphorylation, and the coarse granules circumscribed in the cristae are probably the residues of degradation products of large biomolecules. There are seldom seen in ordinary lesions. The increased autophagosome formation, reticulum may indicate the disturbance of metabolism and the corresponding compensatory processes.

The above results show that the mitochondria damage is particularly severe which might be the main cause of cell death as Coppola [8] pointed out. On the other hand, the nuclear injury is also very important and may be correlated with variation in sensitivity to photodynamic action at different stages of cell cycle. The membrane change is also profound which may bear some relation to the viability of the cell.

Further work is urgently required in order to reveal the exact role of photodynamic action on the tumour cells.

CONCLUSIONS

The photodynamic action of He-Ne laser and HpD causes extensive changes of cell membrane, nucleus, mitochondria etc, which may be roughly interpretated in light of the photodynamic action on the biomolecules. As to what causes the change of ultrastructure of the cell and the cell reactivity is closely correlated with the cell cycle, very little is known at present.

REFERENCES

1. J. D. Spikes, Dye-sensitized photooxidation of protein, Ann. N.Y. Acad. Sci. 171:149 (1970).
2. J. D. Spikes, Porphyrin and related compound as photodynamic sensitizers, Ann. N.Y. Acad. Sci. 496:243 (1975).
3. T. W. Sery, Photodynamic killing of retinoblastoma cell with Hematoporphyrin and light, Cancer Res. 39:96 (1979).

4. D. A. Bellnier, and T. J. Dougherty, Membrane lysis in Chinese hamster ovary cells treated with Hematoporphyrin and light, Photochem. Photobiol. 36:42 (1982).
5. S. Christian, Photodynamic effects of Hematoporphyrin on respiration and calcium uptake in isolated mitochondria, Int. J. Radiat. Biol. 39:227 (1981).
6. J. F. Robert, Induction of DNA damage by porphyrin photosensitizer, Cancer Res. 41:3543 (1981).
7. T. Christensen, Photodynamic inactivation of synchronized human cells in vitro in presence of Hematoporphyrin, Cancer Res. 39:3735 (1979).
8. A. Coppola, Ultrastructural changes in lymphoma cells treated with Hematoporphyrin and light, Am. J. Path. 99:175 (1980).
9. Tao Hong "Ultrastructure in Biology, Medicine and the Electron Microscopy Technology", Sci. Pub. House, China (1980), in Chinese.

Chapter 3

Studies on Experimental and Spontaneous Animal Tumors

HEMATOPORPHYRIN DERIVATIVE PHOTOTHERAPY IN EXPERIMENTAL ONCOLOGY

Gianfranco Canti, Laura Ricci, Paola Franco, Angelo
Nicolin[X], Alessandra Andreoni[¨], Rinaldo Cubeddu[¨]

Dept. of Pharmacology, School of Medicine, Milan, Italy
xI.S.T., Genoa, Italy; ¨Center for Quantum Electronics
Milan, Italy

INTRODUCTION

Photoradiation therapy is currently under investigation as a new form of treatment for solid malignant tumors in human. The method involves photosensitization of drugs and fluorescent dyes, such as Hematoporphyrin[1]. This dye has been shown to accumulate with a certain degree of specificity in tissues with a high mitotic index[2]. Moreover, neoplastic tissue might be identified by the fluorescence emitted from cancerous lesions that have incorporated the dye in larger amounts than normal tissues[3]. The photodynamic action has implicated singlet oxygen (a short-lived excited molecular state of ground-state triplet oxygen) as the effective cytotoxic agent[4].

This property has assumed in recent years therapeutic significance due to its applicability to the treatment of experimental[5] and human tumors[6,7,8,]. Although promising applications in the therapy of superficial metastatic foci of human tumors and bronchial neoplasia[9] have been obtained by a combined treatment with Hpd and light exposure, a number of basic characteristics of Hpd, namely the optimal schedule of treatment, possible interactions with classical antineoplastic agents, toxic effects, biological alterations of normal and neoplastic cells have not yet been studied in detail.

In our laboratory we decided to study the Hpd properties in two different ways:

1. Hpd without light exposure.   2. Hpd and light exposure.
We studied the Hpd effect on immune system and its cytocidal activity
with laser light.

RESULTS AND DISCUSSION

In our laboratory a long lasting, although reversible inhibition of DNA synthesis in Hpd treated leukemic cells, maintained in
the dark, has been observed. (Table 1).
In these experiments, leukemic cells from L1210 murine leukemia
were treated with Hpd at the indicated concentrations for 45' in the
dark.[3]H-thymidine was added 18h before the culture sacrifice.   The
Hpd treatment shows an uptake inhibition of thymidine dose-dependent.
These doses (also twenty times more) were not cytotoxic for the leukemic cells.   The recovery of DNA synthesis is in 72h.   Hpd inhibition of DNA synthesis was also observed, in a different manner, in
normal and PHA stimulated lymphocytes (Table 2).

Table 1. Hpd-inhibition of ^{3}H-thymidine uptake by L1210 cells
pretreated with Hpd in vitro.

Hpd µg/ml	% uptake inhibition
–	0
0.5	7
1	51
2.5	68
5	80
12.5	83
25	92
50	92

L1210 cells, 10^7/ml were treated with Hpd at the indicated concentrations. ^{3}H-thymidine, 0.8µCi/20µl, was added 18h before the culture sacrifice. Hpd was prepared as described[7].

Table 2. Hpd-inhibition of ^{3}H-thymidine uptake by unstimulated and PHA stimulated lymphocytes.

Hpd μg/ml	% uptake inhibition	PHA
-	0	0
0.5	48	51
1	49	77
2.5	41	79
5	59	94
12.5	77	97
25	97	100

10×10^6 C57 spleen cells were incubated for 1h at 37°C with Hpd diluted in HBSS at the indicated concentrations and washed in excess HBSS. 5×10^5 cells suspended in 100 μl conditioned medium were incubated for 48h, with or without PHA, in microculture wells and (^{3}H)-thymidine was added 18h before culture sacrifice.

An almost complete inhibition of thymidine incorporation was obtained in both lymphocyte populations with the highest Hpd dose (25μg/ml). When Hpd concentration was decreased to 12.5, 5 and 2.5 μg/ml, the inhibition of thymidine incorporation is lower in resting lymphocytes than in PHA stimulated cells and this could be confirmation of the Hpd preferential incorporation by large and fast metabolizing cells such as PHA stimulated lymphocytes and neoplastic cells; this preferential incorporation has been exploited to selectively remove upon light exposure blast lymphocytes from resting lymphocytes[10].

Since immunity is important in the control of tumor growth and spreading, we decided to examine the effect of Hpd-treatment on lymphoid cells, evaluated by a number of in vitro assays commonly used to study humoral and cell mediated immunity. One important function of T lymphocytes is the cellular cytotoxicity that can be measured in vitro with the cell mediated cytotoxic assay. Constituents of the cell-mediated cytotoxic assay, namely target cells and effector cells, were pretreated with Hpd and the results of the lytic reaction are reported in Table 3.

Table 3. Effects on the CML of an Hpd treatment of effector
cells or target cells.

Target cells	Effector cells	CPM $\pm$ SE	% Cytotoxicity E/T 100 : 1
L1210	✶ I	1027 $\pm$ 101	40.2
"	I_{H20}	589 $\pm$ 49	0.4
"	I_{H5}	652 $\pm$ 53	6.1
"	I_{H1}	890 $\pm$ 68	27.7
✶✶ $L1210_{H20}$	I	1039 $\pm$ 98	41.3
$L1210_{H5}$	"	1033 $\pm$ 96	40.8
$L1210_{H1}$	"	1049 $\pm$ 96	42.2

✶ C57 lymphocytes immune against L1210 cells treated with Hpd at
   the indicated concentrations.
✶✶ L1210 cells treated with Hpd (μg/ml).

Hpd treated C57 lymphocytes, previously sensitized to L1210
cells did not have any cytotoxic activity on the relevant target
cells. Highly effective cytotoxic cells were completely inhibited
as a consequence of Hpd treatment. In contrast, target cell susceptibility to cell-mediated lysis was not affected by Hpd treatment.
The unchanged susceptibility to cell-mediated lysis by treated cells
appears to exclude indiscriminate Hpd damage of cell surface structures. Cell mediated lysis of target cells proceeds through two
fundamental steps: the recognition phase and the lethal hit phase.
Table 4 shows that effector recognition was inhibited while the relevant characteristic of target cells to be recognized was not modified. Inhibition was dose-dependent and the viability of neither
the effector cells nor the target cells was damaged.

In other experiments of absorbing capacity and lysis susceptibility we did not observe any Hpd alteration of target molecules
like surface receptors. Gross and non specific chemical modifications of cell surface molecules seem not be responsible for the
effector cell loss of recognition capacity.

Table 4. Effect of an Hpd treatment on immune lymphocyte binding to target cells.

Target cells	Immune Lymphocytes	^No. of positive cells ± SE	% binding
[x] L1210	[xx] I	242 ± 29	48
"	I_{H20}	90 ± 18	18
"	I_{H5}	136 ± 9	27
"	I_{H1}	222 ± 12	44
$L1210_{H20}$	I	255 ± 28	51
$L1210_{H5}$	"	240 ± 20	48
$L1210_{H1}$	"	250 ± 23	50

[x] see footnote Table 3   [xx] see footnote Table 3
^ Immune cells and target cells in a ratio of 40:1 incubated 1h at 4°C were counted under a light microscope by two independent observers. Fivehundred small lymphocytes were counted and cells with 3 or more tumor cells bound were considered positive cells.

Another set of experiments reported in Table 5 were directed at seeing whether Hpd might influence the lateral mobility of molecular structures on cell surface with the Con A agglutination of cancer cells test.

Hpd treatment of the cells caused an almost complete inhibition of lectin agglutination. Inhibition was dose-dependent. Studies are in progress to elucidate the nature of membrane modifications and, possibly, the specific structure damage. The inhibition of some immune cell activities reported here appeared to be dependent on Hpd alterations of the movement of cell surface structures rather than an alteration of the chemical integrity of cell surface molecules, since the intimate mechanism of many cellular interactions is still obscure, detection of specific Hpd alteration of membrane properties might help to elucidate some characteristics of immune cell interations and, more generally, to study some properties of eukaryotic cells.

Table 5. Reduced Con A agglutinability of Hpd treated L1210
cells.

Tumor cells	Con A µg/ml	Agglutination index
L1210	50	++++
L1210$_{H20}$	"	+
L1210$_{H5}$	"	++
L1210$_{H1}$	"	++
L1210	100	++++
L1210$_{H20}$	"	+
L1210$_{H5}$	"	+
L1210$_{H1}$	"	+

2×10^6 Hpd treated L1210 cells were incubated with Con A (50-100
µg/ml) 30' at 37°C and then 10' at 4°C. The agglutination index
was evaluated under the light microscope by two independent observers with arbitrary scores from 0 to ++++.

        Regarding the results of Hpd activity on tumor cells after
light activation with laser, Hpd treated leukemic cells, undamaged
in the dark, have been completely lysed upon exposure to the red
light of an He-Neon laser (Table 6).

        Light mediated cytocidal activity was dependent on Hpd con-
centration. A low Hpd dose such as 2.5 µg/ml devoid of any cytotoxic activity in the absence of light, exhibited the maximum cytocidal effect.

Table 6.   Cytocidal effect of Hpd and laser on L1210 tumor
cells.

Hpd	Cell viability		Specific ^{51}Cr release		
μg/ml	− Laser	+	−	Laser	+
−	87	91	0		0
0.5	85	87	3		1
1	91	38	1		44
2.5	90	0	4		86
5	85	0	3		91
12.5	73	0	11		93
25	68	0	14		93

L1210 cells treated with Hpd at the indicated concentrations, after
extensive washing were exposed for 45' to an He-Neon laser light or
maintained in the dark. Cell viability was checked by the Trypan
blue dye exclusion test. In a parallel experiment, $Na_2{}^{51}CrO_4$, 200
μCi/ml (specific activity 200mCi/mM, Amersham England) was added to
samples under treatment with Hpd, washed and treated with laser as
described. Specific ^{51}Cr release in supernatant by Hpd-laser-treated
samples was calculated as follows:

$$\frac{\text{CPM in experimental samples - CPM in control samples}}{\text{CPM in detergent treated samples - CPM in control samples}} \times 100$$

The potent cytocidal activity of light activated Hpd was further
confirmed by injection of Hpd-laser treated L1210 cells in syngeneic
animals and data are reported in Table 7.

The time of death of syngeneic animals challenged with Hpd-
laser-treated L1210 cells was registered. The large majority of
mice challenged with viable 10^5 L1210 cells treated with 5γ/ml and
light survived indefinitely, in spite of the fact that an L1210
inoculum as low as 10^2 cells is lethal. In contrast the survival
of L1210 leukemic mice was not improved by the Hpd treatment alone.

Table 7. Survival of mice challenged with L1210 cells pretreated with Hpd and laser.

HPD	Laser −		Laser +	
γ/ml	MST	D/T	MST	D/T
-	10	8/8	10	8/8
50	12	8/8	-	0/8
25	11	8/8	-	1/8
12.5	11	8/8	-	1/8
5	9	8/8	-	2/8
2.5	10	8/8	12	7/8
1	10	8/8	12	8/8

L1210 cells, untreated or treated with Hpd were maintained in the
dark or exposed to laser light as indicated for Table 6. $CD2F_1$
mice were challenged with 10^5 cells ip and the time of death registered. MST, median survival time (days); D/T, dead animals/treated
animals.

The Hpd-laser cytocidal activity in vivo was studied in mice
bearing MS-2 sarcoma derived from murine Moloney Sarcoma Virus
(MSV-M) (Table 8).

Table 8. Antitumor activity of Hpd + Laser

Treatment	Exp.1 Hpd 5mg/kg ip		Exp.2 Hpd 25mg/kg ip	
	MST	D/T	MST	D/T
-	43	6/6	46	6/6
HPD	45	6/6	49	6/6
HPD X3 ✴ LASER X3	45	6/6	89	6/6
HPD + LASER	45	6/6	69.5	6/6
LASER	52	6/6	ND	

$CD2F_1$ mice challenged id with 10^6 sarcoma MS-2.
✴ = $50mW/cm^2$ x45'.

Treatment of mice with Hpd and exposure of the tumor mass to laser light prolonged the median survival time in respect to the control animals untreated or treated with Hpd or with laser (dye-laser) $P=50mW/cm^2 \times 45'$ only. The problem regarding relapse around the scar area is probably due to some microscopic neoplastic cells that had already spread into normal tissues. As presently applied however, the major limitation of this method is the limited effective penetration of the light through tissues, estimated to be approximately 2 cm. This limitation can be eliminated by delivering the light through a quartz fiber optic, imbedded directly into the tumor mass. Indeed results using this technique are the same as other external techniques.

After these encouraging results we decided to carry out some experiments with another solid tumor, the B16 melanoma, that quickly metastatizes to the lung. Infact, in clinical oncology, the metastases are the most important problem, therefore we tried to apply this new methodology on one experimental metastatic tumor. For these experiments the laser light was delivered through a quartz fiber optic imbedded directly into the tumor mass. (Table 9).

We observe from this table that the phototherapy is quite active on the metastatic tumor.

In conclusion these preliminary results are encouraging in view of the clinical applications. Studies are in progress to compare

Table 9. Antitumor activity of Hpd + laser on a tumor with established metastases.

[x] Treatment	MST	D/T
	23	6/6
[xx] Hpd	25	6/6
[xx] Laser	24	6/6
Hpd x 3 + Laser x 3	46	5/6

BDF_1 challenged id with 10^6 B16 melanoma. [x] Treatment was started when tumor had lung metastases. [xx] 200 mW (fiber output) x 10'.

the photoradiation methodology with the conventional surgical excision, to explore new and eventually more active cancer therapies
and furthermore to combine different modalities of treatment.

These studies, infact, might improve the efficacy of the photoradiation therapy and, more important, could be interesting for
better clinical approaches.

REFERENCES

1.   T.J.Dougherty, Activated dyes as antitumor agents, J.Natl.
     Cancer Inst. 52:1333 (1974)
2.   F.H.H. Figge, G.S.Weiland, L.O. Manganiello, Cancer detection
     and therapy affinity of neoplastic embryonic and traumatized
     tissues for porphyrin and metalloporphyrin. Proc.Soc.Exp.Biol.
     Med. 68:640 (1948)
3.   H.B.Gregorie, E.O.Horger, J.L.Ward, J.F.Green, T.Richards, H.C.
     Robertson, T.B.Stevenson., Hematoporphyrin derivative fluore-
     scence in malignant neoplasma. Ann.Surg. 167:820 (1968)
4.   K.R.Weishaupt, C.J.Gomer, T.J.Dougherty, Identification of
     singlet oxygen as the cytotoxic agent photoinactivation of
     murine tumors. Cancer Res.36:2326 (1976)
5.   T.J.Dougherty, G.B.Grindey, R.Fiel, R.R.Weishaupt, D.G.Boyle.
     Photoradiation therapy: Cure of animals tumors with hemato-
     porphyrin and light. J.Natl.Cancer Inst. 55:115 (1975)
6.   T.J.Dougherty, J.E.Kaufman, A.Goldfarb, K.A.Weishaupt, D.Boyle,
     A.Mittelman. Photoradiation therapy for the treatment of
     malignant tumors. Cancer Res. 38:2628 (1978)
7.   T.J.Dougherty, G.Lawrence, J.E. Kaufman, D.G.Boyle, K.R.
     Weishaupt, A.Goldfarb. Photoradiation in the treatment of
     recurrent breast carcinoma. J.Natl.Cancer Inst. 62:231 (1979)
8.   A.Dahlman, A.G.Wile, R.G.Burns, G.R.Mason, F.M.Johnson, M.W.
     Berns. Laser photoradiation therapy of cancer. Cancer Res.
     43:430 (1983)
9.   Y. Hayata, K.Harubruni, C.Konaka, J.Ono, M.Takizawa. Hema-
     toporphyrin derivative and laser photoradiation in the treat-
     ment of lung cancer. Chest 81:269 (1982)
10. G.Canti, O.Marelli, L.Ricci, A.Nicolin. Hematoporphyrin-treated
     murine lymphocytes:in vitro inhibition of DNA synthesis and
     light mediated inactivation of cells responsible for GVHR.
     Photoch. and Photobiol. 34:589 (1981)

PHOTORADIATION THERAPY (PRT) OF LEWIS LUNG CARCINOMA IN B_6D_2 MICE,

DOSIMETRY CONSIDERATIONS

R. Ellingsen, L. O. Svaasand and A. Ødegaard[*]

Division of Physical Electronics, University of Trondheim
N-7034 Trondheim-NTH, Norway

[*]Department of Pathology, University of Trondheim
N-7000 Trondheim, Norway

INTRODUCTION

In tumor therapy there will presumably exist an optimum of the optical dose rate and the photosensitizer dose. This work discusses the PRT of Lewis lung carcinomas in mice performed at low optical power levels combined with rather high doses of photosensitizer. The light and temperature dosimetry is of great importance in photo-therapy, consequently those parameters have been monitored during the irradiation period. Equally important is the drug dosimetry. Reported values of administered drug concentrations vary over almost two orders of magnitude [1].

In this work the HpD concentration is varied by one order of magnitude. The response to treatment was evaluated by visual inspection for 2-6 days. The animals were then sacrified and pathological sections prepared for histological examination.

MATERIALS AND METHODS

Tumor

Rapidly growing Lewis lung carcinomas were used. Tumor cells were injected subcutaneously and grew up in the shape of spheroids. The tumor bearing animals were 6-8 week old female mice of the hybrid B_6D_2. Some preliminary trials showed that 6-9 days time lapse from tumor cell injection to the start of treatment gave the best compromise between the tumor dimension and the spontaneously developed necrosis of the center region. The typical tumor dimension at the time of treatment was 6-10 mm in diameter.

Experimental Series

6 experimental series are reported. Each series was composed
of one control and two HpD-injected animals, 5 mg/kg and 50 mg/kg,
respectively. The initial experiment was designed for 100 mV optical dose rate at 630 nm. However, this dose rate was reduced to
45 mW in our treatment scheme for reasons that will be discussed
later. The irradiation period was of 60 min. duration, i.e. 160-
-360 J was delivered. One final experiment was performed in order
to obtain hyperthermal conditions of treatment: 300 mW of green light
(514.5 nm wavelength) was irradiated for 15 minutes (270 J). The
purpose of non-treated controls in each series was to represent a
typical basis of spontaneously developing necrosis for the following examination by histology.

HpD, Light, Irradiation/Detection system

The commercially available HpD was manufactured by Oncology
Research & Development, Inc. (Cheektowaga, N.Y., USA). The drug was
injected into the subcutaneous tumor 24 hours prior to irradiation.
Red light at 630 nm wavelength was delivered by an argon-ion laser
pumped dye-laser from Spectra Physics (Mountain View, CA, USA).
Green light at 514.5 nm wavelength was delivered by the argon-ion
laser. The laser beam was coupled into an optical fiber that was
centrally inserted into the tumor through the lumen of a 21-gauge
(0.8 mm outer diameter) hypodermic needle. No multiple excitation
fiber insertions were used. Another needle with axis parallel to
the first one's, with the same length and mechanically fixed to-
gheter was also inserted. Through its lumen was threaded either
an optical fiber or a thermocouple. This way it was possible to
monitor light intensity or temperature in the tumor during treatment. Measurements of optical penetration depths of those tumors
were performed "in vivo". See Ref. 3 for a definition of penetration depth and experimental method. Excitation and detection fibers were silicone clad fused silica core fibers, core diameter
200 μm, from Quartz & Silice (Pithivers, France). The fiber ends
were cleaved optically flat. The thermal sensor was a sheathed
chromel-alumel thermocouple wire of outer diameter 250 μm from
Sodern, Thermocoax (Suresnes, France). Light picked up by the detection fiber was transmitted through approximately 1 m of fiber
and measured by a silicon PIN detector. Further analysis of signals
were performed by standard lock-in amplifier technique (chopping of
light).

Treatment evaluation

The animals were observed for some days post-treatment. In
the cases referenced in this report the animals were sacrificed

2-6 days later. During this observation period the tumor response
was described by visual inspection and measurement of tumor diameter. In order to attain a description of tumor cell development,
a post-treatment histological evaluation was performed. A slice of
3-4 mm thickness of tumor tissue was dissected and fixed for 12
hours in a solution of 80% EtOH, 15% formaldehyd and 5% acetic acid.
Subsequently the specimens were kept in 80% EtOH in H_2O until the
final preparations (sectioning and staining) for light microscopy
took place.

RESULTS

Some preliminary experiments showed that 14 days old tumors
(time measured from subcutaneous injection of tumor cells) developed a central necrosis of 1/2-3/4 of the total tumor volume (tumor
diameter approx. 15 mm). This natural necrosis problem was reduced
to an acceptable level when the animals were entered into treatment
6-9 days after tumor cells injection.

Temperature measurements

Figure 1 shows measured temperatures at 4 mm distance in 3 cases.
The measurements are performed with the thermal sensor situated at
the body side of the subcutaneously growing tumor. Both cases of

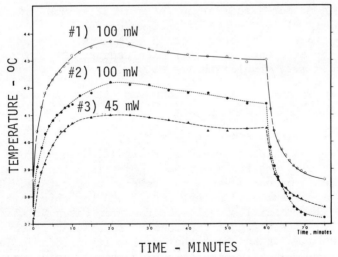

TIME - MINUTES

Fig. 1.   Tumor temperature at 4 mm distance from fiber end versus
          time. Irradiation period of 60 min. Two cases irradiated
          by 100 mW transmitted power: No. 1) initial body tempera-
          ture of 38.6°C (o); No. 2) initial body temperature of
          37.3°C (•). One case irradiated by 45 mW: No. 3) initial
          body temperature of 37.2°C (▲). Wavelength λ = 630 nm.

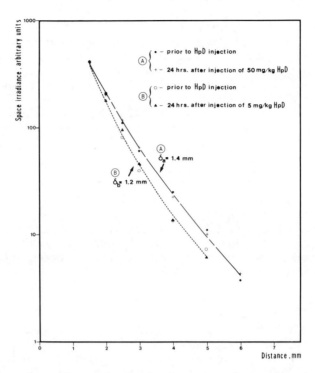

Fig. 2. Space irradiance in Lewis lung carcinoma in mice versus
         distance from fiber end. "In vivo" measurements. Two cases,
         both measured before and 24 hours after HpD injection.
         (A) (●,+) - injected with 50 mg/kg HpD.
         (B) (o,▲) - injected with 5 mg/kg HpD.
         Calculated optical penetration depths: δ_a = 1.4 mm, δ_b =
         = 1.2 mm. Wavelength λ = 630 nm.

100 mW optical power (No. 1 and No. 2) show maximum temperature
rises of approximately 5.0°C above initial body temperature at 4 mm
distance from the light source. This situation may induce hyperthermal effects in the region close to the fiber end. Whether this
will be the case or not depends on the body temperature. Hyperthermal effects are assumed to appear at 42-43°C for this irradiation
duration [2]. The initial body temperature for cases No. 1 and 2
differs by 1.3°C (see figure captions). Approximately the same difference is retained throughout the 60 min. irradiation. This difference will consequently result in a greater tumor volume receiving hyperthermal treatment in the case of the highest initial body
temperature. However, even the temperature rise of case No. 1 is
not sufficient for an adjuvant therapy of the total tumor volume;
the growing border region will experience a temperature too low
for adequate hyperthermia.

Case No. 3 (45 mW) shows a temperature rise of only 3.8°C above body temperature at 4 mm distance. This dose rate should undoubtedly give phototherapy-dominated treatment.

Light intensity measurements

The space irradiance measurements versus distance (Fig. 2) are used for optical penetration depth calculations (see Ref. 3 for details). The penetration depth equals a distance along the negative photon flux density gradient that gives a space irradiance attenuation of e^{-1} (37%). Both cases shown in Fig. 2 verify that no significant change of optical penetration depth or optical absorption is introduced by injection of HpD-doses of those concentrations. Note, the measurements were performed immediately before 24 hours post injection, i.e. a situation that is coincident with that of the treatment scheme.

Light intensity measurements in the tumors as a function of time during 60 min. were carried out at 3 mm distance from the light source. The intensity was monitored for transmitted optical power levels between 150 and 45 mW (630 nm). At this wavelength 3 mm distance represents approximately 2 penetration depths (see Fig. 2).

Repeated experiments gave typically these results: in the 45 mW cases space irradiance was kept constant throughout 60 min.; 90 mW or higher gave a reduction of 2-3 orders of magnitude of the space irradiance during the 60 min. period, the main drop took place within 10 min. from the start. Actually it has been found that 50 mW represents a maximum limit for transmitted optical power (630 nm) if one wants to be sure that light intensity should not be severely reduced in the tumor mass during irradiation. The reason for this increased light absorption is assumed to be a charring/carbonization process at the fiber end. Those arguments are applied when the light delivery system is a single optical fiber with no optical light scattering arrangement at the output. For this reason all treated cases reported in this paper are irradiately by the rather low optical dose rate of 45 mW.

Treatment evaluation, visual observations

During the observation period succeeding phototherapy the animals were kept away from direct daylight, otherwise they were given the normal laboratory conditions. 2-6 days post treatment are certainly a short term. However, the intention of the experiment was to search for early celllular damage that could be demonstrated histologically. Table 1 summarizes the visual observation of 6 series.

Table 1.   Summary of Visually Observed Results of HpD-phototherapy
            of Lewis Lung Tumors in Mice.

Injected HpD-dose [mg/kg]	Optical dose rate [mW] Wavelength [nm]	Number of animals	Tumor volume relative to control at sacrifice	Time from irradiation to sacrifice [days]
0 (Control)	0/-	6	1	2-6
5	45/630	6	1	2-6
50	45/630	6	3 cases - 0.7 2 cases - 0.5 1 case - 0.2	2 3 6
0	45/630	3	1	2-3
0	300/514.5	1	0.1 - 0.2	2

Treatment evaluation, histology

      Figure 3 presents micrographs of: A) non-treated control, and
4 treated animals; B) -5 mg/kg HpD; C) -50 mg/kg HpD; D) -50 mg/kg
HpD; E) - No HpD. B), C) and D) were all irradiated for 60 min.
with 45 mW transmitted optical power at 630 nm wavelength. E) was
irradiated for 15 min. with 300 mW transmitted optical power at
514.5 nm. A), B), C) and E) were sacrificed 2 days post treatment.
D) was sacrificed 6 days post treatment. The maximum measured temperature in case E) was 52.2°C at 3 mm distance from the light source.

      The observations summarized in Table 1 are mainly supported by
these micrographs. The extensive tumor necrosis and inflammatory
reaction of C) is specific. A) (control) and B) (5 mg/kg HpD) show
some differences. While little or no necrosis can be observed in
A) there can be seen both necrotic areas and an acute inflammatory
reaction in B); this situation gave no distinct differences in the
visual observations. D) shows a situation where similar conditions
as in C) have developed for 6 days. The area is dominated by an
acellular, post-necrotic part of the original tumor with distinct
fibroblastic activity. However, a focus of proliferating tumor
tissue is still present. Whether this is a viable tumor rest or not
is left unanswered since no long term follow-ups have been performed. The hyperthermally treated tumor was observed to be considerably reduced within 2 days post treatment (bottom row of Table 1).

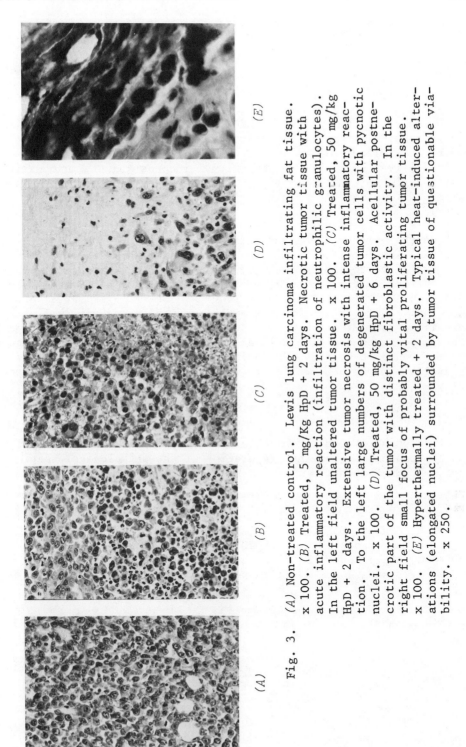

(A)   (B)   (C)   (D)   (E)

Fig. 3.   (A) Non-treated control. Lewis lung carcinoma infiltrating fat tissue.
x 100. (B) Treated, 5 mg/Kg HpD + 2 days. Necrotic tumor tissue with
acute inflammatory reaction (infiltration of neutrophilic granulocytes).
In the left field unaltered tumor tissue. x 100. (C) Treated, 50 mg/kg
HpD + 2 days. Extensive tumor necrosis with intense inflammatory reaction. To the left large numbers of degenerated tumor cells with pycnotic
nuclei. x 100. (D) Treated, 50 mg/kg HpD + 6 days. Acellular postne-
crotic part of the tumor with distinct fibroblastic activity. In the
right field small focus of probably vital proliferating tumor tissue.
x 100. (E) Hyperthermally treated + 2 days. Typical heat-induced alterations (elongated nuclei) surrounded by tumor tissue of questionable viability. x 250.

However, with reference to Fig. 3.E), the rest of this tumor may be viable with regrowth as a possible result if no sacrifice took place.

CONCLUSION

Initially this "in vivo" experiment was designed to be performed with approximately double the optical dose rate actually used. It became clear that for this specific tumor and the light delivery system consisting of one single fiber, the optical power at 630 nm has to be limited to 50 mW. Because of the local temperature rise, an initially higher optical power level induces clotting and possibly carbonization at the fiber tip. Consequently, light absorption is increased to a non-acceptable level for HpD phototherapy of the tumor.

Further, it is found that this situation of rather low optical dose rate may be effective if the HpD-dose is increased by a factor of 10 relative to the one usually used, 5 mg/kg. This treatment scheme is shown to give curative tumor response both by visual observation and by histology. The low HpD-dose (5 mg/kg) gave no significantly different response from the control case by visual observation; some difference was observed histologically. The temperature measurements give evidence that this low optical dose rate scheme should be regarded as dominated by photodynamic mechanisms. An increase of optical dose rate will definitely increase the extent of hyperthermally treated tumor.

ACKNOWLEDGEMENTS

The authors wish to thank Barbara Reitan for her expert typing and Eli Johannesen for the preparation of the pathological sections for light microscopy.

REFERENCES

1. J. H. Kinsey, D. A. Cortese, H. L. Moses, R. J. Ryan and E. L. Braum, Cancer Res. 41:5020 (1981).
2. J. G. Short and P. F. Turner, Proc. IEEE 68:133 (1980).
3. L. O. Svaasand and R. Ellingsen, Photochem. Photobiol. (1983) in press.

STUDY OF IRRADIATION PARAMETERS IN HPD PHOTOTHERAPY OF MS-2 TUMOR MODEL [°]

R. Marchesini, F. Zunino, E. Melloni, G. Pezzoni,
G. Savi, L. Locati, G. Bandieramonte, P. Spinelli,
H. Emanuelli and G. Fava

Istituto Nazionale Tumori, Via Venezian, 1
20133 Milano, Italy

INTRODUCTION

In phototherapy treatment with hematoporphyrin derivatives (HpD) and laser[1], the beam intensity distribution is usually not uniform on the target area. Thus an average irradiance is defined as ratio between the laser output power (emitted directly or by optical fiber) and the brightened area. Moreover, it is well known that in the case of ionizing radiation treatment, tumor response is related to the absorbed dose, and to avoid local relapses, the irradiated area, which has a homogeneous dose distribution, must include the tumor peripheral border. The same principles can be applied to photoradiationtherapy (PRT). Nevertheless, as the irradiance distribution in phototherapy is non-homogeneous and bell-shaped, recurrencies near the field border may occur. In contrast, a hyperthermic effect due to overdose may occur in the center of the exposed area. In these cases evaluation of the mechanism of phototherapy effectiveness is questionable.

This study was undertaken to evaluate the tumor response in PRT following HpD administration to different light dose rate, using MS-2 tumor as the experimental model. The efficacy of PRT on this tumor is of general interest, since this model shows a biological behaviour similar to that of some human tumors, i.e., slow and progressive growth, invasive character, ability to metastasize to lungs and low antigenicity.

[°] This investigation was supported by the Italian National Research Council, Grant No. 82.01754.98.

MATERIAL AND METHODS

Light delivery system. Light was delivered from a Dye laser (Model 375 Spectra Physics) with Rhodamine B dye, pumped with an 18 W Argon ion laser (Model 171 Spectra Physics). The efficiency of the laser pumping system was tipically 17% and the maximum output power at 630 nm wavelength was about 3 W. The beam wavelength smoothly drifted during the whole experiment, ranging between 628 and 631 nm. The optput of the Dye laser was coupled into the proximal end of an optical fiber 600 μm in diameter. Surface irradiation of the tumor was not performed with a lens placed at the exit of the Dye laser because the best ratio is obtained between the 80% light intensity diameter and the total beam diameter (defined at $1/e^2$). By using the optical fiber, the ratio was 0.5, whereas it was only 0.25 with the lens. If we assume that the useful area is enclosed in that part of the beam where light intensity is greater than 80% of the maximum, the use of an optical fiber gave a greater effective field with the same laser output power.

Tumor model. MS-2 sarcoma was produced in BALB/c mice by transplant of in-vitro-cultured cells derived from a primary MSV-M tumor in mice[2]. The tumor model was maintained by serial i.m. passages of a tumor cell suspension into a right hind leg. For PRT treatment, tumor cells (2.5×10^6) were injected into a right foot pad.

Treatment procedure. HpD was supplied as a sterile solution containing 5 mg/ml by Oncology Research and Development (Cheektowaga, New York) and stored frozen in the dark until use. PRT was initiated on day 3 after tumor transplantation (tumor mass not palpable). Mice were given HpD i.v. (25 mg/kg) 24 h before exposure to light. The irradiated area was 6.5 mm in diameter, corresponding to the 80% intensity diameter, whereas the surrounding area was masked by a diaphragm. Irradiance and exposure time for three different groups of mice were: 200 mW/cm^2 for 10 min, 100 mW/cm^2 for 20 min, and 50 mW/cm^2 for 40 min. The total delivered dose was 120 J/cm^2 for all the animals. The effectiveness of the treatment was evaluated by measuring the relative tumor size in the mice that did not show complete response at the indicated days after exposure to light.

RESULTS AND DISCUSSION

We made preliminary measurements of light attenuation and scattering at 630 nm in an egg white and gelatine mixture, which has the same optical characteristics of cytoplasm[3]. At this wavelength, light intensity was reduced by a factor of 3 in passage

through 2.5 mm of a sliced sample of the egg white and gelatine mixture. The 80% relative intensity diameter at 2.5 and 5 mm depths
was increased only by a factor of 1.3 compared to 80% relative intensity at zero depth. From these data it is possible to conclude
that strong absorption and moderate broadening in tissue occur.
Thus in the experimental design on MS-2 experimental tumor treatment, the aforementioned data were taken into account. This solid
tumor was used, since a previous work[4] indicated that the best
conditions for the treatment of MS-2 tumor after 8 days from transplantation were laser irradiation at 160 mW/cm^2 average irradiance
for 10 min, 24 h after 25 mg/kg i.v. injection of HpD (Fig. 1).
At this stage of tumor development (i.e., 8-day-old tumor), tumor
mass (30-50 mg) is too large if uniform irradiation in depth and
width is required.

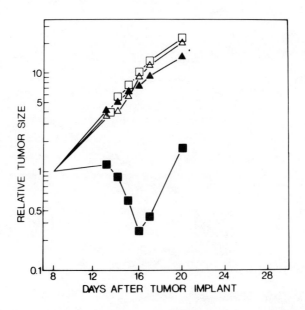

Fig. 1. MS-2 tumor growth following treatment with HpD and light
    ■   or light alone △   or HpD alone □   .Eight-day-
old tumor was exposed to light at 165 mW/cm^2 average irradiance for 10 min. Complete responses were observed in 3/6
mice treated with HpD and light. Control mice ▲   [4].

Thus we treated this experimental tumor at an early stage of development 3 days after transplantation. The results are shown in
Fig. 2. The treatment with 50 mW/cm^2, for 40 min or 100 mW/cm^2 for
20 min provided similar effects; a more marked inhibition of tumor
growth was obtained with 200 mW/cm^2 for 10 min.

Although light itself did not provided a terapeutic effect
under our previous experimental conditions (Fig. 1) a synergistic
interaction between photodynamic effect mediated by HpD and hyperthermal effect produced by light irradiation cannot be excluded.
The occurence of a hyperthermal effect is also suggested by the
observation that under our exposure conditions (160 mW/cm^2 for
10 min) light induced, to a variable extent, phototoxic damage to
normal tissue in the absence of HpD treatment, probably as a consequence of the temperature rise during treatment, even if no therapeutic results were obtained in the irradiated tumors without HpD.

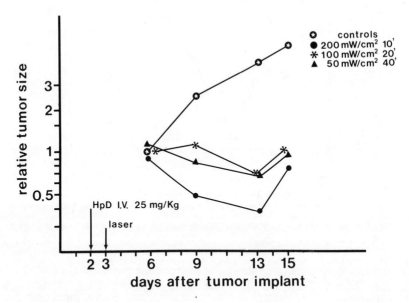

Fig. 2.   MS-2 tumor growth following treatment with HpD and light
          at different dose rates. The curve obtained at 200 mW/cm^2
          for 10 min refers to only one mouse. The other mice showed
          complete response.

Thus, although the effectiveness of the combined treatment with
HpD and visible light appears dependent on two factors:
1) preferential localization of HpD components at tumor sites,since
   pure hematoporphyrin did not produce appreciable tumor necrosis
   and
2) photochemical reactions of porphyrins, since light alone has no
   effect,
our results suggest that, using a relatively high light dose rate
(> 100 mW/cm^2), tumor destruction may be the result of both photodynamic and hyperthermal effects.

REFERENCES

1. T. J. Dougherty, K. R. Weishaupt, and D. G. Boyle, Photosensitizers, in:"Cancer:principles & practice of oncology", C. T. Devita,
   S. Hellman, and S. A. Rosenberg,eds., J. B. Lippincott, Philadelphia (1982).
2. A. Di Marco, T. Dasdia, F. Giuliani, A. Necco, A. M. Casazza,
   P. T. Mora, S. W. Lubowrsky, and L. Waters, Biological properties of cell lines derived from Moloney virus-induced sarcoma,
   Tumori 62:415 (1976).
3. J. R. Baker, Cytological technique, in:"Principles of biological
   microtechnique: a study of fixation and dyeing", Methuen,London
   (1958).
4. F. Zunino, R. Marchesini, E. Melloni, G. Savi, G. Pezzoni, L.
   Locati, and G. Fava, Effectiveness of laser photoradiation
   therapy following hematoporphyrin derivative administration
   in the experimental MS-2 tumor model, Tumori 69:305 (1983).

EXPERIMENTAL ENU INDUCED BRAIN TUMORS WITH HpD AND DYE LASER LIGHT

S. Pezzotta, G. Spanu, R. Cubeddu[*], A. Andreoni[*] and
M.T. Giordana[¤]

Dipartimento di Chirurgia-Sezione di Clinica
Neurochirurgia, Università di Pavia, Italy

[*]Centro Elettronica Quantistica e Strumentazione
Elettronica, CNR, Milano, Italy

[¤]Clinica Neurologica II, Università di Torino, Italy

INTRODUCTION

It is well know that the Hematoporphyrin Derivative (HpD) accumulates preferentially in tumor tissues as compared with the normal tissues (Leonard and Beck, 1971; Lipson et al., 1961; Dougherty
et al., 1976).

A sizeable reduction in tumor mass for a number of different
types of non-neural tumors was obtained by the irradiation of the
tumor mass with light in animals that had received HpD at the doses
of from 2 to 5 mg/kg of body weight (Dougherty et al., 1975, 1978;
Gomer and Dougherty, 1979).

Diamond et al. (1972) demonstrated that glioma cells, which
are grown in cell culture or implanted subcutaneously in rats,
could be destroyed by exposure to laser light if they had been photosensitized previously by treatment with Hematoporphyrin.

Tumor necrosis induced by HpD photosensitization seems to function on a basis of resonant energy transfer between triplet HpD and
the endogenous molecular oxygen. After the HpD molecules that accumulate in the tumor are brought to their first excited singlet
state by the absorption of light, most of them decay to the long-
-lasting triplet state. When triplet HpD collides with an oxygen

227

molecule, the oxygen molecule is excited to its first or singlet state. The singlet oxygen produced by this photodynamic action, is known to be radical and is likely to be the cytotoxic agent responsible for this tumor necrosis. The most effective results of this tumor phototherapy are achieved using red light (631 nm wavelength) at doses of 100 J/cm^2.

MATERIALS AND METHODS

Tumor Induction

A single dose of Ethylnitrosourea (ENU) (20 mg/kg i.v.) was given to pregnant Fisher-344 rats on the 16th day of gestation according to Grossi-Paoletti et al. (1972).

A systematic diachronic study of the brain was begun on the 15th day of extrauterine life (Shiffer et al. 1978, 1980).

Hematoporphyrin Determination

Hematoporphyrin was extracted from tissues and then measured according to a modified procedure of Lemberg and Legge (Spanu et al., 1983).

The Hematoporphyrin concentration in the HCl solution was determined with a Perkin-Elmer MPF 4 spectrophotofluorimeter. An estimate of the amount of Hematoporphyrin was obtained by calculating the sum of the emission intensities at 630 nm, proportional to the integrated area of the emission spectrum in the 550-750 nm wavelength range and amount of Hematoporphyrin in 1M HCl solution (Jori et al., 1979).

Laser Irradiation

Sixty animals were divided into three groups and, starting on the 90th day of extrauterine life, treated as follows: one control group (Group 1) underwent laser treatment only, the second control group (Group 2) underwent combined treatment with HpD + laser, while the group treated with ENU (Group 3) also underwent combined treatment with HpD + laser. The Hematoporphyrin Derivative (Photofrin, 5 mg HpD per ml) was administered i.p. at a dose of 5 mg/kg. All animals were irradiated 48 hours after HpD injection. Each group received 2 laser treatments 3 days apart.

Ten animals of each group were sacrificed 24 hours after the first treatment and the remaining animals were sacrificed 15 days after the second treatment.

Carnoy at 0° was used to fix the brains which were then dehy-

drated, paraffin embedded and cut into 4 μm thick serial sections.
The following stains were employed: hematoxylineosin (HE), PTAH,
luxol fast blue B for myelin.

The following zones were examined with progressing development:
germinal zone, cortex, mantle zone, basal ganglia, medullary center,
paraventricular white matter and subependymal plate. Cell count was
performed in microscope fields of 160 μm^2 x 110 μm^2.

The irradiation source was cw (continuous wave) dye laser
(Coherent 599) pumped by Argon ion laser (Coherent CR-18). The lasing
dye Rhodamine B (Exciton Rhodamine 610) dissolved in Ethylglycol
was used. The dye-laser output was split into two beams of the same
power and coupled into two optical fibers of 400 micron diameter.
A craniotomy of 2 mm in diameter was performed and each single fiber
was placed on the dura using a sterotaxic device. All irradiation
was performed using 200 mW per fiber for 10 minutes.

Table 1. Uptake of HpD in Normal and Tumoral Brain

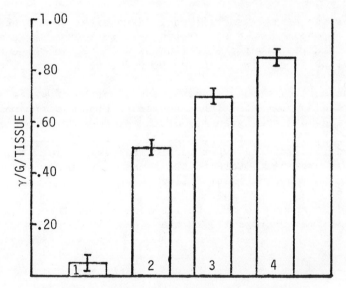

1 = NORMAL TISSUE; 2 = ISOMORPHIC OLIGODENDRO-
GLIOMA; 3 = POLIMORPHIC OLIGODENDROGLIOMA;
4 = GASSER NEURINOMA

EACH VALUE REPRESENTS THE MEAN ± S.E.M. OF LAST
FIVE DETERMINATIONS.

RESULTS

The uptake values of HpD in the brain tissues of the control
rats in different oncotypes induced with ENU are shown in Table 1.
The values referring to normal brain tissues present a much lower
uptake of HpD. We can consider this value equal to zero since if
refers to tiny traces of substances still present in the blood and
in the capillaries included in the tissue homogenate. Contrarily,
the values found in the three oncotypes evaluated are at least 5
times higher than in the controls: isomorphic oliogodendroglioma
incorporates .50 gamma/gr of tissue, polymorphic oliogodendroglioma
.72 gamma/gr and neurinoma .81 gamma/gr.

Six animals died between 6 and 12 hours after the second application of the laser. In 2 cases, the cause of death was attributed
to an intracranial hematoma and in 4 cases to a diffuse brain edema.

Histological Observation

In the rats sacrificed 24 hours after the first laser treatment,
in proximity of the hole of the craniotomy, there was a non-delimit-
ed necrosis, characterized by eosin pallor and nuclear phyknosis of
the cortex and while matter.

As for the animals sacrificed 15 days after the second laser
treatment, Group 1 showed a necrotic cyst surrounded by a moderate
gliomesodermic reaction; the lesion was situated in the cortex and
subcortical white matter close to the point of laser application.

In the rats of Groups 2 and 3, localization and size of the
necrosis were approximately the same as in Group 1; the most striking difference was the intensity of the gliomesodermic reaction,
consisting of abundant macrophages, vessel proliferation with endo-
thelial hyperplasia, and hypertrophic reactive astrocytes. Mitotic
activity was prominent, both in the reactive elements and in the
immediately surrounding glial cells.

We had no chance to observe laser effect on tumors, since the
tumor lesions were very small at the age of 90 days.

CONCLUSIONS

In the 60's and 70's various authors demonstrated the accumulation of HpD in tumoral tissues (Leonard and Beck, 1971; Lipson et
al., 1961, Weishaupt et al., 1976; Winkelman and Rasmussen-Taxdal,
1960; Carpenter et al., 1977, Dougherty et al., 1976). Moreover,
other authors demonstrated the distribution of this substance in
the tissues of various animal species (Dougherty et al., 1975, Gomer et al., 1979; Laws et al., 1981; Rounds et al., 1982). Although

there is little data from the literature regarding HpD determination
in spontaneous brain tumors, various studies have attempted to determine the presence of HpD in subcutaneously transplanted glial
tumors.

Our data on brain tumors, which were induced with ENU, show
a significant accumulation of HpD in different oncotypes. This data
are similar to the preliminary experiments conducted on man using
fluorescence to determine HpD by Perria et al., 1980; and Laws et
al., 1981.

In the cases presented by Perria et al., three of which underwent both bioptic and autopsic histologic diagnosis after treatment,
the authors found necrotic areas near the tumor which they relate
to photoradiation treatment.

In the cases reported by Laws et al., which were only investigated by CT scan, wide necrotic-hemorrhagic-cystic cavities were
shown.

Our data, on the other hand, which refers to a limited period
of observation, show that the use of HpD + laser in this experimental mode with this technique, tends to stimulate a very marked cellular response with respect to tissue damage as the quantity of mi-
toses in the reaction tissues demonstrates. The biologic potential
of this intense proliferative activity caused by this treatment requires further investigation and an evaluation of its effects after
longer periods of time. It is difficult to compare histological
data reported up to now because of the difference in the intervals
at which the determinations were performed.

In order to evaluate the efficacy of this treatment, in our
opinion, it is necessary to perfect the parameters used (duration
and potency of therapy, exposition time, determination of itracel-
lular location of HpD) and to learn more about the mechanism of cell
destruction. These are open problems which must be solved at an
experimental level before this treatment, which must still be prov-
ed to be effective in the therapy of brain tumors, may be applied
in man.

SUMMARY

The authors describe HpD determination in normal brain tissue
and in experimental brain tumors induced by ENU in rats. In the
same study the animals were treated with laser irradiation (HpD +
dye laser).

Histological evaluation were made of the following: 1) the effects of the therapy with laser light only in animal controls,
2) the effects of HpD + laser in another group of animal controls,

and 3) the effects of HpD + laser in a group of animals with tumors induced by ENU.

The histologic evaluations refer to a brief period of observation; therefore data on tissue alterations caused by HpD + laser cannot be considered definitive.

REFERENCES

Carpenter, R. J. III, Neel, H. B., Ryan, R. J., Sanderson, D. R., 1977, Tumor fluorescence with Hematoporphyrin Derivative, Ann. Otol. Rhinol. Laryngol., 86:661.

Diamond, I., Granelli, S. G., McDonogh, A. F., Nielson, S., Wilson, C. B., Jaenicke, R. , 1972, Photodynamic therapy of malignant tumors, Lancet, 2:1175.

Dougherty, T. J., Grindey, G. B., Fiel, R. , Weishaupt, K. R., Boyle, D. G., 1975, Photoradiation therapy, II, Cure of animal tumors with Hematoporphyrin and light, J. Nat'l Cancer Inst., 55:115.

Dougherty, T. J., Gomer, C. J., Weishaupt, K. R., 1976, Energetics and efficiency of photoinactivation of murine tumor cells containing Hematoporphyrin, Cancer Res., 36:2330.

Dougherty, T. J., Kaufman, J. E., Goldfarb, A., Weishaupt, K. R., Mittleman, D., Mittleman, A., 1978, Photoradiation therapy for treatment of malignant tumors, Cancer Res., 38:2628.

Gomer, C. J., Dougherty, J. D., 1979, Determination of ^{3}H and ^{14}C Hematoporphyrin Derivative distribution in malignant and normal tissue, Cancer Res., 39:146.

Grossi-Paoletti, E., Paoletti, P., Pezzotta, S., Schiffer, D., Fabiani, A., 1972, Tumors of the nervous system induced by ethylnitrosourea administered either intracerebrally or subcutaneously to newborn rats. Morphological and biochemical characteristics, J. Neurosurg., 37:580.

Jori, G., Pizzi, G. B., Reddi, E., Tomio, L., Salvato, B., Zorat, P., Calzavara, F., 1979, Time dependence of Hematoporphyrin distribution in selected tissues of normal rats in ascites hepatoma, Tumori, 65:425.

Laws, E. F. Jr., Cortese, A. N., Kinsey, J. H., Eagan, R. T., Anderson, R. E., 1981, Photoradiation therapy in the treatment of malignant brain tumors: A phase I (feasibility) study, Neurosurg., 9:672.

Lemberg, R., Legge, J. W., 1949, "Hematin Compounds and Bile Pigments", Interscience Publishers Inc., New York.

Leonard, J. R., Beck, W. L., 1971, Hematoporphyrin fluorescence: and aid in diagnosis of malignant neoplasm, Laryngoscope, 81:365.

Lipson, R. L., Baldes, E. J., Olsen, A. M., 1961, The use of a derivative of Hematoporphyrin in tumor detection, J. Nat'l Cancer Inst., 26:1.

Perria, C., Capurso, T., Cavagnaro, G., Datti, R., Francavilla, N.,

Rivano, C., Tacero, V. E., 1980, First attempt at the photo-
    dynamic treatment of human gliomas, J. N. Science, 24:119.
Rounds, D. E., Jaques, S., Shelden, C. H., Shaller, C. A., Olson,
    R. S., 1982, Development of a protocol for photoradiation
    therapy of malignant brain tumors; Part 1, Neurosurgery,
    11:500.
Schiffer, D., Giordana, M. T., Pezzotta, S., Lechner, C., Paoletti,
    P., 1978, Cerebral tumors by transplacental ENU; a study of
    the different tumoral stages, particularly of early neoplas-
    tic proliferations, Act. Neuropathol. (Berl), 41:27.
Schiffer, D., Giordana, M. T., Mauro, A., Racagni, G., Bruno, F.,
    Pezzotta, S., Paoletti, P., 1980, Experimental brain tumors
    by transplacental ENU. Multi-factorial study of the latency
    period, Acta Neuropathol. (Berl), 49:117.
Spanu, G., Pezzotta, S., Cubeddu, R., Andreoni, A., Giordana, M. T.,
    1983, HpD and laser applied to ENU induced brain tumors,
    Phronesys (in press).
Weishaupt, K. R., Gomer, C. J., Dougherty, T. J., 1976, Identifica-
    tion of singlet oxygen as agent in photo-inactivation of a
    murine tumor, Cancer Res., 36:2326.
Winkelman, J., Rasmussen-Taxdal, D. S., 1960, Quantitative determi-
    nation of porphyrin uptake by tumor tissue following paren-
    teral administration, Bull Hopkins Hosp., 107:228.

STUDIES WITH HEMATOPORPHYRIN DERIVATIVE

IN TRANSPLANTABLE UROTHELIAL TUMORS

M. Kreimer-Birnbaum[1,5]*, J.E. Klaunig[2], R. Keck[3],
P.J. Goldblatt[2], S.L. Britton[4], and S.H. Selman[3]

[1]Research Department and Porphyrin Laboratory
St. Vincent Hospital and Medical Center, Toledo OH 43608 USA
Departments of [2]Pathology, [3]Surgery (Div. of Urology), [4]Physiology
[5]Biochemistry, Medical College of Ohio, Toledo OH 43699 USA

INTRODUCTION

HpD is a mixture of dicarboxylic porphyrins with tumor localizing as well as photosensitizing properties. The active component(s)
of HpD and the alkali solubilized HpD, hereafter referred to as
HpD(Inj.), have been under intense study in many laboratories
(general ref.: Kessel and Dougherty, 1983).

The mechanisms of porphyrin uptake by cells, their apparent
preferential uptake (retention?) by tumors, and the photosensitization mechanisms remain to be elucidated. This communication summarizes our attempts to characterize the component porphyrins in HpD
and various HpD(Inj.) preparations. It also describes the interactions of HpD(Inj.) with cultured rat bladder cells in vitro, and
with transplantable tumors in vivo.

Abbreviations; HpD = Hematoporphyrin derivative; HpD(Inj.) =
Hematoporphyrin derivative (Injectable); Hp = Hematoporphyrin;
HVD = Hydroxyethyl vinyl deuteroporphyrin; Pp = Protoporphyrin;
HEPES = N-2-hydroxyethylpiperazine-N'-2-ethanesulfonic acid;
PBS = Phosphate buffered saline; TLC = Thin layer chromatography;
FANFT = N-(4-(5-nitro-2-furyl)-2-thiazolyl)formamide; NRBL =
Normal rat bladder cells

---

*To whom correspondence should be addressed at St. Vincent Hospital
and Medical Center

MATERIALS AND METHODS

Porphyrins

Hp, HVD, and Pp were obtained from Porphyrin Products (Logan, Utah, USA). "Photofrin"[R] and Hematoporphyrin diacetate were obtained from Oncology Research & Development, Inc. (Cheektowaga, NY, USA). HpD(Inj.) was prepared from HpD (Porphyrin Products) as per Kessel (personal communication).

Cell Cultures. Two types of cells were used: Normal rat bladder cells = RBL-01 were developed in one of our laboratories (Klaunig et al., manuscript in preparation). AY-27 Cells were kindly supplied by Dr. R. Chaplowski (U. of Mass., Worcester, MA, USA) and are derived from a FANFT-induced transitional cell carcinoma.

Both cultured cell types showed no apparent changes in growths when maintained in serum-free media for up to 48 hrs. Cells were grown in a humidified 3% CO_2:97% air atmosphere, at 36.5°C. For the individual experiments, cells were trypsinized and plated. Prior to the HpD(Inj.) uptake experiments, the culture media were removed. All subsequent processing was done in dimmed lights. Incubations with HpD(Inj.) in Dulbecco's PBS (GIBCO, Grand Island, NY, USA), in concentrations ranging from 10 to 25 µg/ml, were run for 1 hr. After the incubations were completed, media containing porphyrins were removed, and the cells washed 3 or 4 times with PBS. Porphyrins were extracted from the cells with Triton X-100:50 mM HEPES, pH 7.0 (0.6% v/v). Quantitation of the extracted porphyrins was done by fluorometry, using appropriate standards. Cell viability was determined by Trypan Blue exclusion, before and after incubations with HpD(Inj.). Cell counts were done on aliquots of trypsinized suspensions with the aid of a Hemocytometer. Protein was determined by the method of Lowry et al. (1951), using bovine serum albumin as the standard. From the relative fluorescent intensities and the protein levels, porphyrin uptake per mg of protein was calculated. Each value represents the average of at least triplicate plates.

Chromatographic Procedures: For identification of porphyrins, two analytical TLC systems were used: System A on Silica Gel G (Ellfolk and Sievers, 1966; and Henderson et al., 1980) and System B, reverse phase chromatography on KC_{18} plates, as per Kessel (1982).

In vivo studies: Transplantable AY-27 urothelial tumors were propagated in syngeneic Fischer 344 rats (Charles River, Boston, MA, USA) by trocar technique. In each animal two tumors were grown on the midline of the abdominal wall, one below the xiphoid process (A tumor) and the other above the pubis (B tumor). Further details on the HpD(Inj.) and light treatments, as well as the blood flow determinations by a radioactive microsphere technique are given in Selman et al. (1983).

RESULTS AND DISCUSSION

TLC Characterization of HpD and HpD(Inj.) Preparations

Resolution of the HpD(Inj.) major components by System A was satisfactory. Mixtures of Pp, HVD and Hp were clearly separated and the individual components identified. However, this system worked less than satisfactorily when the HpD preparations were analyzed. Acetyl derivatives of Hp and HVD were found to have Rf coinciding with some of the tertiary alcohol markers. The HpD(Inj.) preparations, having been subjected to alkaline hydrolysis, were supposed to have lost all their acetylated derivatives (Dougherty et al., 1978; Bonnett et al., 1981). That this is indeed the case was clearly shown by reverse phase TLC (System B). HpD(Inj.) showed as its four major components Hp, HVD (isomers) and to a lesser extent Pp. HpD, on the other side, showed at least 3 main additional components that disappear during the solubilization process. One of these components runs with an Rf very close to one of the HVD isomers and it has been identified as diacetyl Hp by comparison with the compound kindly supplied by Dr. A. Smith (L.S.U. Med. Center, New Orleans, LA, USA) and prepared according to Bonnett et al. (1981).

When the HpD(Inj.) prepared from various HpD powders and Photofrin[R] were compared, their TLC profiles were found to be similar and comparable to reported profiles obtained by HPLC (Moan et al., 1982; Cadby et al., 1982; Dougherty et al., 1983). However, one HpD(Inj.) preparation showed no obvious changes in its TLC profile yet was lacking in biological activity when tested in vivo (see below). Our observations are consistent with the remarks of Dougherty (1982) that it is not clear how the biological phenomena of localization and photosensitization are related to the porphyrin components in the mixtures, or why apparently similarly prepared injectable solutions show variable biological activity.

In vitro Uptake of HpD(Inj.) Components by Cultured Rat Bladder Cells

Table 1 summarizes the apparent uptake of HpD(Inj.) components by AY-27 and NRBL cells, after incubation for 1 hr. Extracts from NRBL cells showed levels of about 50 to 60% from those found in the transformed cells. For AY-27 cells, the porphyrin uptake was 0.80 µg per mg of protein, while the comparable uptake by the NRBL was 0.47 µg per mg protein. Henderson et al. (1983) have reported porphyrin uptake by four different cell lines ranging from 0.06 to 0.1 (1 hr) and from 0.15 to 0.25 µg porphyrins per mg of protein, after 2 to 4 hour incubations and essentially no differences between transformed and normal cells. Our experiments were conducted with serum-free media and this may account for the apparently higher rate of uptake by both cell lines, as suggested by Chang and Dougherty (1978). The protection afforded to cells by added serum has been

Table 1. In vitro uptake of HpD(Inj.) components by rat bladder cells[*]

Cell Type	Extraction Solvent	ng porphyrins /plate	µg protein /plate	µg porphyrins /mg protein
AY-27	Triton:HEPES	976+95	1220	0.80
NRBL	Triton:HEPES	488+64	1043	0.47

[*]AY-27 cells derived from a transitional cell carcinoma and NRBL, normal rat bladder cells, were exposed to HpD(Inj.) in PBS (10 µg/ml) at 36.5°C for 1 hr. Incubation media was removed, 3 washes with PBS followed and the porphyrins were later extracted as described in Materials and Methods. Values represent mean+S.D. of 3-6 plates.

reported by other laboratories and confirmed by us (Klaunig et al., unpublished). With respect to the apparently higher levels of porphyrins found in malignant versus non-transformed cells, our results tend to confirm Mossman's et al. (1974) observations. Moan et al. (1981) also found slightly higher uptake of porphyrins per unit volume of malignant cells, but in spite of the difference in uptake, degrees of photosensitivity were comparable for both cell types.

We do not feel these short time incubations completely explain the observed higher content of porphyrins found in tumors in vivo after systemic administration of HpD(Inj.). This differential uptake or retention phenomenon constitutes the basis for photoradiation therapy. One may postulate that other mechanisms such as poor lymphatic drainage are operational in vivo as suggested by Bugelski et al. (1981). Another mechanism may be the preferential retention of porphyrins by tumors through the intracellular transformation of those porphyrins with hydrophobic side chains into more hydrophilic ones that would preclude their excretion (Kessel, 1982).

Further studies of the porphyrins extracted from cultured rat bladder cells after short term incubation (in serum free media) were conducted by spectro-fluorometric analysis and TLC. It was found that an apparently higher proportion of the most hydrophobic porphyrins in the HpD(Inj.) preparations such as HVD and Pp had been retained by the cells (Kreimer-Birnbaum et al., 1983). These data would support the conclusions arrived at by Kessel (1982) and Moan et al. (1982).

Treatment of Transplantable AY-27 Urothelial Tumors in vivo

Our early experiments using HpD(Inj.) and phototherapy for the treatment of subcutaneous transplantable FANFT-induced tumors in syngeneic Fischer 344 rats demonstrated histologic evidence of early post-treatment hemorrhagic necrosis. From these observations we

Table 2.   Blood flow determinations in 4 groups of animals

Group [*]	Treatment [¤]	A Tumor Flow (ml/min/g)	B Tumor Flow (ml/min/g)
I	No HpD(Inj.) No Light	0.684+0.226	0.575+0.127
II	HpD(Inj.) only No Light	0.477+0.153	0.432+0.117
III	A: Light (B Control)	0.266+0.082	0.213+0.036
	B: Light (A Control)	0.295+0.080	0.281+0.062
IV	A: HpD(Inj.)+Light (B Control)	0.022+0.009	0.195+0.044
	B: HpD(Inj.)+Light (A Control)	0.294+0.101	0.046+0.018

[*]Four groups, I–no treatment; II–HpD(Inj.) only; III–light only; IV–HpD(Inj.) + light. All animals had two subcutaneous tumors on the abdominal wall; in animals receiving light treatment one tumor served as a control. Light source: 500 watt Kodak projector fitted with red 2418 filter; light intensity 200 mW/cm^2. [¤]Treatment for 30 minutes, 24 hr after intravenous HpD(Inj.) (10 µg/g b.w.). Blood flow determined by radioactive microsphere (15 µ) technique 10 minutes after phototherapy in animals receiving light treatment. Only HpD(Inj.) + phototherapy treated tumors showed significant ($p < 0.05$) difference in blood flow over light-shielded controls. Values represent mean $\pm$ S.E., n = 6. (Selman et al., 1983)

hypothesized that HpD(Inj.) and phototherapy disrupted blood flow rendering these tumors anoxic. This hypothesis was tested and results are summarized in Table 2. HpD(Inj.) and phototherapy resulted in a statistically significant decrease in blood flow within ten minutes of completion of therapy, while HpD(Inj.) or phototherapy alone were without significant effect. Twenty-four hours after completion of phototherapy (data not shown), reductions in blood flows were similar to the ones observed after 10 minutes. Thus disruption of blood flow may be a key mechanism in the photo-destruction of tumors.

Acknowledgements: Supported in part by grants from the F. M. Douglass Foundation, the American Cancer Society (Ohio Division,

Inc.), and B.R.S. SO-7-RR 05700-12, -13. Special thanks to Ms.
K. E. Schultz for preparation of the manuscript, to Mr. B. Barut
for assisting with the cell cultures, and to Mr. M. Lust for
excellent technical assistance.

REFERENCES

Bonnett, R., Ridge, R. J., Scourides, P. A., and Berenbaum, M. C.,
    1981, On the nature of 'haematoporphyrin derivative.' J.
    Chem. Soc. Perkin Trans. I 37:3135.
Bugelski, P. J., Porter, C. W., and Dougherty, T. J., 1981, Auto-
    radiographic distribution of hematoporphyrin derivative in
    normal and tumor tissue of the mouse, Cancer Res. 41:4606.
Cadby, P. A., Dimitriadis, E., Grant, H. G., Ward, A. D., and Forbes,
    I. J., 1982, Separation and analysis of haematoporphyrin
    derivative components by high-performance liquid chromato-
    graphy, J. Chromatogr. 231:273.
Chang, C. T., and Dougherty, T. J., 1978, Photoradiation therapy:
    kinetics and thermodynamics of porphyrin uptake and loss in
    normal and malignant cells in culture, Radiat. Res. 74:498.
Dougherty, T. J., Boyle, D. G., Weishaupt, K. R., Henderson, B. A.,
    Potter, W. R., Bellnier, D. A., and Wityk, K. E., 1983,
    Photoradiation therapy - clinical and drug advances, in:
    "Porphyrin Photosensitization," D. Kessel and T. J. Dougherty,
    eds., Plenum Press, New York.
Dougherty, T. J., Kaufman, J. E., Goldfarb, A., Weishaupt, K. R.,
    Boyle, D., and Mittelman, A., 1978, Photoradiation therapy
    for the treatment of malignant tumors, Cancer Res. 38:2628.
Dougherty, T. J., 1982, Variability in hematoporphyrin derivative
    preparations, Cancer Res. 42:1188.
Ellfolk, N., and Sievers, G., 1966, Thin layer chromatography of
    free porphyrins, J. Chromatogr. 25:373.
Henderson, R. W., Bellnier, D. A., Ziring, B., and Dougherty, T. J.,
    1983, Aspects of the cellular uptake and retention of hemato-
    porphyrin derivative and their correlation with the biologi-
    cal response to PRT in vitro, in: "Porphyrin Photosensiti-
    zation," Plenum Press, New York.
Henderson, R. W., Christie, G. S., Clezy, P. S., and Lineham, J.,
    1980, Haematoporphyrin diacetate: a probe to distinguish
    malignant from normal tissue by selective fluorescence,
    Brit. J. Exper. Pathol. 61:345.
Kessel, D., 1982, Components of hematoporphyrin derivatives and
    their tumor-localizing capacity, Cancer Res. 42:1703.
Kessel, D., and Dougherty, T. J., 1983, "Porphyrin Photosensitiza-
    tion," Plenum Press, New York.
Kreimer-Birnbaum, M., Baumann, J. L., Klaunig, J. E., Keck, R.,
    Goldblatt, P. J., and Selman, S. H., 1983, Chemical studies
    with hematoporphyrin derivative in bladder cell lines, in:
    "Clayton Symposium on Porphyrin Localization and Treatment

of Tumors," D. R. Doiron and C. J. Gomer, eds., Alan R. Liss,
    New York, in press.
Lowry, O. H., Rosebrough, A., Farr, A. L., and Randall, R. J.,
    1951, Protein measurement with the Folin phenol reagent, J.
    Biol. Chem. 193:265.
Moan, J., McGhie, J. B., and Christensen, T., 1982, Hematoporphyrin
    derivative: photosensitizing efficiency and cellular uptake
    of its components, Photobiochem. Photobiophys. 4:337.
Moan, J., Steen, H. B., Feren, K., and Christensen, T., 1981, Uptake
    of hematoporphyrin derivative and sensitized photoinactiva-
    tion of C3H cells with different oncogenic potential, Cancer
    Lett. 14:291.
Mossman, B. T., Gray, M. J., Silberman, L., and Lipson, L., 1974,
    Identification of neoplastic versus normal cells in human
    cervical cell culture, J. Obstet. Gynaecol. 43:635.
Selman, S. H., Keck, R., Klaunig, J. E., Kreimer-Birnbaum, M.,
    Goldblatt, P. J., and Britton, S. L., 1983, Acute blood flow
    changes in transplantable FANFT-induced urothelial tumors
    treated with hematoporphyrin derivative and light, Surgical
    Forum, in press.

TIME DEPENDANCE OF 3H HEMATOPORPHYRIN DERIVATIVE DISTRIBUTION
IN THE DIGESTIVE TRACT IN THE RAT

G. Sabben, A. Bosshard and R. Lambert

Hepatogastroenterology and INSERM U.45

Pav. H bis Hospital E. Herriot 69374 Lyon, France

Application of Laser irradiation with Hematoporphyrin Derivative to the destruction of digestive tumors in the humans require preliminary studies of the method in animals. The HPD distribution is to be determined in normal tissues and in digestive cancers. Thereafter if HPD levels are higher in the digestive tumor than in normal tissues, this method would be safe.

This study concerns the labelled HPD distribution in the digestive tissues of normal rats.

MATERIAL AND METHOD

In this experiment, HPD (Photofrin I) from Oncology Research Development (Cheektowaga N.Y.) was triatiated by catalytic exchange (Center of Atomic Study - Saclay - France)with a specific activity of 135 mCi/mmol. Thin layer chromatography of labelled and unlabelled HPD were identical. Male Fischer rats (weight 300 g) were choosen because they are syngenic animals and then potential receivers of transplanted digestive tumors. Following an IV injection of triatiated HPD (10 mg/kg) the rats were sacrificed at 1-2-4-6-12-48-72 hours with 6 animals at each time. Duplicate samples were taken at each interval of time in blood (sera - red cells) esophagus, fundus, antrum, small intestine and colon. For digestive tissues, the mucosa was separated from the muscular layer before analysis. The following tissues samples were collected as controls : lung, liver, spleen and kidney. The radioactivity of each wet-weighted sample was determined after combustion using a Packard Tricarb Model 306 oxidizer and then expressed after calculation as μg/g of wet tissue.

RESULTS

The mean half-life of triatiated HPD in the serum is 3 hours. In all tissues the maximum HPD concentrations are obtained at 4 hours followed by a slow decrease till 72 hours.

The highest levels are detected in lung (at 4 hours : 185 μg/g, liver 183 μg/g), spleen (119 μg/g) and kidney 23 μg/g) while very low HPD concentrations are obtained in the digestive tract. Level measured in the esophagus and the colon are lower than in the small intestine (Table I).

Table. 1, HpD Concentrations in Digestive Mucosae
Mean + SEM μg/g

	1 h	4 h	72 h
Esoph.	2.10 + 0.23	2.94 + 0.70	2.01 + 0.29
Fundus	3.16 + 0.16	2.52 + 0.15	1.34 + 0.11
Antrum	3.05 + 0.18	5.25 + 0.39	2.36 + 0.21
Small intest.	6.28 + 0.46	8.10 + 0.56	4.53 + 0.54
Colon	2.27 + 0.13	2.40 + 0.26	1.76 + 0.10

Furthermore the distribution of HPD is similar to the digestive mucosae and the muscular layer in the different organs of the digestive tract. The ratio of mucosal/muscular concentrations of HPD does not vary from 1 with the time factor (4 - 72 h). Thenceforth not dependy of the cell turn over in epidermoid vs glandular mucosae.

On histoautoradiography Kuppfer cells are labelled in the liver and macrophagic cells are labelled in the lung and the spleen. The detection of labelled cells in the digestive mucosae is more difficult (low activity) however labelled macrophagic cells are detected at 4 hours in the small intestine.

CONCLUSION

Following an IV injection in Fischer rats the serum half-life of triatiated HPD is 3 hours with a maximum uptake at 4 hours in tissues. HPD concentrations in the digestive mucosae are low when compared to the liver. The affinity to normal digestive mucosae does not differ whatever the structure of the mucosae, epidermoid or glandular. These results speak for the reasonnable safety at 72 hours of the phototherapy method for the surrounding normal tissues when a digestive cancer is to be treated.

Moreover two hypothesis are suggested. An enterohepatic circulation may exist because of the high HPD levels in liver and small intestine. A detoxication mechanism may occur by RES cells.

REFERENCES

GOMER CJ, DOUGHERTY TJ
Determination of 3H and 14C hematoporphyrin derivative distribution in malignant and normal tissue.
Cancer Research, 1979, 39, 146-151

TOMIO L, ZORAT PL, JORI G, REDDI E, SALVATO B, CORTI L, CALZAVARA F
Elimination pathway of hematoporphyrin from normal and tumor bearing rats.
Tumori, 1982, 68, 283-286

Nd YAG DESTRUCTION OF TUMOR SENSITIZED

OR NON SENSITIZED BY HPD

Thierry Patrice, Marie-Françoise Le Bodic, Christos
Roussakis, Yves Le Tourneux, Louis Le Bodic

Department Laser CMB
2ème étaqe Hôtel-Dieu
Nantes - France

For 2 years in Pr. Le Bodic Laser Department we have tried
to improve the efficiency of the Nd-Yag Laser in the laser treatment especially in the destruction of tumors.

In order to reach this aim we studied the Nd-Yag laser action
on solid tumours sensitized by HPD. In the same way we were
interested by the action mechanism of the Nd-Yag laser. So we
made a study in which in used culture cells as experimental model
and we can give now the preleminary résults.

I - Action of the Nd-Yag laser on solid state tumours sensitized by HPD.

Materials and methods:

1 - Material : the energy was a Nd-Yag laser(Cilas) emitting
in the near infra-red (1,06 μm). The beam is transmitted by an
optic fiber of 600 μm diameter and surrounded by a teflon sheath
through wich a coaxial azote stream circulates under a pression
of 4 bars. The divergence is of 10° and the distance fiber-tissue
is constant (5 mm). A system, combining a thermopile 101 and 1
energy meter 102 is used to measure the power at the end of the
optic fiber. The He-Ne laser visualisation beam was off during
all the experiment. The hematoprophyrim derivated is prepared
according to Lipson and Gregory method :
   - the experiment animal is the male nude albino mouse
   - the tumour graft is carried out by under cutaneous injection of a crushed tumour colic adenocarcinoma in a culture solution. This solid state tumour usually has a spontaneous necrosis

247

rate inferior to 5 % and is maintained in vivo according to the NCI standards.

2 - Methods : the mice are divided into 5 groups.

Group I : 14 mice bearing adenocarcinoma received 9 days after the graft an injection of HPD (5 mgkg IV). The tumour is irradiated at a power of 45 W with an exposure time of 1,5 s on the tenth day.

The shots are joined (AV number of shots per tumour is 5).

Gr. IIa : The grafted tumours are not treated and are used to check the spontaneous necrosis rate.

Gr. IIb : The tumours were irradiated according to the condition described above, but without preliminary HPD sensibilisation.

Gr. IIc : The 8 tumours of this group received only an HPD injection without laser irradiation.

Gr. IId : After an HPD injection the eight tumours of the group were exposed to the daylight for 10 mn in order to show that the surrouding light doesn't interfere in the reactions we observed. Tumours of the 5 groups are 48 hours after the irradiation (D 12), fixed by formoldehyde 12 %, then colored with hemalum safran eosin to proceed to an anatomic examination.

Results : Whereas the Gr. IIa tumours don't show necrosis the 11 G. I tumours show a huge acidophilic necrosis, destructing all the tissue and cellular structures (nuclei ++). The other three tumours from this group show in incomplete acidophilic necrosis by covering nearly 90 % of the tumour. As far, the IIb group tumours,show an considerable necrosis but different at the qualitative level. Actually it means a non acidophilic coagulation necrosis showing an important oedema and a visible picnosis of nuclei. The frame remains the same. The IIe and IId groups have a necrosis never superior to 15 % of the tumour (3 photos).

To sum up, in Gr. I, in which the tumours were sensitized by HPD and irradiated by Nd Yag-Laser, we can observe a total necrosis more important than with the laser only and acidophilic. The reaction leading the necrosis varies in Gr. I and Gr. IIb, at the same power. This suppose that the reaction is altered after HPD sensibilisation.

II - At this stage we wanted to know whether laser effect was similar to those described with laser emitting in 632 mn (photochemical effect) or the heat could intervene in the reaction. So, we used a cell line in suspension, the P 388 cell. We irradiated the P 388 cell after HPD sensitisation or not, but maintaining heat rise at 3° c. The cells come from a lymphoblastic leukemia induced by the methyl cholanthren and conserved in culture according to the NCI standards especially as far as the increase rate is concerned.

Material and methods : The laser source and HPD are similar, such as the optic fiber. The irradiation system only is different.

The distance optic fiber-target is 17 cm and the power 10 W.
The attenuation of the beam by the flask wall was 0,5 W. The
energy was varying from 60 to 400 J/cm^2 by modification of the
time exposure. Each flask contained a ml of Cl Na 0,9 °/oo, 3 ml
of cell suspension with 0,66 10^5 cell/ml of RPMI. For the HPD
sensitisation we added 25 g/ml HPD 30 minutes before the laser
irradiation.

The temperature of the room was 22° c during the irradiation
and the heat rise caused by the laser inferior to 4° c (measured
by thermocouple). We made 2 measures per flask of the cellular
inhibition rate obtained in these conditions for a constant laser
power. Simultaneously we took measures in two flasks without laser
but with incubation with HPD and two flasks irradiated by laser
without HPD.

The exposure and temperature were similar for all the flasks.

Results : We notice at once that in these conditions the Nd-
Yag laser, induces an inhibition compared to HPD only.

HPD may be toxic for the cell line we used. But the Nd-Yag laser irradiation mechanism is different from the lasers emmitting
in the red, since for a similar power, no noticable reaction in
vitro and even a reduction of the inhibition are observed. The
heat rise even weak makes enter the P 388 cells into mitosis
(which have a reduced metabolism at 22° c). The longer is the
exposure time, the more obvious is the phenomenon.

In conclusion, we can assert that the Nd-Yag laser is active
in vivo on solid state tumours. This activity is increased after
HPD sensitisation but the phenomenon is not observed when we
reduce the heat rise. The Nd-Yag laser irradiation mechanism is
different from the lasers emmitting at 632 nm.

HpD PHOTOTHERAPY ON SPONTANEOUS TUMORS IN DOG AND CAT

Renato Cheli, Flaminio Addis, Carlo M. Mortellaro, Diego
Fonda, Alessandra Andreoni[*], and Rinaldo Cubeddu[*]

Clinica Chirurgica Veterinaria, Unversità degli Studi
di Milano, Italy

[*]Centro Elettronica Quantistica e Strumentazione
Elettronica del C.N.R., Istituto di Fisica del Politecnico
Milano, Italy

INTRODUCTION

Phototherapy with Hematoporphyrin Derivative (HpD) was performed in 26 clinical cases on 11 types of spontaneous tumors in
dog and in cat, in most cases untreatable by conventional means.
The tumors consisted in 7 squamous cell carcinomas of the mouth
and tonsils, 5 mastocytomas of the skin, 4 eosinophilic granulomas
of the lip and the skin, 2 adenocarcinomas of the nasal glands, 2
reticulum cell carcinomas of the lip, 1 osteolytic sarcoma of the
radius, 1 carcinoma of circumanal glands and in the oral cavity 1
hemangiopericytoma, 1 liposarcoma, 1 melanoma, and 1 fibrosarcoma.

METHODS

48 hours after intravenous injection of HpD, the tumor masses
were treated with the light. HpD (Photofrin I) was provided by
Oncology Research and Development Inc. (Cheektowaga, N.Y., USA) and
was administered at the dose of 2.5 mg/kg body weight in the first
set of animals and 5.0 mg/kg body weight in the second set. As a
light source, we used a Rhodamine B dye laser continuously pumped
by an argon laser and tuned at 631 nm wavelength with an output
power up to 2 watts. The irradiations were carried out coupling the
light to an optical fiber usually applied externally, sometimes
inserted into the tumor mass and in three cases introduced completely into the nasal cavities. Subsequent irradiations were performed

251

Table 1.   Phototherapy after I.V. Injection of 2.5 mg/kg HpD.

HISTOLOGICAL TYPE	LOCATION/SIZE	ENERGY FLUENCE $(\frac{mW}{cm^2} \times min)(\frac{J}{cm^2})$		RESPONSE (follow-up)
1. MASTOCYTOMA (dog)	dorsal skin (1 cm^2)	300 x 45'	810	NR
2. MASTOCYTOMA (dog)	preputial skin (0.8 cm^2)	225 x 20'	270	NR
3. HEMANGIOPERICYTOMA (dog)	oral cavity (2.5 cm^2)	240 x 15'	192	NR
4. OSTEOLYTIC SARCOMA (dog)	distal radio (2 cm^2)	150 x 60'	540°	PR
5. EOSINOPHILIC GRANULOMA (cat)	lip (1 cm^2)	300 x 7'	126	CR (6 months)
6. EOSINOPHILIC GRANULOMA (cat)	thigh skin (6 cm^2)	83 x 24' 83 x 22'	120 110*	PR
7. LIPOSARCOMA (dog)	oral cavity (17.5 cm^2)	46 x 60'	165	NR
8. MELANOMA (dog)	hard palate (8 cm^2)	75 x 30' 80 x 30'	135 144	PR
9. MASTOCYTOMA (dog)	lip (8.7 cm^2)	171 x 10' 274 x 10' 274 x 7' 103 x 30'	103 165 115* 185	CR (7 months)
10. EOSINOPHILIC GRANULOMA (cat)	lip (0.3 cm^2)	667 x 10' 667 x 30"	400 40*	CR (28 months)
11. RETICULUM CELL SARCOMA (dog)	lip (3 cm^2)	167 x 15' 400 x 15' 400 x 35' 400 x 30'	150 360 840*° 720°	SR
12. SQUAMOUS CELL CARCINOMA (dog)	oral cavity (6 cm^2)	400 x 10' 267 x 15' 500 x 15' 233 x 30'	240 240 450* 420	SR, LR
13. NASAL GLAND ADENOCARCINOMA (dog)⁰	nasal cavities (2.5 cm^2)	76 x 10'	49	CR (7 months)

⁰ Tumor treated after surgical exeresis.

* Irradiation 15 days after HpD injection.

° With inserted fiber into tumor mass.

within 10 days from HpD injection.

These results of therapeutic effects were evaluated on the ground of histological and clinical features. Histologically we reported the positive or negative biopsies obtained in every case from tissue sections. The clinical evaluation was divided into the following grades: no remission (NR) = less than 20% of the original tumor volume disappeared; partial remission (PR) = more then 20% but less than 60% of the original tumor disappeared; significant remission (SR) = 60% or more of the original tumor mass disappeared; complete remission (CR) = no tumor was evident; early recurrence (ER) = a new local tumor appeared in a month after the treatment; late recurrence (LR) = a new local tumor appeared in more than a month after the treatment.

RESULTS

Table 1 and 2 show the therapeutic results of the phototherapy with HpD. In the first set of animals, injected intravenously with 2.5 mg/kg body weight of HpD, we treated 13 neoplasms without encouraging results or with a low therapeutic effect (Table 1): we had no remission (NR) in 30% of the cases, partial reduction (between 20%-70% of the original tumor volume) in 40% of the cases and complete remission (CR) in about 30% of the cases. The longest follow-up that was of 28 months in a surviving cat, after two treatments (n. 13); the others were that of 7 months in a dog with a large neoplasia (n. 9), and that of 6 months in a cat (n. 5). The fourth tumor, an adenocarcinoma of the nasal glands, had been surgically removed by a previously rhinotomy and the residual part of nasal cavities was positively irradiated, obtaining a clinical follow-up to 7 months after the last treatment.

About the other cases reported in Table 1 it must be noted that: (i) the four tumors without remission (n. 1,2,3,7) had only one treatment; (ii) the light intensity used in the first nine cases (n. 1-9) was near that used by other researchers[1,2,3,4], while in the cases n. 10, n. 11 and n. 12 we used higher intensities in shorter time. This gave the advantage of reducing the irradiation times and seemed to improve the clinical effect. So we treated almost all the tumors of the second group of animals at high intensities.

In front of these results, in the second set of tumors, we doubled the HpD dosage (5.0 mg/kg body weight) on the treatment of 13 neoplasms, with high positive therapeutic effects (Table 2): we obtained complete remission in 100% of the cases, though we had four recurrences and one case of regional metastasis. As these treatments begun 10 months ago, the longest follow-up to date were those of 9 months (n. 10) in the tumors previously treated with

Table 2. Phototherapy after I.V. Injection of 5 mg/kg HpD.

HISTOLOGICAL TYPE	LOCATION/SIZE	ENERGY FLUENCE $(\frac{mW}{cm^2}$ x min$)(\frac{J}{cm^2})$		RESPONSE (follow-up)
1. SQUAMOUS CELL CARCINOMA (dog)	tonsil (6 cm^2)	600 x 10' 900 x 15'	360 810	CR (2 months) metastasis
2. SQUAMOUS CELL CARCINOMA (dog)	oral cavity (2 cm^2)	325 x 15'	293	CR, ER untreated
3. RETICULUM CELL SARCOMA (dog)	lip (4 cm^2)	650 x 15' 1000 x 2'	585 120	CR, LR (2 months)
4. SQUAMOUS CELL CARCINOMA (dog)	gum (2 cm^2)	600 x 15' 1600 x 3'	540 288	CR (5 months)
5. MASTOCYTOMA (cat)	lips (1 cm^2)	1800 x 3' 1800 x 3'	324 324	CR, LR (1 month)
6. EOSINOPHILIC GRANULOMA (cat)	lips (2 cm^2)	600 x 5' 1000 x 1'	180 60	CR (3 months)
7. FIBROSARCOMA (dog)	gum (0.8 cm^2)	1000 x 5'	300	CR (5 months)
8. SQUAMOUS CELL CARCINOMA (dog)	oral cavity (2 cm^2)	900 x 16' 1200 x 9' 670 x 15'	900 648 600	CR, LR (1 month)
9. CIRCUMANAL GLAND CARCINOMA (dog)	perianal skin (10 cm^2)	367 x 20' 80 x 30' 169 x 20'	400 144 203	CR (2 month)
10. NASAL GLAND ADENOCARCINOMA (dog)[o]	nasal cavities (6 cm^2)	67 x 10'	40	CR (9 months)
11. MASTOCYTOMA (dog)[o]	lip (7 cm^2)	343 x 5'	103	CR (2 months)
12. SQUAMOUS CELL CARCINOMA (dog)[o]	nasal cavities (6 cm^2)	83 x 10'	50	CR (2 months)
13. SQUAMOUS CELL CARCINOMA (dog)[o]	oral cavity (2 cm^2)	500 x 10'	300	CR (2 months)

[o] Tumor treated after surgical exeresis.

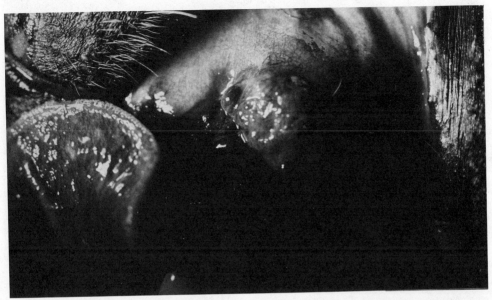

Fig. 1.   Case n. 4 of Table 2.   Squamous cell carcinoma.   Before
the first treatment.

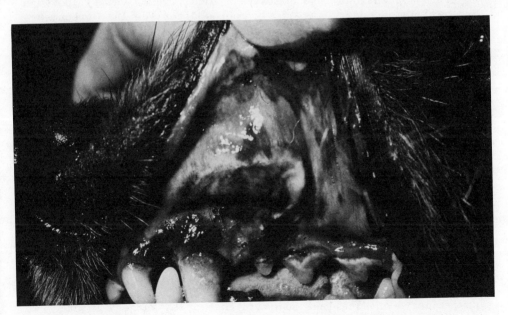

Fig. 2.   The same case.   5 days after the last treatment.

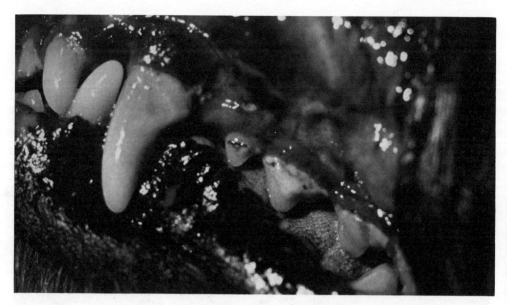

Fig. 3.   The same case.   30 days after the last treatment.

surgical exeresis, and of 5 months (n. 4 and n. 7) in the neoplasms
treated only by phototherapy (Fig.s 1,2,3). Only two cases had
negative conclusions: the dog with a tonsil tumor (n. 1) showed a
regional lymphonode metastasis 2 months after the last treatment
and was sacrificed; a squamous cell carcinoma (n. 2) after complete
remission had an early recurrence, but further treatments were not
allowed by the owner. We had also three cases of late recurrences
after 3 months (n. 3), 5 months (n. 5) and 4 months (n. 8): these
tumors were retreated with a new complete disappearence. In the
four cases treated after surgical excision (n. 10-13), only one
treatment of previous neoplastic area was necessary using lower
light intensities.

CONCLUSIONS

     On the basis of the results shown in the two Tables, it seems
that HpD phototherapy results to be a very promising therapy of
spontaneous tumors in cats and dogs, once the drug and light dosages are optimized. In fact, most of the tumor types treated by
other techniques (conventional surgery or CO_2 laser surgery) have
shown a higher recurrency, in our experience. Moreover HpD phototherapy avoids all the problems connected with surgery, like operating wounds, scars and healing problems. In a few cases phototherapy appears an excellent adjuvant therapy to surgery in order to
control residual neoplastic areas and further local recurrences.

Table 1. Hystological Type of Tumors and HpD Doses.

HYSTOLOGICAL TYPE	TOTAL CASES	HpD	
		2.5 mg/Kg	5.0 mg/Kg
SQUAMOUS CELL CARCINOMA	7	±	+ + + + + +
MASTOCYTOMA	5	- - +	± +
EOSINOPHILIC GRANULOMA	4	+ ± +	+
RETICULUM CELL SARCOMA	2	±	±
NASAL GLAND ADENOCARCINOMA	2	+	+
HEMANGIOPERICYTOMA	1	-	
OSTEOLYTIC SARCOMA	1	±	
LIPOSARCOMA	1	-	
MELANOMA	1	±	
FIBROSARCOMA	1		+
CIRCUMANAL GLAND CARCINOMA	1		+

+ complete remission

± partial reduction of the tumor mass

- no remission

A larger number of cases will allow a more accurate evaluation of the response to HpD phototherapy of each histological type of tumor (Table 3): the only thing we can say safely is that phototherapy with HpD administered at 5.0 mg/kg body weight has a high therapeutic effect on spontaneous tumors.

REFERENCES

1. K. R. Weishaupt, C. J. Gomer, and T. J. Dougherty, Energetics and efficiency of photoinactivation of murine tumor cells containing Hematoporphyrin, Cancer Res. 36:2326 (1976).
2. T. J. Dougherty, J. E. Kaufman, A. Goldfarb, K. R. Weishaupt, D. G. Boyle, and A. Mittleman, Photoradiation therapy for the treatment of malignant tumors, Cancer Res. 38:2628 (1978).
3. T. J. Dougherty, G. Lawrence, J. E. Kaufman, D. G. Boyle, K. R. Weishaupt, and A. Goldfarb, Photoradiation in the treatment of recurrent breast carcinoma, J. Natl. Cancer Inst. 62:231 (1979).

4. T. J. Dougherty, R. E. Thoma, D. G. Boyle, and K. R. Weishaupt,
    Photoradiation therapy of malignant tumors: role of the la-
    ser, in: "Lasers in Photomedicine and Photobiology", R. Pra-
    tesi and C. A. Sacchi, eds., Springer-Verlag, Berlin - Heidel-
    berg - New York (1980).

Chapter 4

Light Dosimetry and Instrumentation for Tumor Diagnosis

THERMAL AND OPTICAL DOSIMETRY FOR PHOTORADIATION THERAPY OF

MALIGNANT TUMORS

Lars O. Svaasand

Division of Physical Electronics
University of Trondheim
Trondheim, Norway

INTRODUCTION

Successful development of photoradiation therapy into an efficient clinical modality requires knowledge of the drug distribution [13] and photosensitization of the neoplastic tissue as well as information of the optical and thermal distribution [1,2].

Typical reported doses of HpD in clinical or preclinical procedures are in the range 2.5-5 mg drug per kg bodyweight administered 24-72 hours prior to irradiation at 625-640 nm wavelength. The optical dose delivered during surface irradiation is typically in the range 10-200 J/cm^2. Most researchers report necrosis of tymor cells for doses 50-200 J/cm^2, blistering and formation of eschar for doses 25-100 J/cm^2 and little or no reaction for doses smaller than 10 J/cm^2 [3-7].

The duration of the exposures has been in the range 15-60 min with a typical value 20-30 min. The corresponding dose rates vary from 15-300 mW/cm^2 with a typical value 100-200 mW/cm^2. The distinction between optical dose and optical dose rate is of fundamental importance for the interpretation of the therapeutic result. The photodynamic effect is primarily dependent on the accumulated number of excited molecules; thus it is dependent on the total optical dose. The hyperthermal contribution which depends exponentially on the temperature rise is primarily dependent on the dose rate [2]. The temperature rise is also of importance for possible synergism or thermal enhancement of the photodynamic effect [3,11].

Detailed analysis of the exact optical and thermal distribution in a high inhomogeneous medium as a vascular tumor is, however, an

impossible task. It is therefore important to simplify the description to a level where it will meet the requirements for accuracy
during clinical procedures, and simultaneously be of reasonable
mathematical complexity. The optical distribution will be approximated by optical diffusion theory [8,12] and the analysis of the thermal distribution will be based on thermal conduction and diffuse
blood perfusion [2]. The validity of this approach is limited proximal to highly anisotropic optical sources and in the vicinity of
larger blood vessels. But is should, hopefully, be adequate for the
regions which require the most precise dosimetry, i.e. the diffuse
boundaries between the normal and the invasive malignant tissue.
These regions will normally be some millimeters from the interface
between the tissue and the light source, and the blood will be distributed through capillary blood flow.

OPTICAL DISTRIBUTION

The propagation of light in tissue is governed by scattering
from inhomogeneities of the cellular structure and by absorption in
absorbing constituents such as hemoglobin, myoglobin and melanin.
The light is scattered into a more isotropic distribution after
propagating some tenths of a millimeter in most tissues. This isot-
ropy is in particular valid for the regions some millimeters from
the source.

The quantity of light may be characterized by several parameters as the radiance L, the irradiance E and the space irradiance Φ.
The radiance L is defined as the flux of optical energy in a particular direction per unit solid angle and per unit area oriented
normal to the direction $\vec{\ell}$ of propagation. The energy flux incident
on an infinitesimally small surface element dA oriented normal to
the unit vector $\vec{\ell}$ from rays within the solid angle $d\Omega$ is thus
$LdAd\Omega$. The irradiance E is defined as the total energy flux per
unit area incident on one side of a plane area. The space irradiance or the radiant energy fluence rate Φ is defined as the light
flux incident on an infinitesimally small sphere divided by the
cross-sectional area of that sphere. The relation between the irradiance, space irradiance and radiance may thus be expressed

$$E = \int_{\Omega=0}^{2\pi} L\vec{\ell}\cdot\vec{n}d\Omega \tag{1}$$

and

$$\Phi = \int_{\Omega=0}^{4\pi} Ld\Omega \tag{2}$$

where $\vec{n}$ is the unit surface normal. An exact isotropic light distribution is defined by a constant radiance in all directions. Eqs. (1) and (2) then define

$$\Phi = 4\pi L = 4E \tag{3}$$

The radiance in a region with almost isotropic irradiance may be expressed by [12]

$$L = L_m + \frac{3}{4\pi} \vec{j} \cdot \vec{\ell} \tag{4}$$

where L_m is the average radiance and $\vec{j}$ is the diffuse energy flux vector. The diffuse energy flux vector represents the net flux of diffuse energy. This energy flows in the direction of decreasing space irradiance and it may be expressed

$$\vec{j} = - \zeta \, \text{grad} \, \Phi \tag{5}$$

where ζ is defined as the diffusion coefficient. The absorbed optical power is dependent on the flux of optical energy incident from all directions onto an absorbing spherical molecule. The steady state energy balance requires that this power must be transported into the particular element of volume by the diffuse energy flux vector. This balance may thus be written

$$-\text{div} \, \vec{j} = \beta \Phi \tag{6}$$

where $-\text{div} \, \vec{j}$ is the influx of energy per unit volume, $\beta \Phi$ is the absorbed power and β is the absorption coefficient. Substitution of Eq. (5) in Eq. (6) gives

$$\text{divgrad} \, \Phi - \frac{\Phi}{\delta^2} = 0 \tag{7}$$

where the optical penetration depth δ is

$$\delta = \sqrt{\frac{\zeta}{\beta}} \tag{8}$$

The solution of Eq. (7) for the one-dimensional case where a broad optical beam is incident upon the plane surface of the tissue, may be expressed

$$\Phi = \Phi_{op} e^{-\frac{x-\delta}{\delta}} \tag{9}$$

where x is the distance from the surface and Φ is defined as the
space irradiance at a distance corresponding to the penetration
depth. This expression does not relate the space irradiance to the
incident optical power density. The expression might of course be
extrapolated to the surface. But the validity of the diffusion
theory is limited in the regions proximal to the source and the
relation may better be expressed by a semi-empirical relation.
This may be written

$$\Phi_{op} = k_p I \tag{10}$$

where I is the incident optical power density and k_p is a semi-
empirical dimensionless coupling coefficient. The solution of Eq.
(7) for the spherically symmetrical case may be written

$$\Phi = \Phi_{os} (\frac{\delta}{r}) \; e^{-\frac{r-\delta}{\delta}} \tag{11}$$

where r is the distance from the center and Φ_{os} is defined as the
space irradiance at a distance corresponding to the optical penetration depth. The relation between this irradiance and the total radiant power P may be written

$$\Phi_{os} = k_s \frac{P}{4\pi\delta^2} \tag{12}$$

This equation defines k_s as a dimensionless semi-empirical quantity.
The coupling coefficients k_p and k_s are both dependent on the properties of the source and of the tissue. The should in principle
be determined for each particular source, tissue and wavelength.
The coupling coefficients have been determined for red light penetrating into normal and neoplastic human brain tissue. The measurements on the normal brain were done on human cadavers 1-2 days post
mortem [8]. The measurements on neoplastic brain tissue were done on
surgically resected tumor 1-2 hours after surgery. The coupling
coefficient k_p for a broad collimated optical beam at normal incidence to the surface of the tissue was found in the region $k_p = 0.8-$
$- 1.0$ for the wavelength region $\lambda = 610$ nm to $\lambda = 710$ nm. The coupling coefficient k_s for an inserted optical fiber with core diameter 200 μm* and numerical aperture NA = 0.2 was determined to $k_s =$
$= 1.8 - 3.2$ for the same wavelengths. The coupling coefficient
varied somewhat for different insertions and no systematic difference was found for normal adult, neonatal or neoplastic tissue.

---

*Quartz et Silice, S.A.

The coupling coefficient was however significantly reduced if the radiant optical power was sufficiently high to introduce clot formation and carbonization proximal to the end-surface of the fiber. This phenomenon was observed for radiant power down to P = 50 mW of green or blue light. But it was never observed below P = 100 mW of red light in the "in vitro" measurements. The coupling coefficient for the "in vivo" case was, however, found to be significantly below the "in vitro" values. The "in vivo" measurements were done on Lewis lung tumors in B_6D_2 mice. The coupling coefficient k_s for the wavelength $\lambda = 610 - 710$ nm was here reduced to $k_s = 0.3 - 0.5$. The coupling coefficient for the same tumors measured after sacrifice of the animal was $k_s = 1.8$, i.e. close to the values for the human brain tissue. The reason for the lower values for the "in vivo" case was presumably seepage of blood into the lesion resulting from the insertion of the fiber [9].

The threshold power level for clot formation and carbonization at the fiber tip was also significantly reduced in the "in vivo" case where radiant power of red light down to P = 50 mW easily initiated clot formation. The coupling coefficient k_s was subsequently reduced by two to three orders of magnitude within a few minutes. The optical penetration depth was, however, not found to be significantly different for the "in vivo" and the "in vitro" case. The reason for this is presumably that the penetration depth is dependent on the mean distribution of blood within the tissue itself and is independent of the conditions proximal to the fiber end. The penetration depth will thus be unchanged if the tissue blood content is maintained after sacrifice of the animal.

Typical optical distribution in neoplastic intracranial tissue is shown in Fig. 1. The light was coupled into the tissue and the space irradiance was evaluated with the same type of 200 μm core diameter fibers. The tumor was a large ($\sim$ 20 cm^3) meningioma from a 67 year old woman. The broken lines in Fig. 1 represent the best fit between the measured values and the functional relationship from Eq. (11). The space irradiances for the three different wavelengths are all normalized to the same limiting value at the origin. The penetration depth varies from $\delta = 0.8$ mm at $\lambda = 514$ nm, $\delta = 1.8$ nm at $\lambda = 635$ nm and to $\delta = 5.4$ nm at $\lambda = 1060$ nm wavelength.

Typical results for the optical penetration depth in normal and neoplastic human brain tissue at $\lambda = 635$ nm wavelength are summarized in Table 1. The values are measured in a total number of 7 normal human brains; 4 adult and 3 neonatal. The penetration depth in the neonatal brain is typically 2-3 times larger than the corresponding value for the adult brain. This difference is attributed to the increased scattering in the fully myelinated adult brain[8].

The results indicate that the penetration depth of primary brain tumors is in the region between the corresponding values for

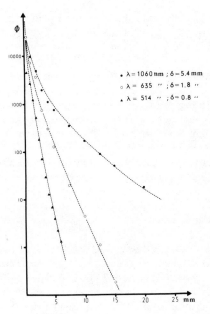

Fig. 1. Space irradiance versus distance from fiber end. Meningioma
         from 67 year old woman; measured 1-2 hours after surgical
         resection.

Table 1. Optical Penetration Depth at λ = 635 nm Wavelength in Nor-
         mal Human Brain and Intracranical Tumors.

Tissue	Penetration depth in mm
Normal adult brain*	0.8 - 1.5
Metastasis, OAT-cell from lung*	1.2
Astrocytoma degree I-II, 51 year old male**	1.7
Meningioma, 67 year old female**	1.8
Astrocytoma, degree III, 68 year old male **	2.5
Astrocytoma, degree III, 59 year old male **	2.6
Glioblastoma multiforme, 40 year old male**	2.6
Normal neonatal brain*	3 - 4.5

*   measured 1-2 days post mortem
** measured 1-2 hours after surgery.

the normal adult and the neonatal brains, i.e. up to 2 times larger
than the value for the normal adult brain.   The highest values are
found in highly malignant rapidly growing tumors as glioblastoma
multiforme, and the lowest values are found in slowly growing tumors
as astrocytoma degree I-II.   The penetration depth in the metastasis
(OAT-cell from lung) was slightly lower than the penetration dept
in the surrounding white matter.

THERMAL DISTRIBUTION

The thermal balance is determined by four mechanisms; heat
transported by thermal conductivity, heat transported by the capillary blood flow, heat generated by absorption of optical irradiation and finally heat which is released or accumulated due to change
in the local temperature.   The balance may thus be expressed [2]

$$\operatorname{div} \vec{j}' + \rho C Q (T - T_A) - \beta \Phi + \rho C \frac{\partial T}{\partial t} = 0 \tag{13}$$

where $\vec{j}'$ is the heat flux vector, ρ is the mass density, and C is
specific heat per unit mass.   The specific heat per unit volume,
ρC is taken to be the same for blood and for tissue.

The capillary blood flow Q is measured in volume of perfused
blood per unit volume of tissue per unit time.   The local temperature is T and T_A is the arterial blood temperature, i.e. the normal
body temperature.   It is convenient to normalize the body temperature to zero.   Thus, if T_A is put equal to zero, the temperature T
in Eq. (13) must be interpreted as the temperature rise above normal
body temperature.   The first term $\operatorname{div} \vec{j}'$ in Eq. (13) now represents
the amount of thermal energy which is transported out of an element
of volume per unit time by thermal conduction.   The second term
$\rho C Q T$ is the amount of thermal energy which is convected out of the
unit element per unit time by increasing the capillary blood temperature from $T_A = 0$ and to T.   The third term $\beta \Phi$ is the conversion
rate of optical energy to heat by absorption, and the last term
$\rho C \, \partial T / \partial t$ is the rate of change of heat content per unit volume.
The magnitude of the heat flux vector is proportional to the maximum
decrease in temperature per unit length and the vector is directed
in the direction of maximum decrease, i.e. the vector is proportional to the vector -grad T.   The heat flux vector is thus

$$\vec{j}' = -\kappa \operatorname{grad} T \tag{14}$$

where κ is the thermal conductivity.

Substitution of Eq. (14) in Eq. (13) gives

$$\text{divgrad } T - \frac{1}{\chi} \frac{\partial T}{\partial t} - \frac{T}{\delta_V^{\ 2}} = - \frac{\beta \Phi}{\kappa} \tag{15}$$

where the thermal diffusivity χ is defined

$$\chi = \frac{\kappa}{\rho C} \tag{16}$$

and the thermal penetration depth δ_V is

$$\delta_V = \sqrt{\frac{\chi}{Q}} \tag{17}$$

The thermal penetration depth characterizes the ability of the blood perfusion to suppress any temperature rise. The contribution to the local temperature rise from a source located at a distance equal to the thermal penetration depth will be suppressed by a factor $1/e$ (37%) by the blood perfusion. The thermal penetration depth varies from about $\delta_V = 1$ mm in tissue with very high blood perfusion such as the choroid layer of the eye to $\delta_V = 10$ mm in tissue with low blood flow as a resting muscle. The penetration depths in the gray and the white matter of the human brain are about $\delta_V = 4$ mm and $\delta_V = 8$ mm, respectively [2].

The steady state temperature rise from a spherical emitter of radius a embedded in a vascular tissue with optical penetration depht δ and thermal penetration depth δ_V is thus [Eqs. (5), (6) and (15)] [2]

$$T = \frac{P_t}{4\pi\kappa(1 - (\frac{\delta}{\delta_V})^2)r} \left\{ \frac{1}{1 + \frac{a}{\delta_V}} e^{-\frac{r-a}{\delta_V}} - \frac{1}{1 + \frac{a}{\delta}} e^{-\frac{r-a}{\delta}} \right\} \tag{18}$$

where P_t is the transmitted optical power. The optical diffusion theory is in this expression extrapolated to the interface between the source and the tissue. Deviations from this theory proximal to the fiber end will have negligible influence on the thermal distribution in the distal region. The result is illustrated in Fig. 2 where the shaded region shows the temperature rise versus distance from the center of the emitter. The transmitted optical power is put equal to $P_t = 300$ mW, the optical penetration depth $\delta = 2$ mm and the emitter radius is $a = 0.1$ mm. The upper limit of the shaded region corresponds to low flow, i.e. $\delta_V = 10$ mm and the lower limit corresponds to medium blood flow, i.e. $\delta_V = 5$ mm. The lower limit

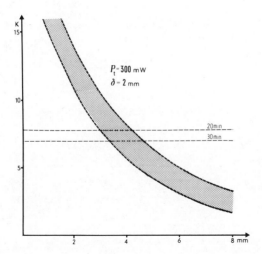

Fig. 2.   Steady state temperature rise versus distance from fiber
end. The upper and the lower part of shaded region correspond to low blood flow (δ_V = 10 mm) and medium blood
flow (δ_V = 5 mm), respectively. Total radiant optical
power P_t = 300 mW, optical penetration depth δ = 2 mm.

thus corresponds to typical blood flow in skin, the cortex of the
brain and the gastro-intestinal tract. The temperature rise for
this idealized emitter should be close to the actual case when a
single fiber is inserted in the tissue. The amount of light which
is reflected back into guiding rays in the fiber is very small and
the transmitted power P_t will thus be almost equal to the power
coupled into the fiber. The upper and the lower horizontal broken
lines in Fig. 2 correspond to the temperature rises which are required to obtain a hyperthermal therapeutic result during 20 min.
and 30 min. exposure, respectively [10]. The normal body temperature
is here taken to be 37°C. The thermal conductivity κ = 0.4 W/mK
and the thermal diffusion χ = 1.2 10^{-7} m^2/s. These results indicate
that a hyperthermal contribution to the cell kill is expected in the
region up to about r = 4 mm in radius during 20-30 min. exposure with
300 mW optical power. This value for the radius r is, as follows
from Eq. (18), rather independent of the optical penetration depth
provided that this depth is in the range δ = 0-2 mm.

The experimental results are shown in Fig. 3. Optical power
P = 300 mW was coupled into the center of a subcutaneous Lewis lung
tumor in mice through a fiber. The temperature was monitored with
a micro-thermocouple with 250 μm outer diameter. Fig. 3 shows the
temperature rise versus time at a position r = 4 mm from the fiber

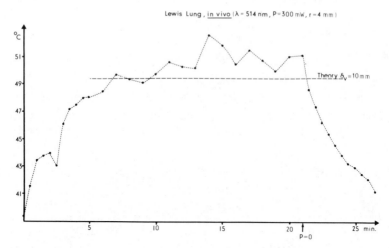

Fig. 3.   Temperature rise versus time.   Subcutaneous Lewis lung
          tumor in B_6D_2-mice.   Total radiant optical power P_t = 300 mW,
          wavelength λ = 514 nm.

end.   The optical radiation is reduced to zero after 21 min.   The
rapid irregularities in the temperature are due to motions of the
animal.   The tumor which was about 12 mm in diameter had a sluggish
blood flow due to spontaneous necrosis.   The horizontal broken line
corresponds to the steady state temperature rise predicted in accordance with Eq. (18) (T = 10 K).

    The temperature rise in small subcutaneous tumors with linear
dimensions comparable or smaller than the thermal penetration depth
will be higher than the value predicted from the infinitely large
tissue model in Eq. (18).   The temperature rise in a small tumor
with a hemispheric elevation of the skin might, as follows from
Eq. (15), be up to twice as large as for the same tumor embedded
into surrounding tissue.

    The temperature rise during transcutaneous or transmucosal ir-
radiation with a plane optical beam will be dependent on the cooling conditions of the surface.   The steady state temperature rise
for the case with no surface cooling is [Eq. (15)]

$$T = \frac{\delta I_t}{\kappa(1 - (\frac{\delta}{\delta_V})^2)} \{ \frac{\delta_V}{\delta} e^{-\frac{x}{\delta_V}} - e^{-\frac{x}{\delta}} \} \qquad (19)$$

where I_t is the transmitted optical power density. The corresponding temperature rise for the case where the surface temperature is
kept at a constant temperature T_0 by forced air cooling or liquid
flow is

$$T = \frac{\delta I_t}{\kappa(1 - (\frac{\delta}{\delta_V})^2)} \{ e^{-\frac{x}{\delta_V}} e^{-\frac{x}{\delta}} \} + T_0 e^{-\frac{x}{\delta_V}} \qquad (20)$$

The transmitted optical power density I_t is defined by

$$I_t = (1 - \gamma)I \qquad (21)$$

where γ is the reflection coefficient. Typical values for this
coefficient for red light in whitish tissues as brain and Caucasian
skin are about $\gamma = 0.5 - 0.6$.

The results from Eqs. (19) and (20) are shown in Fig. 4. The
upper shaded region corresponds to the case with no heat loss from
the surface into the air, and the lower shaded region corresponds
to the case where the surface is kept at the normal tissue temperature by the forced cooling ($T_0 = 0$). The upper and lower parts of
both shaded regions correspond to low blood flow ($\delta_V = 5$ mm), respectively. The upper and the lower horizontal broken lines correspond again to the temperature rises which are required to obtain
a hyperthermal therapeutic result during 20 min. or 30 min. exposure,
respectively. The normal body temperature is taken to be 37°C.
These results indicate that a transmitted optical power density
$I_t = 50$ mW/cm^2 of red light may introduce a hyperthermal therapeutic
result at depths up to about 5 mm from the surface in a tissue with
low blood flow. But the temperature rises in the case of normal
blood flow in the skin or in the case of forced cooling at the surface are both well below the required values. A transmitted power
density of 50 mW/cm^2 corresponds to an incident optical power density in the range $I = 100 - 130$ mW/cm^2, dependent on the coefficient
of reflectivity.

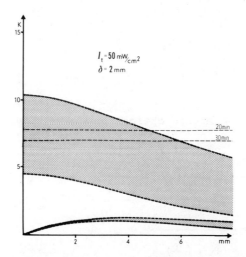

Fig. 4.   Steady state temperature rise versus distance from surface.
The upper shaded region corresponds to no cooling at the
surface.   The lower shaded region corresponds to a constant
surface temperature equal to the normal body temperature.
Transmitted radiant power density I_t = 50 mW/cm^2, optical
penetration depth δ = 2 mm.

DOSIMETRY

The minimum reported optical dose for any tissue reaction for
an HpD dose in the range 2.5 - 5 mg/kg is, as discussed in the introduction, about 12 J/cm^2. The corresponding optical dose for total tumor necrosis is up to one order of magnitude higher. If the
reciprocality is valid for the optical and the drug dose, an optical
dose 12 J/cm^2 should result in a complete tumor necrosis for an HpD
dose of 25-50 mg/kg.

The maximum distance from the surface for obtaining this dose
during 30 min. irradiation is shown in Fig. 5. This distance is
shown versus incident optical power density in a collimated beam.
The coupling coefficient k_p [Eq. (10)] is put equal to k_p = 1 and
the broken lines correspond to the various penetration depths δ =
1.0; 1.5; 2.0; 2.5; 3.0 and 3.5 mm (from lower to upper broken line).
A collimated beam with power density 100 mW/cm^2 will thus deliver
the optical dose 12 J/cm^2 during 30 min. exposure at a distance
3-5 mm from the surface in the normal adult brain. But the same incident power density and exposure time may administer this dose at
a distance 10 mm from the surface in a gliobastoma.

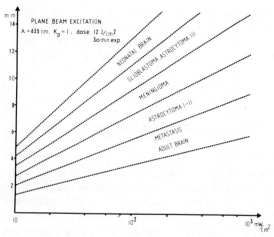

Fig. 5. Maximum distance from surface for an optical dose 12 J/cm^2 during 30 min. exposure versus power density of incident collimated beam.

The corresponding results for interestitial photoradiation therapy are shown in Fig. 6. This figure shows the maximum distance from the end of a single inserted fiber where an optical dose 12 J/cm^2 is delivered during 30 min. exposure versus total radiant optical power. The coupling coefficient k_s is put equal to the value measured

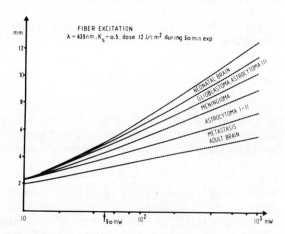

Fig. 6. Maximum distance from fiber end for an optical dose 12 J/cm^2 during 30 min. exposure versus total radiant optical power.

"in vivo" in Lewis lung tumors in mice, i.e. k_s = 0.5. If the total
radiant power is kept below the power limit 50 mW for clotting, the
maximum radius of the region with a therapeutic optical dose will
be about 3-4 mm in the normal adult brain. The radius of the region
with the corresponding dose will, however, be close to 5 mm for the
glioblastoma. If the design of the applicator allows the radiant
power to be increased to 500 mW without clot formation and carbonization, the radii of the regions will be 5-6 mm and 9 mm for the
normal brain and for the gliobastoma, respectively.

The clot formation will, however, only have a minor influence
on the temperature rise at distances larger than the optical penetration depth. The hyperthermal contribution to a therapeutic result will thus remain almost unchanged. The exposure time which
is required to obtain a hyperthermal therapeutic result is reported
to be halved for each degree centigrade temperature rise above
42.5°C. Typical reported exposure times are 240 min. at 41°C and
15 min. at 45°C [10]. The necessary exposure Δ' time in seconds may
thus be expressed

$$\Delta' = E'e^{-\zeta(T + T_n)} \tag{22}$$

when the constants E' = $3.2 \cdot 10^{16}$ s, ζ = $- \ln 0.5$ K^{-1}, T is the temperature rise and T_n is the normal tissue temperature in °C. The ther-
apy rate $(\Delta')^{-1}$ in hyperthermia is thus exponentially dependent on
the temperature rise and therefore also exponentially dependent on
the radiant optical power.

The photodynamic effect is dependent on the total number of
photons absorbed by the Hematoporphyrin molecules and is thus dependent on the total radiant energy. The required exposure time Δ" in
seconds may be written

$$\Delta'' = \frac{D}{\Phi} \tag{23}$$

where the optical dose D = 12 J/cm^2 and Φ is the space irradiance
at λ = 625 - 640 mm wavelength in W/cm^2. The therapy rate $(\Delta'')^{-1}$ in
phototherapy is hence only linearly dependent on the radiant optical
power. Eqs. (22) and (23) are illustrated in Fig. 7 which gives the
therapy rate as a function of the radiant power from an inserted optical fiber. The optical penetration depth is here δ = 1.4 mm, which
corresponds to the value for Lewis lung tumor in mice at λ = 635 nm.
The thick broken lines give the therapy rate for phototherapy at
various distances from the fiber end. The coupling coefficient is
k_s = 0.5. The parallel thinner broken lines give the corresponding

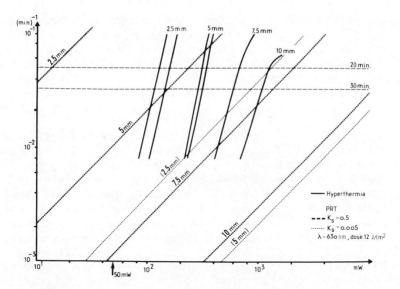

Fig. 7.   Photodynamic and hyperthermal therapy for inserted fiber.
Therapy rate, i.e. reciprocal required exposure time, versus total radiant optical power. Optical penetration depth
δ = 1.4 mm, coupling coefficient k_s = 0.5, optical dose
12 J/cm^2.

therapy rate after a possible clot formation has reduced the coupling coefficient by two orders of magnitude, i.e. k_s = 0.005. The
solid line give the hyperthermal therapy rate [Eq. (22)] for various
distances from the fiber end. The thermal penetration depth is
δ_v = 10 mm and the normal body temperature is T_n = 37°C. The left
hand lines of the double lines at the distances r = 2.5 mm and r =
5 mm correspond to the case where clot formation has occurred. The
right hand lines corresponds to no clot formation. The difference
between the two cases is insignificant at distances larger than
5 mm. The clot formation which is highly disastrous to the phototherapy results in a minor enhancement of the hyperthermia.

The temperature rise distal to the fiber end is somewhat delayed due to the finite velocity of the thermal waves. The required
total exposure time Δ_t' during hyperthermia is therefore somewhat
larger than the effective exposure time Δ'. The total time may be
found by solving the time dependent Eq. (13). The mathematical
solution of this equation is rather composite; but an approximate
expression may be written [2]

$$\Delta_t' = \Delta' + \frac{r^2}{\chi} \qquad\qquad (24)$$

where the second term on the right hand side is the thermal relaxation time. This relaxation time has a minor influence on the required exposure time for distances smaller than 5 mm. But the influence is of importance for distances larger than 5 mm for the case with small total exposure times. The curvature of the upper part of the solid lines for distances 7.5 mm and 10 mm is due to this phenomenon.

A total radiant power P = 10-15 mW will give an optical dose 12 J/cm^2 during 20-30 min. exposure about r = 2.5 mm from the fiber end. These is no hyperthermal effect at this distance, the radiant power must be increased to about P = 100 mW for obtaining this. A radiant power P = 150-200 mW will administer the optical dose 12 J/cm^2 at a distance up to r = 5 mm. The hyperthermal effect is enhanced and extends to about 3.5 mm from the fiber end. A hyperthermal therapeutic result at 5 mm distance during 20-30 min. exposure requires about P = 300 mW radiant power. An optical dose 12 J/cm^2 at 7.5 mm during 20-30 min. requires a total radiant power P = 1000-2000 mW. The hyperthermal contribution will now be dominant and it extends beyond r = 10 mm; a hyperthermal therapeutic result at r = 7.5 mm requires only radiant power P = 500-600 mW. The photodynamic and the hyperthermal contributions are equally important at a distance r = 6 mm; a radiant optical power P = 375 mW will administer 12 J/cm^2 during 30 min. exposure and simultaneously heat the tumor to 44°C. This optical power must be radiated into the tissue without clot formation at the fiber end. The hyperthermal contribution will be dominant in all space if clotting occurs. An enhancement of the photodynamic effect over hyperthermia at distances larger than r = 6 mm may be done by increasing the exposure time or by using an intermittent exposure where the length of each exposure period is much smaller than the thermal relaxation time for the relevant distance. It should, however, be emphasized that the distance for equal importance of the two therapeutic modalities is strongly dependent on the optical penetration depth. If the penetration depht is equal to δ = 2.6 mm, i.e. the value found for gliobastoma of the human brain, a radiant power P = 1200 mW will heat the tissue to about 44°C at a distance r = 11 mm from the fiber and simultaneously deliver an optical dose 12 J/cm^2 in this region.

DISCUSSION

The results have been examined in Lewis lung tumor in B_6D_2 mice. A detailed discussion of these results is given in ref. (9). A radiant optical power P = 50 mW at λ = 630 nm wavelength was coupled into the center of tumors during 60 min. exposure. The tumors were 8-10 mm in diameter. An HpD[*] dose 5 mg/kg was injected directly into the tumorous mass 24 hours prior to exposure. Histologic findings

---

[*]Oncology Research and Development Inc.

showed a necrotic mass with viable tumor. But the findings were
almost indistinguishable from spontaneous necrosis in the control
animal. The formation of spontaneous necrosis represented a large
problem for the interpretation of these results. The photodynamic
contribution to the cell kill was therefore enhanced by increasing
the HpD dose to 25 mg/kg and 50 mg/kg for the same optical power
and exposure time. Histological findings now revealed complete
tumor necrosis and formation of granulation tissue to a distance of
about r = 4 mm. The expected distance from the fiber end of an
optical dose 12 J/cm^2 is 4.5 mm in a tissue with δ = 1.4 mm and
k_s = 0.5 [Eqs. (11) and (12)]. The temperature rise at the margins
of the tumor for P = 50 mW radiant power was measured to be in the
range 39–40°C, i.e. well below the threshold for hyperthermia.

     Hyperthermia was, however, enhanced by coupling P = 300 mW op-
tical power at λ = 514 nm wavelength into the center of the tumor
during 15 min. exposure. No HpD dose was given. Visual inspection
1 and 2 days after treatment indicated complete irradiatication of
the tumorous mass.Histological examination did, however, reveal
viable tumor cells in the necrotic mass.

     Comparable results have also been reported for the treatment
of mammary adenocarcinoma in C3H/HeN mice [3]. The light attenuation
at λ = 630 nm wavelength was here reported to be a factor of 10 in
passage through 4 mm of freshly excised tumor. This corresponds to
a penetration depht δ = 1.7. mm. The tumor killing distance from
the fiber end for a radiant optical power of 50 mW during 20–30 min.
exposure and an HpD dose 50 mg/kg administered i.p. 24 hours prior
to irradiation, was reported to be 3.7 mm. A radiant power of 50 mW
during 20–30 min. exposure is expected to administer an optical
dose 12 J/cm^2 up to a distance 3.7–4.1 mm in a tissue with optical
penetration depth δ = 1.7 mm and k_s = 0.5 [Eqs. (11) and (12)].
The same study demonstrates a hyperthermal cure of an 8–10 mm diameter tumor with 300 mW radiant optical power at λ= 630 nm wavelength. The observed temperature rise is here about twice as large
as would be expected from Eq. (18) even for the case with negligible
blood flow; the reason may be the loss of cooling at the hemispheri-
cal elevation of the skin [Eq. (15)]. The study further reports no
cure but eschar of the skin during surface irradiation with 15 mW/cm^2
with a total optical dose of 100 J/cm^2. A radiant optical dose of
100 J/cm^2 is expected to be reduced to 12 J/cm^2 at a depth 5.3 mm
[Eqs. (9) and (10) with δ = 1.7 mm and k_p = 1.0]. Since this depth
is smaller than the tumor thickness (8–10) no cure is to be expected.

CONCLUSIONS

     The required optical dose for a total photodynamic cell kill
at λ = 625–640 nm wavelength and HpD dose 2.5–5 mg/kg is about

50-100 J/cm^2. The temperature rise during surface irradiation of the tumor is dependent on the surface cooling, the blood flow and the dose rate. If the dose 100 J/cm^2 is administered during 15 min. exposure the temperature rise may by sufficient to give a hyperthermal contribution to the cell kill in tumors with sluggish blood flow. The hyperthermal contribution is insignificant if the same optical dose is delivered during 60 min. exposure. Once the conditions for hyperthermia are satisfied in the surface layer, this contribution to the cell kill is expected to penetrate deeper into the tumorous mass than the corresponding penetration of the photodynamic cell kill. This phenomenon occurs because the thermal penetration depth in most tissues is larger than the optical penetration depth. The thermal penetration depth is in the range δ_V = 5-10 mm and the optical penetration depth is typically δ = 1-3 mm. Enhancement of the photodynamic cell kill by increasing the optical dose rate with constant exposure time and drug dose might easily result in a predominant photodynamic cell kill confined to the surface layers only while a hyperthermal cell kill will be dominant in the distal regions. The expected "cross-over distance" for the two modalities for an HpD dose 2.5-5 mg/kg and exposure time 20-30 min. is in the region 3-10 mm. Advances in the research for more potent photosensitizers with less side-effects may result in a significant increase in this distance. These photosensitizers should preferrably be excitable in the 700-800 nm wavelength region where the optical penetration depth is about twice as large as for 630 nm wavelength.

ACKNOWLEDGEMENTS

    The author wishes to thank R. Ellingsen, D.R. Doiron, A.E. Profio and T.J. Dougherty for cooperation and stimulating discussions. The work has been supported by a NATO Research Grant, no. 0342 under NATO Science Programmes. The author is thankful to B. Reitan for competent typing.

REFERENCES

1. A. E. Profio and D. R. Doiron, Dosimetry considerations in phototherapy, Med. Phys. 8:190 (1981).
2. L. O. Svaasand, D. R. Doiron and T. J. Dougherty, Temperature rise during photoradiation therapy of malignant tumors, Med. Phys. 1:10 (1983).
3. J. H. Kinsey, D. A. Cortese and H. B. Neel, Cancer Res. 43:1562 (1983).
4. C. Perria, T. Capuzzo, G. Cavagnaro, R. Datti, N. Francaviglia, C. Rivano, V. E. Tercero, J. Neurosurg. Sci. 24:119 (1980).
5. A. G. Wile, A. Dahlman, R. G. Burns, M.W. Berns, Lasers i. Surg. and Med. 2:163 (1982).
6. T. J. Dougherty, J. E. Kaufman, A. Goldfarb, K. R. Weishaupt, D. Boyle and A. Mittleman, Photoradiation therapy of the treatment of malignant tumors, Cancer Res. 38:2628 (1978).

7. C. J. Gomer, D. R. Doiron, J. V. Jester, B. C. Szirth and A. L.
    Murphree, Cancer Res. 43:721 (1983).

8. L. O. Svaasand and R. Ellingsen, Optical properties of human
    brain, Photochem. Photobiol. in press.

9. R. Ellingsen, L. O. Svaasand and E. Ødegaard, Photoradiation
    therapy (PRT) of Lewis lung carcinoma in B_6D_2 mice, dosimetry
    considerations, This book.

10. G. J. Short and P. F. Turner, Proc. IEEE 68:133 (1980).

11. T. J. Dougherty, Recent advances in photoradiation therapy,
    Proc. of the Clayton Symposium, Alan Liss, in press.

12. A. Ishimaru, in: "Wave Propagation and Scattering in Random
    Media", Academic Press, (1978).

13. C. J. Gomer and T. J. Dougherty, Determination of [^{3}H] and
    [^{14}C] Hematoporphyrin Derivative distribution in malignant
    and normal tissue, Cancer Res. 39:146 (1979).

PHOTOPHYSICS AND DOSIMETRY OF PHOTORADIATION THERAPY

Daniel R. Doiron, Charles J. Gomer, Stanley W. Fountain and Nicholas J. Razum

Clayton Center for Ocular Oncology, Childrens Hospital of Los Angeles and Department of Ophthalmology, USC School of Medicine, Los Angeles, CA 90027

INTRODUCTION

Hematoporphyrin Derivative (HpD) photoradiation therapy (PRT) has been found to be an effective treatment for a variety of tumors [1,2]. In order for PRT to be used optimumly an understanding of the photophysic principles of the photosensitization reaction must be known. It is also important that the light dosimetry be done properly.

To understand the photophysics of HpD-PRT a knowledge of the optical characteristics and photochemistry of HpD must be known. In addition, the optical characteristics of the tissue and its physiological state must be considered in determining accurate therapeutic dosimetry.

PHOTOPHYSICS AND PHOTOCHEMISTRY OF HpD

In order for any photochemical or photodynamic reaction to take place the photoactivating molecule must first absorb one or more light photons. Most photobiological reactions are of the single photon absorption type unless very short pulses with high peak powers are used. Once the photon is absorbed the molecule is raised to an excited state from which it may de-excite by a number of mechanisms. For porphyrins the ground state and initial excited state is a singlet. Measurement of one of the possible de-excitation pathways, fluorescence for example, does not allow direct correlation to the efficiency of the other possible de-excitation pathways. The different pathways are competitive with each other. For this reason the use of fluorescence to assess the potential photosensitization response directly is not valid.

HpD is a mixture of at least four major components and a variety of minor ones [3]. The absorption and fluorescence characteristics of these various components in various solvents or bound states have been studied by different groups [4,5]. At the commercially provided concentration of 5 mg/ml the various porphyrin molecules are extremely aggregated. Upon dilution in saline the larger loosely bound aggregates dissociate into smaller more tightly bound aggregates and monomers. This dissociation is greater in the presence of proteins. The dissociation is evident by the red shift and narrowing of the soret absorption band. Figure 1 shows this shift for HpD in saline and saline plus 10% fetal calf serum.

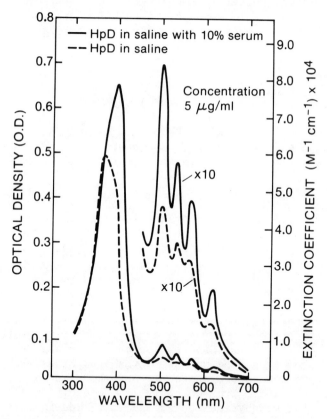

Fig. 1. The absorption spectrum of HpD in saline and saline with 10% fetal calf serum [6]. Extinction coefficient is based on a molecular weight of 600.

It must be remembered that when HpD is used in "in vivo" and
"in vitro" experiments not all of its components, or derivatives
of them, may be responsible for a measured photosensitization or
photochemical response. When considering "in vivo" experimentation
it must be remembered that biological systems may selectively localize and/or retain any of these various components. This process
may take place for a specific component dependently or independently
of the others. The biological system may also alter these components
and thereby change their photophysical characteristics. Caution
must be used in translating "in vitro" experiments directly to the
"in vivo" situation.

HpD Absorption

HpD exhibits what is called an aetio type absorption spectrum
in neutral solutions and when bound to serum proteins. At concentrations greater than 5 µg/ml in saline self and cross aggregation
between the various components does occur. When aggregated, the

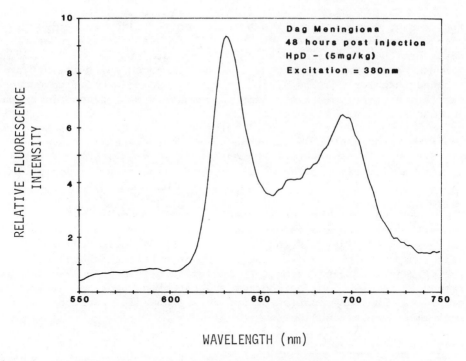

WAVELENGTH (nm)

Fig. 2.   The corrected fluorescence emission spectrum of a spon-
          taneous meningioma specimen from the brain of a dog. Exci-
          tation wavelength is 380 nm. The specimen was a taken 48
          hours post injection of 5.0 mg/kg HpD.

absorption curve exhibits a blue shift and broadening of the soret
band. In the presence of proteins the aggregation is decreased but
may not lead to complete dissociation. The red shift obtained upon
binding with serum proteins is even more pronounced in cells when
dilute concentrations of HpD are used.

HpD Fluorescence

One mode of de-excitation of the porphyrin molecule after absorption of a photon is by fluorescence emission. The HpD solution
exhibits a very broad red fluorescence emission (610-740 nm) with
two major peaks and a minor one. The wavelength of the peak emissions will vary according to the solvent and the environmental conditions, (i.e. binding, aggregation, pH, etc.). In saline the major
peaks are at 615 nm and 675 nm and for saline containing 10% fetal
calf serum they are 625 nm and 683 nm respectively [6]. The minor
peak is around 660 nm and may be hidden by the shoulder of the longer major wavelength peak. The fluorescence emission spectra will
vary depending on the state of the HpD components "in vivo". Figure
2 shows the fluorescence emission of a meningioma from the brain of
a dog 48 hours after the I.V. injection of 5.0 mg/kg of HpD. The
measurement was done on a biopsy specimen shortly after surgery
using a solid specimen holder in an SLM 8000 spectrofluorometer.
Note that the fluorescence emission peaks are now 633 nm and 698 nm
for the major peaks and 670 nm for the minor one which is more pronounced than for the "in vitro" case. Figure 3 is the fluorescence
excitation spectrum for the same specimen. The presence of the major excitation peaks at 385 nm and 410 nm are most likely indication
of both aggregates and monomers being present. It appears that the
state of HpD "in vivo" may not be simply correlated to that found
"in vitro". These spectral shapes "in vivo" may also be expected
to change with time as the porphyrins are removed or biologically
altered.

These various changes is spectral shape from "in vitro" to
"in vivo" may also indicate changes in the fluorescence quantum
yield. Considering this and the fact that the degree of fluorescence may not correlate to the amount of potential photonsensitization reaction, caution must be taken in correlating measured fluorescence "in vivo" to HpD content and potential photonsensitization
response. Photodegradation of HpD during the fluorescence measurement must also be considered.

Photosensitization Reaction

Once a porphyrin molecule is excited one of its possible modes
of de-excitation in an intersystem crossover to a metastable triplet state. It is this triplet state that is thought to be responsible for the vast majority of the "in vivo" PRT response via a

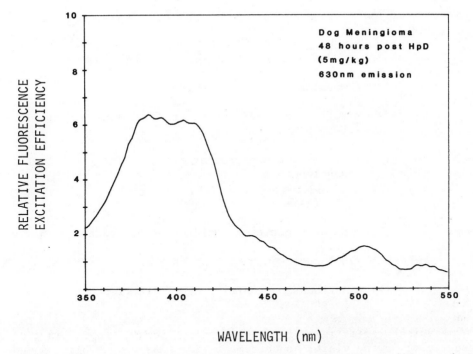

Fig. 3. The fluorescence excitation for the same specimen as in
        Figure 2. Emission wavelength is 630 nm.

type-II, singlet oxygen mechanism [7]. This highly reactive form of
oxygen can oxidize various biological molecules to achieve a net
therapeutic response. In HpD-PRT the response is tissue damage and
eventually cell death. If this mechanism is the truely dominate
one "in vivo" then the effectiveness of HpD-PRT will depend not only
on the HpD active component content, effective light delivery, but
also on the physiological conditions of the tumor, (i.e. O_2 content).
Even if a high HpD concentration and light dose are delivered to
the tissue there is no guarantee that a therapeutic effect can be
obtained. It should also be pointed out that fluorescence is in
direct competition with the photosensitization reaction. If a compound exhibits a large fluorescence quantum yield than it will most
likely have a poor photosensitization yield.

PHOTODYNAMIC REACTION "IN VIVO"

Rate Equation

     For a tissue of thickness X the photoreactive yield, (fluores-
cence, intersystem crossover, etc.) for light of wavelength λ can

be expressed by:

$$R = \frac{[1 - \gamma(\lambda)]\Phi \ \beta(\lambda)}{\alpha_T(\lambda)} \ [\ 1 \ - \ e^{- \ \alpha_T(\lambda)x} \ ]$$

where: Φ = Quantum yield for the reaction.

$\gamma(\lambda)$ = Reflection coefficient of the tissue at wavelength λ .

$\beta(\lambda)$ = Absorption coefficient of the reactive drug at
wavelength λ .

$$\beta(\lambda) = 2.3 \ \epsilon \ (\lambda)C$$

where: $\epsilon(\lambda)$ = Molar excitation coefficient of the drug "in vivo".

C   = Molar concentration of the "in vivo" drug.

$\alpha_T(\lambda)$ = Attenuation coefficient of the tissue at wavelength λ .

Typical reflectivity for tissue range from 0.3 to 0.7 in the
red region of the visible spectrum [8]. For tissue with high pigmentation or large scattering $\alpha_T(\lambda)$ will be significant in magnitude
and thereby decrease the reactive yield. This is one of the reasons
fluorescence is hard to visualize in dark tissues.

Light Penetration in Tissues

Light photons interact with tissues through either scattering
and/or absorption. Most tissues are highly inhomogeneous and scatter light significantly. One exception to this is the ocular media.
This inhomogeneity will reduce any spatial coherence of the light
and thereby allow the use of geometrical optics to describe its propagation [8]. Using this simplification and conservation of energy
considerations solutions for the light space irradiance, ϕ, in the
tissue can be obtained. Two cases are of particular interest, namely when absorption is dominate and when scattering is dominate. The
solution for these two cases are outlined in Table 1.

For the absorption dominated case the attenuation coefficient
equals $\beta + \kappa$, the absorption and scattering coefficient respectively. In the scattering dominated case the attenuation coefficient
equals $\sqrt{\beta/\zeta}$, where ζ is the diffusion coefficient. The attenuation
coefficient is highly wavelength dependent as shown in Table 2.
The attenuation depth, $\delta = 1/\alpha$, is the distance at which the space
irradiance is decreased by a factor of 1/e, 0.37. The space irradiance never goes to zero but is attenuated by the 0.37 factor for
every distance δ. By the use of fiber optic probes α and δ have been

Table 1. Solution for Light Penetration in Tissue Under Absorption and Scattering Dominated Conditions. Based on Concervation of Energy and Isotropic Scattering for a Monochromatic Light of Wavelength λ[8].

Case	Solution*
Absorption Dominate	$\phi(r) = \phi_o (\frac{a}{r})^2 e^{-\alpha(r-a)}$
Scattering Dominate (diffusion)	$\phi(r) = \phi_o (\frac{a}{r}) e^{-\alpha(r-a)}$

*ϕ = Space irradiance at point r. ϕ_o = Space irradiance at r = 0. r = Distance. α = Attenuation coefficient at wavelength λ . a = Source radius.

Table 2. Attenuation Coefficient (α) and Attenuation Depth ($\delta = 1/\alpha$) Measurements for a Cat Brain (White Matter) at Selected Wavelengths.

Wavelength	"In vivo"		"In vitro"	
(nm)	α (cm^{-1})	δ (nm)	α (cm^{-1})	δ (nm)
405-410	44.1	0.23	46.1	0.22
488	-----	----	10.9	0.92
496.5	----	----	13.2	0.76
501.7	----	----	13.2	0.76
514.5	----	----	13.3	0.75
545	34.4	0.29	----	----
577	25.9	0.39	----	----
630/633	5.9	1.7	----	----
	4.4	2.3	----	----
	9.8	1.0	8.9	1.1
	5.0	2.0	5.3	1.9

evaluated for a number of tissues[9-12]. It should be noted that in certain tissues the difference from "in vivo" to "in vitro" measurements may be significant [10]. Particularly at wavelengths where blood absorption is significant.

Physiological Factors

A number of physiological factors must be considered in evaluating the actual therapeutic dosimetry in HpD-PRT. In the following section the terms and considerations of light dosimetry are covered. Other factors must be considered in determining the therapeutic dosimetry. If type-II photosensitization is the dominate mode of action for HpD-PRT then the concentration of O_2 in the tissue and its delivery rate will be of extreme importance. This will be especially important if the light fluence, i.e. power, is high. Both the delivery of the HpD and O_2 to the tumor will depend on its circulation. In addition, the potential for induced thermal rise in the tissue during PRT is also heavily dependent on blood flow [9]. The amount of PRT response obtained in a given tumor may be altered by the mount of HpD injected, the delay time between injection, light delivery geometry and the amount of light dose given. The net comparable effect between various tumors may be highly dependent on their particular physiological state.

LIGHT DOSIMETRY

The important factors in specifying and controlling light dosimetry for PRT are: (a) spectral characteristics of the light source, (b) total light dose delivered, (c) geometry of the light delivery and (d) the rate of its delivery. The light source spectrum must provide significant photons which match the absorption spectrum of the HpD components in the tissue. Light outside the HpD absorption band does not add to the PRT reaction directly but may act synergistically by such mechanisms as hyperthermia [13]. For red dye lasers the spectrum band desired is 625 nm – 635 nm with 630 ± 1 nm being optimum [13]. If a broad spectral lamp source is used its true spectral emission curves should be intergrally weighted with the HpD absorption spectrum "in vivo". This gives an effective power which should be used in light dosimetry so that comparisons can be made between data obtained with various light sources. Spectral characteristics of the light source should always be along with the HpD absorption spectrum used in determining the effective power.

The total delivered light dose should be given in joules, "J", or photons, along with a characteristics geometry parameter for the application technique used. A joule is a watt-sec. The number of photons per joule is $1.99 \times 10-6/\lambda$ (nm) [14]. The geometries for application of light in PRT are surface, interstitial point and interstitial cylinder. For surface illumination the light dose should be given in J/cm^2. For the interstitial point treatment, (an inserted

flat cut optical fiber or point source diffuser), the light dose is
joules. Interstitial cylinder illumination should be stated as
J/cm. The total energy delivered by an interstitial cylinder is
determined by multiplying the J/cm by the total cylinder length.
This assumes that the light is evenly distributed along the cylinder
length.

The rate of delivery of the light appears not to be significant
as long as the threshold for thermal effects are not reached. If
thermal raises in the range of 4 to 10 C are reached then direct
hyperthermia or synergistics effects with PRT may be important [13].
All results should state the rate of light delivery and the total
light dose.

CONCLUSION

An understanding of the photophysics principles of HpD-PRT and
the parameters of light and therapeutic dosimetry are important in
doing basic, preclinical and clinical research in this area. It
must be understood that the basic initiating mechanism of PRT is a
photon absorption process. The spectrum of the light used in PRT
must provide photons that match the absorption characteristics of
the tumor localizing components of HpD "in vivo". This is extremely
important for dye laser systems which can operate over relatively
broad spectral ranges. A shift of 10 nm in a dye laser output would
make a significant difference in the achieved therapeutic response.

Once the photon is absorbed it is not certain that it will add
to the photosensitization reaction. Fluorescence and photosensitization are competing de-excitation mechanisms. A measurement of
the fluorescence intensity may give no information as to what the
potential for inducing a type-II photosensitization reaction. Such
a measurement can give an indication of the porphyrin concentration
in the tissue if care is taken to account for (a) absorption of the
exciting and emitted light by the tissue, (b) variation of the fluorescence signal with distance from the source and detector, (c) variation of the fluorescence quantum yield under the given physiological conditions and (d) potential fluorescence quenching and drug
degradation during the measurements. The porphyrin compound fluo-
rescing may not be the one promoting the photosensitization reaction.

When making comparative studies in light dosimetry the rate of
delivery, geometry of delivery and total light dose must be considered.

The complete therapeutic dose must be measured by the net photosensitization reaction. Not only must the amount of light delivered and absorbed in the localized porphyrin components be considered
but also the physiological factors that are important in obtaining
the therapeutic reaction. Of particular importance is the O_2 content
of the tissue and its blood flow.

ACKNOWLEDGEMENT

This work was performed in conjunction with the Clayton Foundation for Research. We thank Albert L. Castorena for assistance in the prepraration of this manuscript.

REFERENCES

1. T. J. Dougherty, J. B. Kaufman, A. Goldfarb, K. R. Weishaupt, D. G. Boyle, and A. Mittleman, Photoradiation therapy for the treatment of malignant tumors, Cancer Res. 38:2628 (1978).

2. T. J. Dougherty, K. R. Weishaupt, and D. G. Boyle, Photosensitizers, in: "Cancer Principles and Practices of Oncology", V. DeVita, S. Helman, S. Rosenberg, (eds.), J.P. Lippincott, Phil., (1982).

3. M. C. Berenbaum, R. Bonnett, and P. A. Scourides, In vivo biological activity of compounds of Hematoporphyrin Derivative, Cancer Res. 35:571 (1982).

4. J. Moan, T. Christensen, and S. Somer, The main photosensitizing components of Hematoporphyrin Derivative, Cancer Letters 15:161 (1982).

5. J. Moan, and S. Somer, Fluorescence and absorption properties of the components of Hematoporphyrin Derivative, Photochem. Photobiol. 3:93 (1981).

6. D. R. Doiron, Fluorescence bronchoscopy for the early localization of lung cancer, Ph.D. Thesis University of California, Santa Barbara (1982).

7. K. R. Weishaupt, C. J. Gomer, and T. J. Dougherty, Identification of singlet oxygen as the cytotoxic agent in photo-inactivation of a murine tumor, Cancer Res. 36:2326 (1976).

8. D. R. Doiron, L. O. Svaasand, and A. E. Profio, Light dosimetry in tissue: Application to photoradiation therapy, in: "Porphyrin Photosensitization, D. Kessel and T.J. Dougherty, eds., Plenum Press, New York, N.Y., (1983).

9. L. O. Svaasand, D. R. Doiron, and T. J. Dougherty, Temperature rise during photoradiation therapy of malignant tumors, Med. Phys. 10:10 (1983).

10. B. C. Wilson, W. P. Jeeves, D.M. Lowe, and G. Adam, Light propagation in animal tissues in the wavelength range 375-826 nanometers, in: "Porphyrin Localization and Treatment of Tumors", D. R. Doiron and C. J. Gomer, eds., Alan R. Liss, Inc., New York, N.Y. (1983) (in press).

11. F. P. Bolin, L. E. Preuss, and B. W. Cain, A comparison of spectral transmittance for several mammalian tissues: Effects at PRT frequencies, in: "Porphyrin Localization and Treatment of Tumors", D.R. Doiron and C.J. Gomer, eds., Alan R. Liss, Inc., New York, N.Y., (1983) (in press).

12. L. O. Svaasand, and R. Ellingsen, Optical properties of human brain, Photochem. Photobiol. (1983) (in press).
13. T. J. Dougherty, Photoradiation therapy (PRT) of malignant tumors, in: "Critical Reviews in Oncology/Hematology, CRC Press, Boca Raton, FL. (1983) (in press).
14. A. E. Profio, and D. R. Doiron, Dosimetry considerations in photoradiation therapy, Med. Phys. 8:190 (1981).

AN OPTIMISED LASER SYSTEM FOR THE EVALUATION OF HpD THERAPY

John Moore

Coherent Inc.
3210 Porter Drive
Palo Alto, CA 94304

INTRODUCTION

The interest in Photo Radiation Therapy (PRT) has increased dramatically in the last two years. As the requirements for the evaluation of the technique have been established we have responded by designing dedicated laser equipment.

The two key aspects of PRT are:
(1) Generation of medium intensity blue-green light to excite fluorescence in the Hematoporphyrin Derivative (HpD).

(2) Generation of intense red light to initiate a photochemical change in the HpD.

When HpD is injected into the body it selectively accumulates in malignant tissue. Excitation of HpD with blue-green light generates fluorescence in the red part of the spectrum. In this way the HpD can be located. The absorption spectrum of HpD is very broad. Light in the region of 400nm to 525nm will be absorbed and give red fluorescence. The blue-green output of the Argon Ion laser is well matched to this absorption having most energy in the region 488nm to 514nm.

To initiate the photochemical reaction which breaks down the HpD molecule is more difficult. The wavelength region in which HpD absorbs and reacts photochemically is quite broad. However a second requirement is that the body tissues, in which the HpD is located, are sufficiently transparent to allow the light to penetrate to useful depths. 630nm has been selected by most researchers in the field as a best compromise. This wavelength can be reached using a

293

combination of Argon and Dye lasers. The Argon laser is used to
excite a second laser in which the active gain medium is a free
flowing stream of dye in a viscous solvent - usually ethylene glycol.
The dye absorbs energy from the Argon laser in the blue-green and
fluoresces in the red. By proper design of the Dye laser the energy
in the dye fluorescence can be concentrated at 630nm.

Both the blue and red light exit the lasers in a narrow collimated beam which can be very efficiently collected and focussed into
an optical fibre.

We have designed a range of PRT equipment to meet the above
requirements. The key elements being an Argon Ion laser, Dye laser
and fibre optic delivery system.

THE ARGON ION LASER

The key requirements for the Argon Ion laser are power, ease of
use, reliability and cost. Consideration of power and cost allows us
to offer two versions of the INNOVA series of Argon lasers. Both
incorporate Tungsten-ceramic technology for performance and realia-
bility. The smaller laser is rated at 5 watts while the larger laser
has a rating of 20 watts. Both lasers benefit from the many years of
product development to give stable power and long life. A choice
between the two can be made on a cost basis alone.

THE DYE LASER

The Dye laser, for the user, should meet the same requirements.
However the nature of the Dye laser imposes more stringent requirements on the design engineer. The Dye laser is optically pumped by
the Argon laser. The performance of the Dye laser is thus intimately
connected to that of the Argon laser and the interface between the
two in addition to its inherent performance.

The Dye laser is built on a solid Invar steel bar to ensure
optimum mechanical and thermal stability. Heavy aluminum is used
to mount all optical components to the Invar bar. High resolution
orthogonal screw adjustments allow simple and reliable optimisation
of the Dye laser optical cavity.

The wavelength at which the Dye laser operates depends on several key elements.
First is the dye used.
Different dyes have different fluorescence curves and for PRT it is
important to choose a dye that has a peak fluorescence in the region
of 630nm. A dye with that characteristic has been found which also
has excellent lifetime characteristics when pumped with the high
powers required for this application.

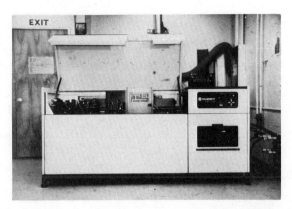

Figure 1. The Coherent PRT 105 system

Second is the optics.
The performance of the dye laser is critically dependant on the
optics used to define the cavity. It is especially important to
optimise the reflectivity and transmission of the optics to ensure
the highest output in the desired wavelength region. The values
chosen will be different from those intended for more general purpose operation of the dye laser.

Third is the wavelength selection.
Whilst the choice of dye and optics limits the region in which the
dye laser can operate, the actual output wavelength will depend also
on the age of the dye, the dye concentration and the reflectivity
of the mirrors. To ensure operation at the desired wavelength it
is important to have an element in the cavity that defines the operating independant of all these variables.
A low loss birefringent filter is used, clamped in position, to
eliminate wavelength drift.

     As a further precaution − and to allow for some controlled
experimentation -- an electronic wavelength readout allows continuous
monitoring of the operating wavelength.

     Any movement of the Argon laser beam with respect to the Dye
laser will cause a drop in power output from the Dye laser. To ap-
preciate how severe this problem can be it must be remembered that
the Argon laser beam is focussed down to a very small spot in the
dye stream. The focussed spot is less than 30 microns. Thus a movement of the Argon laser beam of 5 microns can cause a 10 percent
drop in the Dye laser output power. The most careful mechanical
interface design cannot guarantee 5 percent long term power stability for the Dye laser output without some servo stabilisation
between the Argon and Dye lasers.

To ensure stable long term performance from the Dye laser a
mechanical servo alignment system has been designed to interface
the Argon laser to the Dye laser. A wedge shaped piece of glass
is rotated in front of the Argon laser. This causes the beam to
trace out a small cone shaped surface. In turn the focussed Argon
laser spot in the Dye laser dye stream traces out a small circle.
This is equivalent to a small X and Y dither. Using a phase locked
detector to monitor the Dye laser output an X-Y error signal is
generated. This signal is used in a servo loop to adjust a fold
mirror, which maintains the focussed Argon laser beam at the optimum position in the dye stream. This concept allows long term
operation without the need for operator intervention.

THE FIBRE OPTIC INTERFACE

The first requirements on the fibre optic delivery system is to
select between the blue-green diagnostic beam from the Argon laser
and the red treatment beam from the Dye laser. The second requirement is to allow the red output to be delivered through up to five
independant fibres.

To use the Argon laser output as a diagnostic beam requires
only the insertion of a pick off mirror to direct the blue-green
light through a focussing lens and into a dedicated fibre optic.
To access this beam only requires the operator to select the green
option on the control module. There is no requirement for the operator to physically move or adjust the optical system. Selection
of this option activates a solenoid which moves a pick off mirror
into the Argon laser beam and directs a part of the beam into a
lens. The lens delivers the blue-green beam to a fibre optic. The
remainder of the beam is dumped into a heat sink to ensure that
the diagnostic beam is of a suitably low power.

The optical splitting system uses high quality dielectric
coated mirrors. This ensures minimum loss of laser power and good
control of the amount of energy delivered to each individual fibre.
A series of three beam splitters is used. The front surface of the
first beamsplitter picks off 20 percent of the incoming red beam,
the back surface 25 percent. Only the lower half of the front surface has a 20 percent coating - the top half is antireflection
coated. In this way the beam reflected from the second surface is
transmitted without attenuation back through the first surface
(see figure 2). The second beamsplitter picks off 35 percent of
the beam at the front surface and 50 percent at the back. The last
splitter reflects 100 percent of the remaining energy.

After picking off the five equal intensity beams they are
each focussed by a lens into an optical fibre. The output fibre
ports are individually interlocked to ensure that no light can
escape unless the correct fiber has been inserted into the port.

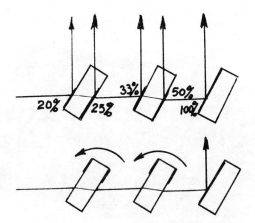

Figure 2.   The optical beamsplitter

The light power going into the fiber optic interface can be monitored
at any time and displayed on the control module.

By rotating the first of the three beamsplitters the dye
laser output can be delivered to only three fibres with an approximate power split of 33/33/33 percent. By rotating the beamsplitters rather than removing them the optical path and alignment remain undisturbed. Alternatively if the second splitter is rotated
the output is again to three fibres with a power distribution 20/
20/60 percent. Rotating both splitters allows all the power output to be delivered through one fibre.

It is possible to remove any fibre from the system without
affecting the performance of those remaining. A safety interlock
ensure that no light leaks from the unused port.

THE REMOTE CONTROL MODULE

The PRT system has been designed with operator convenience in mind
at all times. The mechanical and optical parts are stable enough
to ensure hands off operation over long periods of time. In use it
is possible to locate the console up to 15 metres from the operator through the use of a remote control module. All parts of the
equipment can be controlled with this module. (Fig. 3)

SELECTION OF FIBRES

Using the SPLITTER control on the remote module the red output

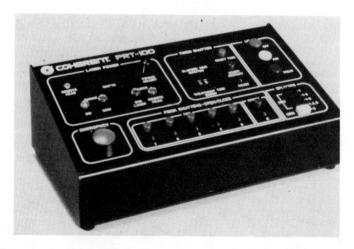

Figure 3. The PRT 105 remote module control system

can be directed through
- All fibres with an equal division of power
- Three fibres with an equal division of power
- Three fibres with a 20/20/60 division of power
- One fibre with all the power

MEASUREMENT AND CONTROL OF INDIVIDUAL FIBRE OUTPUT

The remote module allows the power level from the system to be
continuously monitored and controlled. This facility is for both
the Argon (blue-green) and Dye (red) outputs.

SELECTION OF AIM/TREATMENT MODE

This facility offers a low power output to assist in positioning
the fibres in the best position without risk of overexposure.

SELECTION OF PERIOD OF TREATMENT

The clock feature allows digital selection of the treatment time
with automatic power off at the end of the selected period. A
pause feature is included to allow temporary interruption of the
beam and subsequent continuation of the selected total exposure
time. As a fail safe precaution an emergency off switch on the remote module shuts the system down if needed.

The fibre optic cables are also accessible at the remote module. As a convenience the duration of the treatment can be preset
at the module - and if necessary temporarily interrupted and then

continued using the pause / restart facility.

SUMMARY

An optimised laser system has been described for the evaluation of
HpD therapy. Up to 3.2 watts of continuous power is available at
630nM. This power can be delivered through up to five separate fibres with various power splits between them. In addition a blue-
green diagnostic beam is available for diagnostics. The wavelength
and power level of the output light are continuously monitored at
the remote module. A novel servo system has been included to ensure
long term hands off operation.

A MULTI-LED SOURCE FOR PHOTORADIATION THERAPY

Giulio Jori, Riccardo Pratesi[+], and M. Scalvini[o]

Istituto di Biologia Animale, Università di Padova
Italy

[+] Istituto di Fisica Superiore dell'Università, Istituto
di Elettronica Quantistica, CNR, Firenze, Italy

[o] MASPEC - CNR, Parma, Italy

INTRODUCTION

Light sources emitting at the long wavelength wing of the absorption spectrum of Hematoporphyrin (Hp), between 610 and 640 nm, are currently used in photoradiation therapy (PRT) in order to maximize penetration of light into the tumor mass. Optical output powers of several watts are necessary to ensure the suitable irradiance ($30 \div 100$ mW/cm^2) at the tumor surface. Filtered high-power Xenon or halogen lamps, and ion-laser-pumped dye lasers tuned at $\lambda_p \simeq 630$ nm are the most common sources used so far. The overall electrical-to-optical conversion efficiency of these sources is quite small, typically 0.05% (0.2 for halogen lamps). Flash-lamp-pumped dye lasers are now commercially available at average output power of $10 \div 20$ W; the efficiency is $\sim 0.8\%$ in the red [1]. Their use for photodynamic therapy is under investigation [2]. Gold vapor lasers emitting $1 \div 6$ W at 628 nm with 0.2% efficiency represent another interesting new source for PRT of tumors [3].

A different class of light sources that could find application in the PRT of tumors is represented by Light Emitting Diodes (LEDs). These miniaturized solid-state lamps have been used almost exclusively as very low power indicators and displays untill recently; now the application in several growing fields (such as optical communications) has led to the development of high-efficiency, high-intensity LEDs. Red light emitting diodes are today commercially available at output powers of several milliwatts with an efficiency of $\sim 5\%$, and at low cost. As the emitted wavelengths range from

301

620 to 680 nm a suitably shaped multi-LED system could provide the
necessary power density for the PRT of superficial tumors. The development of tightly-packed arrays of incoherent or coherent high-
-efficiency LEDs may lead to more compact sources for PRT, and, in
particular, to efficient optical fiber systems for endoscopic treatments.

In this paper the possibility of utilizing a multi-LED system
as light source to promote porphyrin-sensitized photoprocesses has
been tested by following the Hp-sensitized photooxidation of the
aminoacid L-tryptophan (Trp) either free or bound with human serum
albumin (HSA), as well as the Hp-sensitized photokilling of HeLa
cells. Both these systems have been previously investigated by using conventional light sources [4,5].

MATERIALS AND METHODS

The H-500 Hi-super bright red LED (GaAlAs) made by Stanley
Electric Co, Ltd (Japan) has been chosen for the experiment. Nominal values of output intensity, peak wavelength and spectral bandwidth at i_f = 20 mA forward current (f.c.) and room temperature are:
I = 500 mcd; λ_p = 660 nm; $\Delta\lambda$ = 60 nm, respectively. All these parameters are strongly temperature dependent. A decrease of the operating temperature produces a blue-shift of the peak wavelength,
and a narrowing of the output spectrum; the total light intensity
increases by several orders of magnitude when the diode is operated

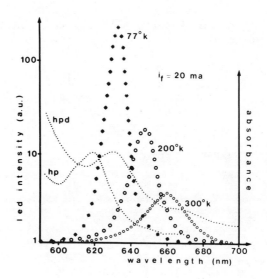

Fig. 1.

at 77°K. Fig. 1 shows the emission spectra (at 20 mA f.c.) of the
H-500 LED at several temperatures, together with the absorption
spectra of Hp and Hp derivative (HpD). As it can be seen, at room
temperature the absorption by Hp is expected to be low due to the
30 nm shift between LED emission and Hp absorption maxima[*]. By reducing the LED temperature, the emission maximum can be brought into
coincidence with the 630 nm peak of HpD: the narrower spectrum and
the much higher intensity should now greatly enhance the efficiency
of the LED to excite HpD molecules.

In the experiment the H-500 LED has been operated at room temperature and at 50 mA f.c.: output powers greater than 3 mW has been
measured in these conditions. The LED collimating capsule provides
a half-intensity full-divergence of 45°, i.e. half power of the LED
can be collected on 1 cm^2 area target placed at 13.5 mm from the
capsule. Thirtythree LEDs have been inserted into closely-packed,
radially oriented holes in a metallic hemisphere with 15 mm inner
diameter. The light intensity distribution over the central 1 cm^2
spot in the equatorial plane was sufficiently uniform with a power
density of $\sim$ 27 mW/cm^2 (at 50 mA f.c.).

RESULTS AND DISCUSSION

Hematoporphyrin-sensitized photooxidation of tryptophan and the
tryptophyl residue of human serum albumin

When 0.7 ml of a 0.1 mM Trp solution in 0.05 M phosphate buffer
at pH = 7.4 was irradiated in the presence of 100 μM Hp at ca. 20°C,
the aminoacid underwent photooxidative modification according to
first-order kinetics (Fig. 2.a,b). Such a behaviour is typical of
porphyrin-promoted photodynamic processes [6]. The rate constant of
the photoprocess was 1.3 10^{-4}s^{-1}, i.e. one order of magnitude lower
than that observed for the same system exposed to a He-Ne laser
emitting ca. 25 mW/cm^2 at 632.8 nm[7]. The rate constant almost doubled (Fig. 2.b) when HSA-bound Hp was used as a photosensitizer for
the modification of the unique Trp residue present in HSA. Under
our experimental conditions, Hp yields a 1:1 ground state complex
with HSA, the porphyrin binding site being at 1.7 nm from the indole
side chain of the Trp redisue [8]. The enhancement of the rate constant for photoprocesses promoted by protein-bound porphyrins has
been previously observed [9] and ascribed to a greater triplet quantum
yield for bound Hp as compared with free Hp and/or a shift in the
overall photooxidation mechanism from a type II ($^1O_2$-involving) pathway to a type I (radical-involving) pathway.

---

[*]
At the time of the experiment the Hewlett-Packard LED HP 3750 emit-
ting 160 mcd at 635 nm was not available. Its better matching of
Hp absorption should compensate for the lower emission power.

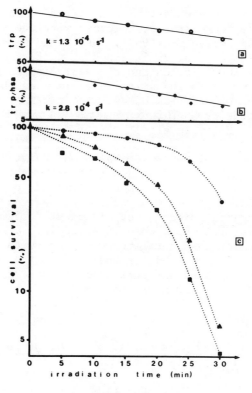

Fig. 2.

The above outline considerations strongly suggest that porphy-
rin-photosensitization induced by irradiation with LEDs follow reaction mechanisms essentially overlapping those promoted by other
types of light sources.

Hematoporphyrin-sensitized photokilling of HeLa cells

The sensitivity of cell cultures to the treatment with LEDs
and Hp was tested by using the heteroploid human cell line (HeLa)
D98/AH$_2$ grown on F$_{12}$ medium (containing 5% calf serum) at 37°C in
Falcon plastic vials saturated with 95% air and 5% CO$_2$. All experiments were performed with cell monolayers from 96 h-aged flasks,
fed 24 h earlier. Cells had been previously incubated in the dark
with Hp (1,10 or 20 µg/ml) for 15 min. at 22°C. After incubation,
the Hp solution was discarded and the cells were rinsed once with
saline. The cell monolayers adherent to the flask were then exposed to the LED for different periods of time.

After illumination, the cells were incubated in the dark at 37°C for 24 hours with sterile HAM solution saturated with air/CO_2. Cell survival was then assayed by the trypan blue exclusion test (0.08% trypan blue solution in saline). Blank studies indicated a ΔE at 580 nm of 0.68 per 10^6 cells under our experimental conditions.

The survival of HeLa cells exposed to red light after incubation with various Hp concentration is indicated in Fig. 2.c. Clearly, increasing the Hp concentration caused both a shortening of the initial lag period and a steeper decrease of the fraction of surviving cells. This finding was expected since under our irradiation conditions there was no total absorption of the incident light, mainly owing to the low molar absorption of Hp in the red spectral region. In any case, the shape of the plots definitely indicates the occurrence of photoinduced irreversible damage of HeLa cells. Once again, the efficiency of the photoprocess is markedly lower than that observed upon irradiation of the same system with white light from a 150 W slide projector [5]. However, the feasibility of cell photokilling using LED systems is apparent.

FUTURE DEVELOPMENTS

The development of high-intensity LEDs at the desired wavelengths, incoherent and coherent LED-arrays, and efficient LED-optical fiber coupling, is only a technological and economic problem, and it may be triggered by a specific application. In this regard, important improvements of active and passive optical components have been recently reported.

<u>Multi-LED System</u>

IR LED sources (λ_p = 880 nm) with 100 mW capability are now available at very low price [10]. Development of 630 nm-high power LEDs would permit the assembly of bidimensional arrays of tightly--packed LEDs capable of producing irradiances suitable for phototherapy of superficial tumors. Because the typical dimension of the LED active area is 300 μm x 400 μm, the high irradiance of a multimilliwatt LED makes coupling to individual optical fiber an attractive possibility for multiple-fiber implantation into tumor masses, and irradiation of internal tumors with large diameter endoscopes (as in gynecology). High coupling efficiency and lower costs are now possible with new LED mountings where in place of the plastic/glass collimating capsule a metal windowed package containing an internal microlensing system is used to project a uniform spot on the can's surface [10]. This structure provides efficient light coupling to optical fibers without the need for expensive precision connectors required with the previous LED-fiber coupling systems.

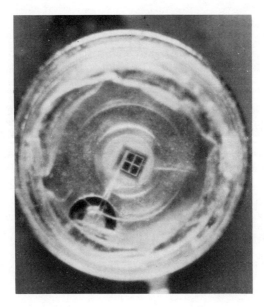

Fig. 3.

LED-Arrays

Straightforward hybrid-circuit fabrication techniques should permit the assembly of single LED chips into tightly-packed arrays capable of producing the irradiance needed for PRT, as already proposed by Epstein et al.[11]. Integrated optical systems could then provide the suitable radiation pattern or efficient coupling to optical fiber delivery systems. Fig. 3 shows a picture of a 2 x 2 array of four IR LEDs already available commercially.

Diode Lasers and Diode Laser Arrays

A number of single-emitter conventional semiconductor diode lasers emit output powers in excess of 50 mW cw from a single facet in the near IR[12]. Far-red diode lasers begin to be produced at lwoer power (10÷20 mW). Future development of high power diode lasers at $\lambda \simeq 630$ nm should permit very compact and efficient multi--element sources for PRT.

Recently, cw operation of multiemitter (40) phase-locked arrays of IR diode lasers has also been demonstrated at output power levels as great as 2.5 W[12]. Because the emission is coherent, the laser light can be focused into a single diffraction-limited spot. When similar powers will be available in the useful porphyrin absorption range, important progresses will be registered in the phototechnology of tumor therapy.

CONCLUSIONS

In this paper evidence has been presented that red light emitting diodes (LEDs) can be used to kill porphyrin-sensitized tumor cells. Multi-LED systems can provide the power density needed for therapy of superficial tumors. Operation of multi-LED (H-500) arrays at 77°K is expected to produce much higher power densities and to allow direct LED coupling to optical fibers for the treatment of internal tumors with large bore endoscopes. The application to PRT of future developments of incoherent LED-arrays, diode lasers, and diode laser arrays has also been discussed.

This work has been supported in part by the CNR Special Project "Laser di Potenza".

REFERENCES

1. P. Mazzinghi, P. Burlamacchi, and V. Rivano, High Efficiency, high energy slab dye laser for photobiological experiments, Submitted for publication.
2. D. A. Belenier, C. W. Lin, and J. A. Parrish, Hematoporphyrin Derivative and pulse laser photoradiation, Symposium on "Porphyrin Locialization and Treatment of Tumors", Santa Barbara, CA, USA, April 24-28 (1983).
3. R. E. Grova, Copper vapor laser come of age, Laser Focus, 18:45 (1982).
4. E. Rossi, A. Van der Vors, and G. Jori, Competition between the singlet oxygen and electron transfer mechanisms in the porphyrin-sensitized photooxidation of L-tryptophan in acqueous micellar dispersions, Photochem. Photobiol. 34:447 (1981).
5. I. Cozzani, and J. D. Spikes, Photodamage of malignant human cells in vitro by Hematoporphyrin-visible light: possible meachanisms for photocytotoxicity, Med. Biol. Environ. 10:269 (1982).
6. J. D. Spikes, Porphyrins and related compounds as photodynamic sensitizers, Ann. N.Y. Acad. Sci. 244:496 (1975)
7. E. Reddi, E. Rossi, G. Jori, L. Tomio, and B. Salvato, Photodamage of biological systems upon irradiation with He-Ne laser in the presence of Hematoporphyrin, Med. Biol. Environ. 10:251 (1982).
8. E. Reddi, F. Ricchelli, and G. Jori, Interaction of human serum albumin with Hematoporphyrin and its Zn (II) and Fe (III) derivatives, Int. J. Peptide Protein Res. 18:402 (1981).
9. E. Reddi, E. Rossi, and G. Jori, Factors controlling the efficiency of porphyrins as photosensitizers of biological systems to damage by visible light, Med. Biol. Environ. 9:337 (1981).

10. T. Ormond, Fiber-optic components, EDN 28:112 (1983).
11. M. E. Mahric, M. Epstein, and R. V. Lobraico, A proposal for light-emitting diode arrays for photoradiation therapy, To be published.
12. D. R. Scifres, R. D. Burnham, C.Lindstrom, W. Streifer, and T.L. Paoli, High-power diode lasers, Paper TUC5, C.L.E.O., Baltimore, USA, May 17-20 (1983).

SIDE RADIATION OPTICAL FIBERS FOR MEDICAL APPLICATIONS

Vera Russo, Giancarlo Righini and Silvana Trigari

Istituto Ricerca Onde Elettromagnetiche - C.N.R.

Firenze Via Panciatichi 64 - Italy

INTRODUCTION

The multimode optical fibers, commercially available, are today a very convenient system for delivering the laser radiation to
the tissue, in surgical as in therapeutic applications. When the optical fibers are used in combination with the endoscopic techniques they represent a powerfull and not destructive method for reaching and treating the tissue situated in inaccessible zones of the
human body.

Generally step-index optical fibers, of relatively large core
diameter (up to 600 µm) are used having a flat end; as a consequence
the output beam presents a limited angular divergence, depending
mostly on the core and cladding refractive indeces.

In some endoscopic or cavitational techniques, it can be difficult to use a conventional flat end fiber radiating moslty forward for the treatment of a sick tissue situated for instance on
the walls and therefore sideways with respect to the fiber. In such
a case an optical fiber able to radiate much more sideways than
forwards could be of effective interest. The danger of a high energy
directed towards healthy tissues could be so avoided and a great
part of the available energy could be used for the treatment.

Modifying the optical characteristics of an optical fiber beam
can be made in different ways. For endoscopic applications the most
convenient technique is that one of giving the fiber tip a differ-

ent shape from the flat end [1,2]. The shaping of the output beam from
a fiber to be used in medicine can be obtained by following techniques similar to that ones used in optical communications for increasing the coupling efficiency between the light sources (L.E.D. or
lasers) and the fiber input.

The first attempt to solve the problem of a side radiation optical fiber in medicine consisted of widening as much as possible
the output angular divergence of the fiber. This has been made by
giving the fiber tip a round shape (arc or bulb type)[3,4] or by frost-
ing the fiber tip, of any shape, so producing a scattering terminal
[2,5].

A different approach to the problem is that one of designing
special terminals having radiation patterns with the intensity maximum in a direction different from the fiber axis.

Two different classes of side radiation terminals can be recog-
gnized. The first one comprehends terminals having a shape symmetric
with respect to the fiber axis and of consequence presenting an output intensity distribution with axial rotation symmetry. The second
class comprehends asymmetric terminals having shape designed in such
a way to have strongly asymmetric radiation patterns. The ultimate
scope is that of obtaining terminals radiating only towards one
side.

Side radiation terminals belonging to both these classes are
presented together a their preliminary characterization. Applications of the differently ended optical fibers are suggested for different medical specialties.

SIDE RADIATION TERMINALS WITH AXIAL ROTATION SYMMETRY

Taper ended optical fibers are characterized by a very wide
radiation pattern having a central minimum [6]. The energy is distributed along cones coaxial to the fiber axis.

Both cone and truncated cone terminals have been constructed
and tested in our laboratory on silica plastic fibers with core
diameter of 600 μm and 300 μm, Fig. 1. Truncated cones are resulted
less brittle than cones and therefore more appropriate for a practi-
cal application if vertex angles very narrow are required.

By varying the geometrical parameters of the taper,end face and
vertex angle, one can vary the direction of the output intensity
maximum [5].

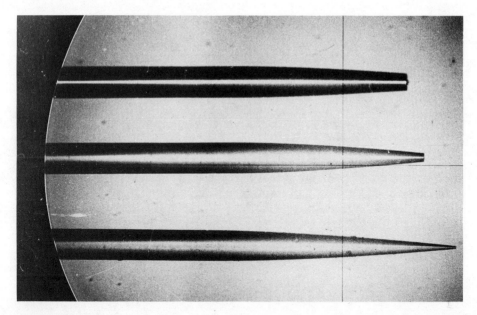

Fig. 1. Cone and truncated cone terminals of optical fibers with
        core diameter of 300 µm.

As an example, Fig. 2 shows the radiation pattern (intensity
distribution detected on a meridional section, plotted versus the
output angle θ) of a truncated cone terminal with α = 15⁰ and
end face   = 30   µm. The intensity maximum has an off-axis direction
of 30⁰ .

A cone ended optical fiber with larger vertex angle (≃60⁰)
is shown in Fig. 3 . It presents the radiation pattern shown in
Fig. 4. Here the maximum has an off-axis direction of 60⁰ .

Truncated cone and cone terminals are obtained with a chemical etching by dipping, for different times, a flat-end fiber suitably prepared in advance in a 40 % fluoridric acid solution. Large
cone terminals need a different preparation from that one for narrow cone terminals.

Cone ended optical fibers with large vertex angles, having
conical output beams at large angles with respect to the fiber,

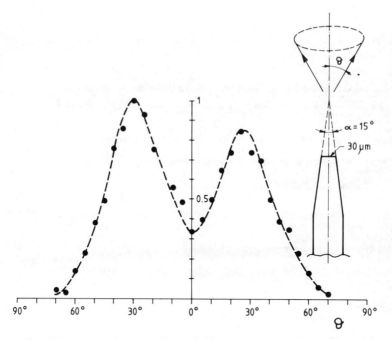

Fig. 2 Intensity distribution from a truncated cone optical fiber
with a small angle α, plotted versus the output angle θ.
The fiber end with the geometrical parameters are sketched
to the right of the radiation pattern together the direction
of the intensity maximum.

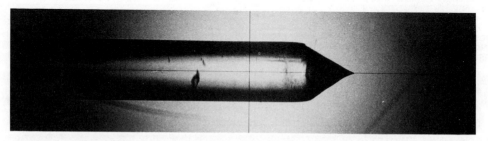

Fig.3 Cone ended optical fiber with a vertex angle of ∼ 60°.

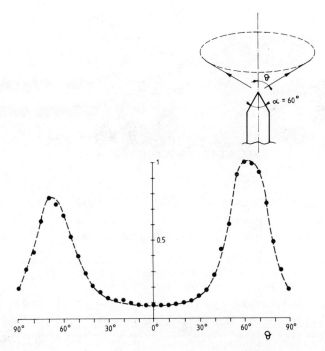

Fig.4 Radiation pattern of the cone ended optical fiber shown in
       Fig. 3

are particularly suitable for laser treatments (surgical or photo-
therapic) of narrow cylindrical cavities. For instance, obstruc -
tions in blood vessels or in bronchos can be easily reached without
damaging the surrounding healthy tissues.

ASYMMETRIC SIDE RADIATION TERMINALS

     Two different types of asymmetric terminals radiating mostly
towards one side are under investigation in our laboratory. The
first type is constituted by optical fibers terminated with a tilted
microlens (bulb type), Fig. 5 a) and b). The second one is constituted by optical fibers having a beveled end, Fig. 5 c) with such an
inclination that the phoenomenum of the total reflection occurs on
this face and the beam get out through the opposite wall of the
fiber. By varying the geometrical parameters, radius of the bulb
and tilting angle or the inclination of the planar end face in the
total reflection terminals, one can obtain different optical per-
formances

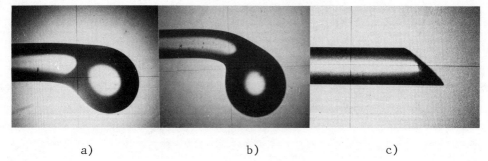

a)   b)   c)

Fig. 5   a) Optical fiber with a bulb terminal having small tilting
         angle. b) Optical fiber with a bulb terminal having large
         tilting angle. c) Optical fiber with a total reflection
         terminal.

As an example,Fig. 6 and Fig. 7 show the radiation patterns of
two bulb terminals having different radius of the bulb, r_b,and different tilting angle. The detection has been made in the meridional
section containing the tilted bulb. Fig. 8 shows the radiation pat-
ter of the total reflection terminal shown in Fig. 5 c).

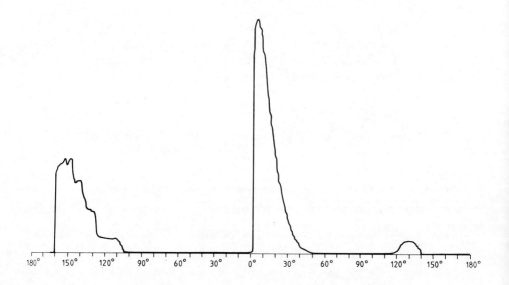

Fig.6 Radiation pattern of a bulb terminal with $r_b=1.7\ r_{fiber}$,shown
      in Fig.5 a). The abrupt cut of the diagram is due to the screen
      ing of the beam from the mechanical support.

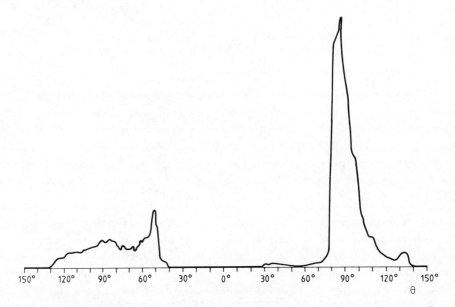

Fig. 7 Radiation pattern of the bulb terminal, with $r_b = 2.25\ r_{fiber}$, shown in Fig. 5b).

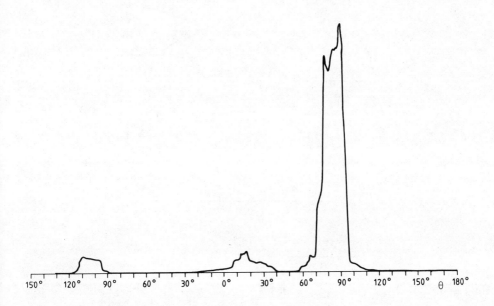

Fig. 8 Radiation pattern of the total reflection terminal with 45° of inclination of the end face.

All the three terminals show a main beam in the expected direction and a secondary beam in the opposite direction. The last two
terminals have the main beam directed at 90° from the fiber axis and
a secondary beam very low, so that they represent, up to now, the
best one side radiation terminals.

Tilted microlens so as total reflection terminals give rise to
output beams at a large angle from the fiber axis. However the two
types of side radiation terminals are characterized by a different
shape of the main beam. In order to have a more complete description
of the behaviour of the above mentioned terminals we carried out another experimental test.

A sheet of photographic paper was rolled around the fiber tip
in such a way as to have a cylindrical surface of 5 cm in diameter
(Fig. 9). The optical fiber, fed by an argon laser illuminated
the photographic paper that, once opened and developed, provided
further information on the shape of the output beam. The intensity
distribution on the meridional section of interest was also detected
on two lines parallel to the fiber axis (dashed lines).

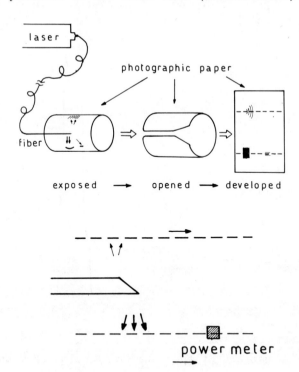

Fig. 9.   Sketch of the experimental test showing the successive steps
          and arrangement of the detector.

The results of the two measurements were collected in Fig. 10, both for a total reflection and for a tilted bulb terminal. The total reflection terminal has the main beam very narrow in the meridional section containing the fiber tip and much larger in the perpendicular section. At the contrary the bulb terminal has the main beam more symmetric.

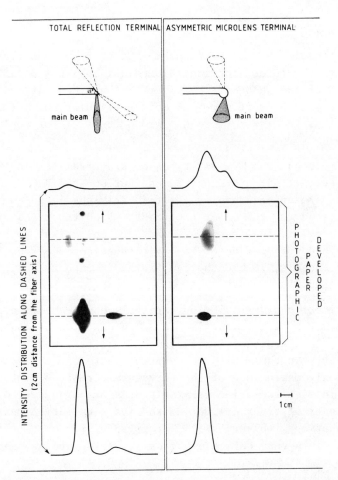

Fig. 10 The photographic paper shows the different shape of the main beam of the two different terminals. The intensity registration along the dashed lines are also reported.

The asymmetric side radiation optical fibers are of particular interest in narrow cavities when one has to irradiate the sick tissue situated on one side of the wall.

Preliminary tests with tilted bulb optical fibers have been carried out in urology for laser surgery of tumors placed in a position inaccessible with the conventional instruments. (In collaboration with the Florence Hospital , Urology Departement).

It is to be noted that microlens terminals can be fabricated[4] in the same operative theatre where a laser is available, withoutto decouple the fiber from the source.

CONCLUSIONS

The shaping of the laser beam exiting from an optical fiber is a subject of interest for many biomedical applications. Simple modifications of the shape of the fiber tip have been already suggested [2,7]. At present more and more particular characteristics are required, as the laser technique widen its field of application in medicine.

In this paper different types of side radiation optical fibers are presented, that are under investigation at I.R.O.E. Terminals with axial rotation symmetry, particularly the large cone terminals, are suggested for the laser treatments of obstructions on the walls of narrow cylindrical cavities. They are convenient to save energy and to avoid irradiation of healty tissues.Applications in treatment of blood vessels, in bronchology, in gastroentherology, in urology are expected.

Asymmetric side radiation terminals can be of interest in cavities where the sick tissue is placed on one side of the wall and therefore inaccessible with a conventional flat end fiber. They are particularly suitable also in cavities where the zone cannot be reached only making use of the curvature permitted by the endoscope. Asymmetric side radiation terminals are more than ever of interest when an optical fiber delivering the laser radiation must be used in combination with very small but rigid vision systems(f.i.Selfoscopes), or in very delicate organs like eye, brain, hearth.

REFERENCES

1. G. C. Righini, V. Russo, and S. Sottini, "Optical fiber device
    for transmitting and focusing laser radiation for medical
    applications", Patent 1/8/1977 filed U.K. 7/4/82.
2. V. Russo, Fibers in Medicine, in: "New directions of guided
    waves and coherent optics", Part I, M. Nijhoff Publishers,
    NATO (1983), in press.
3. V. Russo, G. C. Righini, S. Sottini, and S. Trigari: Characteri-
    zation of a microlens-ended optical fiber, Alta Frequenza
    (1982) in press.
4. V. Russo, G. C. Righini, S. Sottini, and S. Trigari: Microlens-
    -ended fibers a new fabrication technique, in: "Proceedings
    Photon 83", Paris, May 16-19 (1983).
5. S. Trigari, "Terminazioni di fibre ottiche: studio e realizza-
    zione", Thesis University of Florence (1981).
6. C. T. Chang, and D. C. Auth, Radiation characteristics of a
    tapered cylindrical optical fibre, J. Opt. Soc. Am 66:1191
    (1978).
7. K. Eguchi, R. Ono, S. Ikeda, and Y. Doi, J-shaped fiber tip in
    YAG laser cauterization applicable to endobronchial lesions,
    in: "Laser-Tokyo '81", K. Atsumi and N. Nimsakul, eds., Inter
    Group Corp., Tokyo (1981).

FLUORESCENCE OF HEMATOPORPHYRIN-DERIVATIVE FOR DETECTION AND CHARACTERIZATION OF TUMORS

A.E. Profio, M.J. Carvlin, J. Sarnaik, and L.R. Wudl

University of California

Santa Barbara, CA 93106, USA

INTRODUCTION

Hematoporphyrin-Derivative (HpD) is well known for its tumor specificity and its photodynamic effect in photoradiation therapy. HpD is also fluorescent, and can be used to detect and localize tumors such as in fluorescence endoscopy. There is also the possibility that the differential accumulation of HpD may vary not only between benign and malignant states, but at various stages in the transformation of normal cells to malignancy, permitting the fluorescence of HpD to serve as an indicator of the transformation. The concentration of HpD in the tumor and in surrounding nonmalignant tissue is needed to plan the therapy because the absorbed dose in photoradiation therapy is proportional to the concentration of HpD, and the space irradiance or energy flux density of the light at the dose point. Fluorescence may serve as an indicator of HpD concentration if corrections are made for competing absorption.

Techniques are being developed at the University of California, Santa Barbara to image HpD fluorescence (primarily applied to localization of early bronchogenic tumors), to measure the fluorescence yield in vivo and investigate the optimum time after intravenous injection to image or measure fluorescence, and to measure the concentration of HpD in tissues as a guide to photoradiation therapy.

PROPERTIES OF HpD

The absorption and fluorescence emission properties of HpD

321

(Photofrin, Oncology Research and Development Company, Cheek-towaga, NY, USA) have been measured by Doiron.[1,2] More recently, the absorption properties of Photofrin and Photofrin II ("active component") have been measured by one of us (MJC) in the labora-tory of Dr. T.J. Dougherty at Roswell Park Memorial Institute, Buffalo, NY. Figure 1 plots the absorbance as a function of wave-length in CHO cells that had been incubated for 24 hours with medium containing Photofrin. The absorption spectra are of the aetio-type, i.e., four visible bands, I-IV, with relative inten-sities IV > III > II > I, going from short to long wavelength. Different concentrations were investigated, from 10 ug/ml to 50 ug/ml. In all cases the spectrum of Photofrin remained aetio after cellular uptake. Hence, no concentration dependence is expressed in this range. Furthermore, it appears that significant metabolic alteration of the drug does not occur in this system.

Additional experiments were conducted to identify the state of aggregation of porphyrin retained by the cell. The Soret band occurs at 390 nm for monomeric HpD (Photofrin) and is shifted to shorter wavelength for dimers (370 nm) and higher order aggregates or oligomers (365 nm). The absorption spectra of CHO cells that had been incubated with HpD were recorded on a dual-beam spectro-photometer using as a reference a suspension of unlabeled cells of the same density. The spectral measurements were made in a three step process. First, cells were suspended in phosphate buffered saline for 30 minutes and a bulk solution spectrum was measured. Second, the suspension was centrifuged, and the spectrum of the supernatant was recorded. Finally, the cell pellet was resus-pended in new phosphate buffered saline, and the absorption spec-trum measured. The results indicate that the state of aggregation of intracellular porphyrin differs from that of the extracellular porphyrin. The more highly aggregated material appears to be preferentially retained by the cell, while monomeric porphyrin is capable of leaving the cell. This determination is significant in light of other recent results that identify a dimeric species as being the component of HpD having the greatest biological activity.[3,4] A possible explanation for this effectiveness is sugggested by our experiments which indicate a tendency for tissue to sequester aggregated (active) porphyrin while losing porphyrin monomers. Experiments are now being conducted with purified dimeric species isolated from HpD (Photofrin II) to see whether this hypothesis is borne out.

Extinction coefficients are being measured for Photofrin and Photofrin II by serially adding the drug to the appropriate sol-vent, and verifying the Beer-Lambert Law is followed. Some results are listed in Table 1.

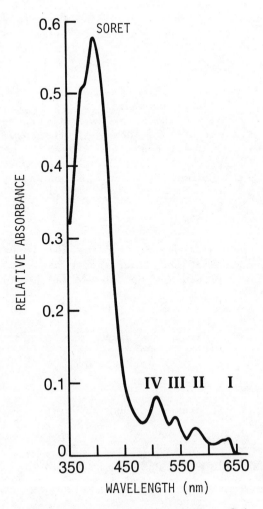

Fig. 1.   Absorbance vs wavelength of Photofrin in cells.

The fluorescence emission spectrum for Photofrin, in 0.9% saline and in saline plus 10% fetal calf serum, is plotted in Figure 2.   The emission spectrum in cells is believed to be similar to that with the saline-plus-serum.   However, the ratios of the peaks in the emission spectrum (625-630 nm, 682-698 nm, and the minor peak at about 665 nm) vary somewhat with the solvent or

cellular environment, and concentration. The fluorescence efficiency (quantum yield, photons emitted per photon absorbed) also
depends on the chemical environment, but is about 4% for HpD in
cells (violet excitation).[1]

Fluorescence excitation follows the absorption spectrum as
long as absorption in other compounds can be neglected. Because
of the large absorption in the Soret band, fluorescence of HpD is
usually excited at about 400 nm. However, other wavelengths could
be used, including the small peak near 630 nm. Inasmuch as this
peak overlaps the emission spectrum, fluorescence can only be
observed at longer wavelengths, and the quantum yield will be
reduced.

TIME DEPENDENCE OF HpD FLUORESCENCE

Experiments are underway in animals and in patients to establish the dependence of the fluorescence as a function of time
after intravenous injection of HpD, hence to guide the selection

TABLE 1

Extinction Coefficients for HpD in Various Solvents

Solvent	Wavelength (nm)	HpD Form	Extinction Coefficient ($M^{-1}cm^{-1}$)
Saline	370	Photofrin	7.70×10^4
	365	Photofrin II	5.84×10^4
Saline + 15% serum	400	Photofrin	9.12×10^4
Sonicated cells	393	Photofrin	7.94×10^4

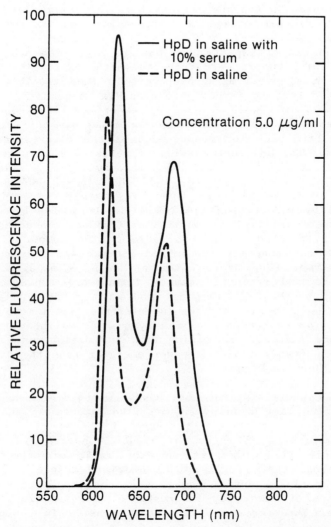

Fig. 2. Fluorescence emission spectra for HpD (Photofrin) in saline plus 10% FC serum (D.R. Doiron).

of the optimum time for detection of small tumors (maximum fluorescence contrast with adequate tumor fluorescence intensity). The
time dependence also impacts on selection of the optimum time for
the photoradiation therapy irradiation, for maximum effect on the
tumor with minimal damage to surrounding nonmalignant tissues.

In one set of experiments, DBA/2Ha mice with subcutaneously
implanted SMT-F tumors were injected in the tail vein with Photofrin at a dosage of 5 mg/kg body weight. Some mice had one tumor
and some had two, to investigate possible errors (the two tumors
on the same animal were in good agreement in fluorescence yield).
At selected times after injection, a mouse was sacrificed and a
skin flap laid back for measurement of the fluorescence of the
tumor and of the adjacent muscle. Fluorescence was excited by a
violet (405 nm) light from a 200 W mercury arc lamp fitted with a
narrowband interference filter and Schott BG-12 absorbing glass
filter to minimize red background (residual background could be
suppressed by subtracting the red light reflected by a suitable
nonfluorescent standard.) The violet light was conducted down one
leg of a bifurcated fiberoptic cable to the tumor. The common
leg, which has randomly intermixed fibers, was in near contact
with the tumor (or muscle) area of about 3 mm diameter. The
fluorescence and reflected source light were conducted up the
other leg, to an S-20 response photomultiplier tube detector,
after passing through a barrier interference filter (695 nm center
wavelength, 40 nm bandpass). The system was calibrated against a
fluorescence standard containing HpD, and measurements were corrected to a standard violet power emerging from the cable. Results are shown in Figure 3.

It is interesting to note that, in this system at least,
there are two time spans when the fluorescence of the tumor is
maximum relative to the fluorescence of the muscle, at about 3
hours (tumor:muscle 5.0) and at about 24 hours after injection
(tumor:muscle 17). This is not the ratio of concentrations,
because among other factors, the tumor and muscle display autofluorescence which adds to the signal from the HpD fluorescence.
In detection of tumors by fluorescence, the autofluorescence of
the tissues interferes and reduces contrast. In photoradiation
therapy, however, autofluorescence is of no consequence and the
optimal time for the irradiation will be determined by other
factors such as retaining sufficient HpD in the tumor for a
reasonable photodynamic dose rate compared to thermal effects or
photodecomposition of the HpD. In either fluorescence detection
or photoradiation therapy, the span in which the tumor: muscle (or
other nonmalignant tissue) ratio is small, should be avoided.

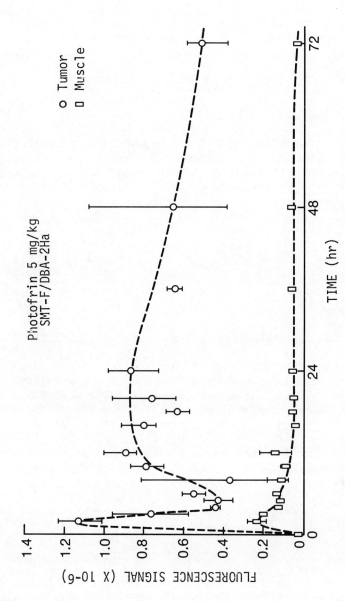

Fig. 3.   Tumor and muscle fluorescence as function of time after injection of Photofrin in mice.

DIFFUSION OF LIGHT IN TISSUE

We have developed a two wavelength-group diffusion theory model for the diffusion of light in tissue, in order to predict light exposure in photoradiation therapy and fluorescence yield and concentration of HpD. The diffusion equations are

$$D_1 \nabla^2 \phi_1 - \mu_{a1} \phi_1 = 0 \tag{1}$$

$$D_2 \nabla^1 \phi_2 - \mu_{a2} \phi_2 + y_{12} \mu_{h1} \phi_1 = 0 \tag{2}$$

where the short wavelength light (excitation or irradiation) is designated by subscript 1, the long wavelength light (average for emission spectrum of fluorescence) is designated by subscript 2, ϕ_1 and ϕ_2 are the corresponding space irradiances (energy fluence rates), D is the diffusion coefficient, μ_a the absorption coefficient of the tissue including any HpD absorption (usually negligible), ∇^2 is the Laplacian operator (equal to d^2/dx^2 in plane geometry), y_{12} is the energy released as fluorescence per unit energy absorbed in HpD at the excitation wavelength, and μ_{h1} is the absorption coefficient of HpD at the excitation wavelength,

$$\mu_{h1} = 2.3 \varepsilon_1 C \tag{3}$$

where C is the concentration and ε_1 the extinction coefficient. These equations can be solved subject to appropriate boundary conditions, e.g., the space irradiance goes to zero at infinity in an effectively infinite medium, or to zero at a boundary, or the partial current density from $J = -D$ grad ϕ may be set equal to the irradiance E_o from a surface source. If there is a volume source, it should be added to the left-hand side of the equation.

The solution for the excitation light, in plane (semi-infinite slab) geometry with a surface source irradiance E_o directed into the slab is

$$\phi_1(x) = \phi_1(0) e^{-\alpha_1 x} \tag{4}$$

where

$$\phi_1(0) = \frac{4E_o}{1 + 2D_1 \alpha_1} \tag{5}$$

and

$$\alpha = \sqrt{\mu_a / D} \tag{6}$$

The solution for the fluorescence is

$$\phi_2(x) = \frac{y_{12}\mu_{h1}\phi_1(0)}{D_2(\alpha_1^2 - \alpha_2^2)} (e^{-\alpha_2 x} - e^{-\alpha_1 x}) \tag{7}$$

If we equate the fluorescence remittance F to the left-directed current density at the surface,

$$F = J_2^- = (\frac{\phi_2}{4} + \frac{D_2}{2}\frac{d\phi_2}{dx}) = \frac{y_{12}\mu_{h1}\phi_1(0)}{2(\alpha_1 + \alpha_2)} \tag{8}$$

then the fluorescence yield for a thick slab is

$$Y = F/E_o = \frac{2y_{12}\mu_{h1}}{(\alpha_1 + \alpha_2)(1 + 2D_1\alpha_1)} \tag{9}$$

Equation 9 can be specialized when $\alpha_1 \gg \alpha_2$, as when the red fluorescence is excited by violet light. For special case of irradiation for photoradiation therapy at 630 nm, while observing fluorescence at 690 nm, we expect $\alpha_1 = \alpha_2$ and

$$Y = \frac{y_{12}'\mu_{h1}}{\alpha_1(1 + 2D_1\alpha_1)} \tag{10}$$

where y_{12}' is different (smaller) than y_{12} because of the overlap of excitation and emission spectra.

In order to evaluate these expressions, one needs to know not only y_{12} which should be characteristic of the HpD, and μ_{h1} which depends on the concentration, but the absorption and diffusion coefficients at the two wavelengths. The diffusion coefficient has been measured in specimens by adding a known amount of absorber in steps, and measuring α at each step by the Svaasand technique.[5] Then from Eq. 6, if we plot the measured α^2 against the known added absorption coefficient, we get a straight line with slope 1/D (as long as absorption is still small enough that D is constant). Knowing D and the α without added absorber, we can get μ_a from Eq. 6. Because it is not feasible to add absorber to tissue in vivo, we are exploring the possibility of deriving D from a measurement of the reflectance, which for a thick slab is given by diffusion theory as

$$R = \frac{1 - 2D\alpha}{1 + 2D\alpha} \tag{11}$$

The attenuation coefficient α might be obtained by measuring the space irradiance at two points.

FLUORESCENCE ENDOSCOPY

The differential uptake and fluorescence of HpD has been applied to detecting and localizing tumors on the linings of body cavities, including bronchogenic lung tumors[6,7,8] and bladder tumors. At present we are mainly concerned with localizing carcinoma in situ and early lung tumors, where the patient has already been diagnosed as probably having lung cancer because of malignant cells in the sputum (positive sputum cytology), but where the lesion is invisible on chest X-ray and under conventional, whitelight illuminated, reflected light bronchoscopy. It is well established that if a bronchogenic tumor is detected and treated while it is yet very small and expecially before metastasis has occured, prognosis for long term survival is markedly improved. These small tumors would be natural candidates for photoradiation therapy.

Figure 4 is a photograph of the image intensifier attachment currently in use by Dr. Oscar J. Balchum at the Los Angeles County-University of Southern California Medical Center. Figure 5 is a diagram of the instrument (note that the periscope assembly that diverts the image around the intensifier appears below the image intensifier in the diagram, and above the intensifier in the photograph). This so-called "flipflop" or alternate fluorescence/ reflectance viewer allows for switching at will between the fluorescence view and the conventional reflected whitelight view in color. The flipflop is attached to the ocular of the bronchoscope (usually an Olympus BF-2T) by means of an adaptor, which now allows for rotation. In the fluorescence viewing mode, the solenoid-actuated flip mirror shown is moved to the $0°$ position, and the fluorescence image is focused onto the photocathode of a microchannel-plate type image intensifier, after passing through a barrier filter to reject reflected violet and as much autofluorescence as possible. The intensified (x45,000) image is presented at the flipflop ocular, and appears green because of the P20 phosphor at the output of the intensifier. The shutter of the violet light source is open, while the shutter on the whitelight source (Olympus CLV xenon arc lamp) is closed during the fluorescence viewing. When desired, the bronchoscopist depresses a switch on the bronchoscope and an electronic controller rapidly moves the flip mirror to the $45°$ position (diverting the image aroung the intensifier), then closes the shutter on the violet source and opens the shutter on the whitelight source. Depressing the switch again switches back to fluorescence mode. In this fashion, the bronchoscopist can examine and compare the regular color view with the fluorescence view. A tumor is indicated by a brighter fluorescence, compared to the immediately adjacent tissue. Figure 6 illustrates the appearance of a small tumor (confirmed by biopsy).

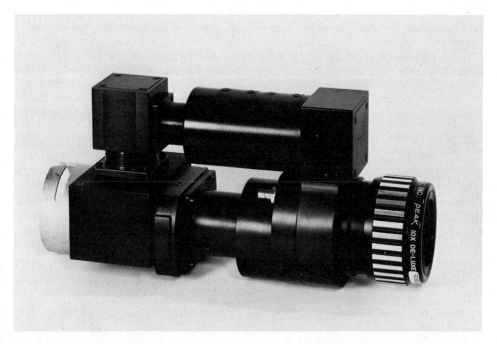

Fig. 4.   Photograph of the alternate fluorescence/reflectance
          viewer (flipflop).

Carcinoma in situ has been detected in fluorescence bronchoscopy, but visualization is difficult because of low contrast
(1.1-1.2). For tumors thinner than the effective depth of penetration of the violet light (typically 0.5 mm), contrast is reduced because some of the fluorescence comes from the underlying
nonmalignant tissue, which has a lower concentration of HpD.
Source background and tissue autofluorescence passed by the
barrier filter add to both tumor and nontumor areas, reducing
contrast. We have found that the source red background is reduced
by an order of magnitude using a fused quartz fiberoptic lightguide inserted in the biopsy channel and coupled through a violet
filter and fused quartz double prism monochromator to a 300 mW
violet krypton ion laser (410 nm, made by Spectra Physics Corporation, Mountain View, CA), compared to a filtered mercury arc
lamp (405 nm) coupled to the fiberoptic lightguide cable of a
bronchoscope. We have added a planoconcave (negative) plastic
microlens to the fiber to diverge the violet and eliminate "hot
spots" in the excitation light field. This lens does increase
background slightly, and may be replaced. Actually, only 10-20 mW
of violet light is needed at the exit of the fiber and lens, using
the high gain image intensifier, which minimizes the photodynamic
effect during the diagnostic examination.

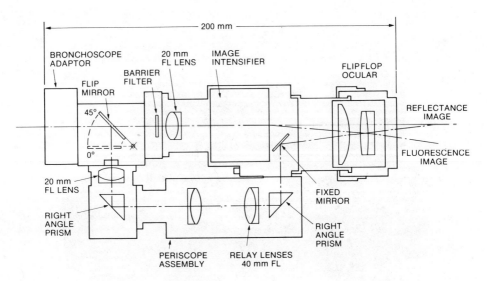

Fig. 5.   Diagram of the alternate fluorescence/reflectance viewer
          (flipflop).

A more serious reduction in fluorescence brightness contrast
comes about because of the autofluorescence of tumor and tissue.
Figure 7 shows the fluorescence spectrum of HpD (major peaks at
630 nm and 690 nm) riding on a tumor autofluorescence spectrum,
which extends from below 450 nm to over 720 nm.[1] The autofluorescence spectrum under the HpD spectrum is approximated by
autofluorescence of muscle, normalized at 590 nm.   The actual
ratio of HpD to autofluorescence intensity is probably lower than
illustrated by this specimen, at the standard human dosage of 3
mg/kg.   The detected or observed ratio of HpD fluorescence to
autofluorescence depends on the barrier filter, and the spectral
sensitivity of the intensifier photocathode.   Figure 7 shows the
response for two barrier filters, "High" transmittance (600 nm at
half-maximum to over 720 nm), and "Low" transmittance (670-710 nm
bandpass at half maximum).   Because the autofluorescence spectrum
decreases with increasing wavelength, the contrast is better with
the Low filter, although the overall brightness is reduced.
Additional measurements of autofluorescence excitation and emission spectra in vivo and in specimens, are in progress.

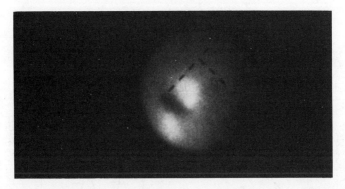

Fig. 6. Photograph of intensified fluorescence image of a small
(carcinoma in situ to minimally invasive) tumor in the
right upper lobe bronchus. (The dashed tee is inscribed
on the intensifier).

We are working on a digital video system that will allow us
to subtract the autofluorescence and source background from the
image. We already have the intensifier coupled through a beamsplitter and fiberoptic imageguide to a sensitive Silicon Intensified Target video camera (Cohu 4410/SIT).[8] The camera is
connected by coaxial cable to a digital image processing computer
with frame-store capability (Quantex DS-20 with 512x512x8-bit
memory). An automated barrier filter slide has been designed for
the flipflop, synchronized to the DS-20 unit. On command, an
image can be stored with filter no. 1 in place, then subtracted
from another image with filter no. 2 in place, and the difference
"freeze-frame" image displayed on the video monitor. We propose
to make filter no. 1 pass some of the autofluorescence spectrum
from, say, 500-600 nm, while filter no. 2 will be our "High"
filter passing the entire HpD spectrum. Then when the autofluorescence spectrum image (scaled to the magnitude under the HpD
peaks) is subtracted from the HpD-plus-autofluorescence spectrum
image, the difference should be the image from HpD fluorescence
alone. By subtracting images, variations in pixel brightness due
only to variations in distance or angular orientation are can-
celed.

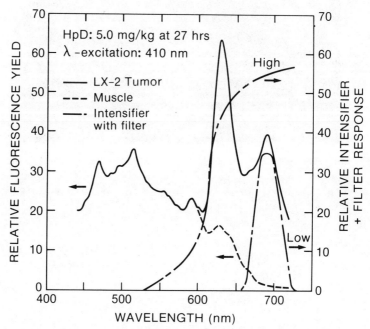

Fig. 7. Example of autofluorescence and HpD fluorescence spectra, and barrier filter transmittances.

NONIMAGING METHODS

We are also investigating a nonimaging method for measuring fluorescence, mainly for quantitative measurements of fluorescence yield where the distance and angular orientation cannot be controlled precisely, as in the lung. This consists of a fiberoptic fiber lightguide inserted in a biopsy channel, and coupled to a dichroic beamsplitter, lenses, filters, and two photomultiplier tubes, one for detecting red fluorescence and the other for detecting reflected violet. The ratio of red-to-violet signals is taken automatically, after autoranging to condition the signals. The ratio is proportional to the fluorescence yield and inversely proportional to violet reflectance, while distance and angle as well as source power variations cancel. The fluorescence yield can be calibrated against a fluorescence standard outside the body. The instrument works well in bench tests on phantoms, and is being prepared for measurements in patients.

A drawback to any nonimaging fluroescence method is field av-
aging. That is, the signal is proportional to the fluorescence
emitted by the whole area contributing to the light collected by
the fiber. If the tumor does not fill this area, its signal will
be averaged or diluted by the signal from nontumor area. While it
is possible to move in close to a small tumor located more or less
straight ahead, e.g., on a spur of the bronchial tree, and thus
fill the area viewed with the tumor, this is not very feasible for
a tumor on the sidewall, unless it is so large that is surrounds
the fiber tip both circumferentially and longitudinally. In search-
ing for a small tumor, we prefer the fluorescence imaging method.

REPORTING DOSE IN PHOTORADIATION THERAPY

In order to interpret and intercompare clinical results in
photoradiation therapy, it is highly desirable to report the effective absorbed dose (J/Kg) for photochemical action [2], and the temperature vs time for hyperthermia or synergistic thermal-photochem-
ical action[10], t key points such as the minimum does and temperature points in the tumor, and the maximum dose and temperature
points in surrounding nonmalignant tissues. It is realized that,
at this stage of development of dosimetry for PRT, it is not easy
to predict or measure the desired quantities. Meanwhile, the important physical and biological parameters should be reported so
that an estimate of dose and temperature can be made as a guide to
explanation of clinical successes and "failures" (incomplete response or regrowth of tumor, or excessive damage to nonmalignant
tissue). The most important parameters are:

1. Light exposure rate

   a. For surface irradiation, give irradiance E_o (W m^{-2}), usual-
      ly calculated from beam power divided by area irradiated.
      Also give distance from irradiator to surface for a diverg-
      ing geometry, angle of incidence for a collimated beam, and
      spot size.
   b. For interstitial point irradiation, give power P(W). Also
      give angular dependence of emission, e.g., for a flat-cut
      fiber, give the numerical aperture or half-angle of emis-
      sion.
   c. For interstitial cylinder irradiation, give power per unit
      length of diffuser P_L (W m^{-1}). Also give length and emis-
      sion characteristics of diffuser.
   d. Describe other irradiation conditions.

2. Wavelength or spectrum

   a. For monochromatic source such as a laser, specify wave-
      length (nm) and how it was set or measured.

b. For a polychromatic source such as a filtered lamp, give
    the spectrum (W or relative units per unit wavelength vs
    wavelength) emerging from the light delivery system.

3. Duration of irradiation

    If source is not steady, give equivalent irradiation time.

4. Light exposure (Exposure rate x duration)

    a. If surface irradiation, energy per unit area ($J\ m^{-2}$).
    b. If point interstitial, energy (J).
    c. If cylinder interstitial, energy per unit length ($J\ m^{-1}$).
    d. Other, give light exposure in energy units.

5. Optical penetration depth

    Estimate distance in tissue concerned, for the space irradiance
    (radiant energy fluence rate) to be attenuated by a factor of
    $1/e = 0.37$, by absorption and scattering[5].

6. Tumor thickness

    Estimate tumor thickness or greatest distance between surface
    or point or line of light delivery, and the boundary of the
    tumor. Also give the thickness of any nonmalignant tissue (and
    tissue type) between light delivery system and tumor.

7. Concentration of photosensitizer

    Give name and origin of photosensitizer and its concentration
    in tumor and surrounding tissue, or dosage (mg/Kg body weight),
    method of administration (usually intravenous), delay time
    between administration and start of irradiation, and tumor type,
    organ, and any other information that may help in estimating
    concentration.

8. Blood flox

    For thermal effects, estimate degree of vascularization, blood
    flow (high, medium, low), and any cooling by other means.

9. Hypoxia

    If hypoxis conditions may apply, describe.

ACKNOWLEDGEMENTS

    The cooperation of Dr. T.J. Dougherty is gratefully acknowledged. The research was sponsored by the U.S. Public Health Service, DHHS, under National Cancer Institute grant CA31865 to Medicine. Instrumentation development was supported in part by the U.S. Department of Energy under subcontract to UCSB from contract DE-AMO3-76SF00113 to the Institute for Physics and Imaging Science, University of Southern California.

REFERENCES

1. D.R. Doiron, Fluorescence bronchoscopy for the early localization of lung cancer, Ph.D. Dissertation, University of California, Santa Barbara (1982).
2. A.E. Profio and D.R. Doiron, Dosimetry considerations in phototherapy, Med. Phys. 8:190 (1981).
3. T.J. Dougherty, Personal communication (1983).
4. D. Kessel and T.H. Chou, Tumor-localizing components of the porphyrin preparation Hematoporphyrin Derivative, Cancer Res. 43:1994 (1983).
5. D.R. Doiron, L.O. Svaasand, and A.E. Profio, Light dosimetry in tissue: Application to photoradiation therapy, in: "Porphyrin Photosensitization", D. Kessel and T.J. Dougherty, eds., Plenum Press, New York (1983).
6. A.E. Profio, D.R. Doiron, and E.G. King, Laser fluorescence bronchoscope for localization of occult lung tumors, Med. Phys. 6:523 (1979).
7. O.J. Balchum, D.R. Doiron, A.E. Profio, and G.C. Huth, Fluorescence bronchoscopy for localizing early bronchial cancer and carcinoma in situ, in: "Recent Results in Cancer Research", Vol. 82, Springer-Verlag, Berlin (1982).
8. A.E. Profio, D.R. Doiron, O.J. Balchum, and G.C. Huth, Fluorescence bronchoscopy for localization of carcinoma in situ, Med. Phys. 10:35 (1983).
9. R.C. Benson, G.M. Farrow, J.H. Kinsey, D.A. Cortese, H. Zincke, and D.C. Utz, Detection and localization of in situ carcinoma of the bladder with Hematoporphyrin Derivative, Mayo Clin. Proc. 57:548 (1982).
10. L.O. Svaasand, D.R. Doiron, and T.J. Dougherty, Temperature rise during photoradiation therapy of malignant tumors, Med. Phys. 10:10 (1983).

IN VIVO FLUORESCENCE EXCITATION SPECTRA OF

HEMATOPORPHYRIN-DERIVATIVE (HpD)

G.H.M. Gijsbers*, M.J.C. van Gemert*, D. Breederveld**,
J. Langelaar** and T.A. Boon***

   * Department of Medical Technology, St. Joseph Hospital
     P.O.Box 988, 5600 ML Eindhoven, The Netherlands
  ** Laser Application and Information Centre (LAICA)
     Laboratory for Physical Chemistry, Nieuwe
     Actergracht 127, 1018 WS Amsterdam, The Netherlands
 *** Department of Urology, Antonie van Leeuwenhoek Hospital
     National Cancer Centre, Amsterdam, The Netherlands

SUMMARY

Fluorescence excitation spectra of HpD in a living animal tumor
are measured. The experiments show that these spectra are different
from the fluorescence excitation spectra of HpD solved in saline.
This can be explained from the presence of blood in the tumor tissue.

INTRODUCTION

It is well known that hematoporphyrin-derivative (HpD) selectively accumulates in tumor tissues. The strong red fluorescence
displayed by HpD when illuminated by violet light, is used as a
tool to detect small tumors in an early stage, which are difficult
to localize with conventional methods. An extensive study has been
presented by Doiron[1].

Up till now light with a wavelength around 400 nm has been
used to excite HpD in vivo, based on the fluorescence excitation
spectrum of HpD solved in saline or saline with a small amount of
serum. This is shown in fig. 1.

In earlier work, Van der Putten en Van Gemert[2,3] found an
indication that in vivo spectra of HpD might be different from
those in vitro. They already found that after excitation with
514.5 nm light from an argon ion laser fluorescence emmission of
HpD in vivo could be observed.

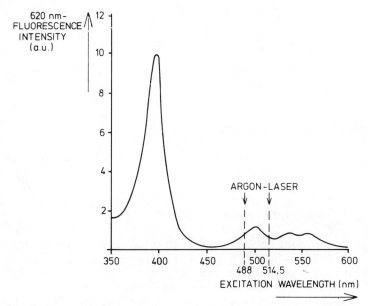

Fig. 1. Fluorescence excitation spectrum of HpD solved in saline.
Concentration of 10 μg/ml. The intensity of the 620 nm
fluorescence light as a function of the excitation wavelength is indicated.

        This work presents measurements of in vivo fluorescence exci-
tation spectra of HpD.

MATERIALS AND METHODS

        Measurements were performed on a RUC-2 squamous cell carcino-
ma which was grown in a rat. The tumor was implanted subcutaneously
ten days before the measurements actually were carried out. During
the measurements the tumors were about 2 cm in diameter. HpD, obtained from Dr. Dougherty (Buffalo) via the Rotterdam Radiothera-
peutic Institute (Dr. Star) was injected intraperitoneally
(20 mg/kg bodyweight).

        After anaesthesizing the rat with Nembutal, the skin above the
tumor was opened and the tumor was positioned in the sample area
of a spectro fluorimeter as schematically given in fig. 2 and described by Langelaar et al[4].

        In order to measure the fluorescence excitation spectrum of
HpD the following procedure was followed:

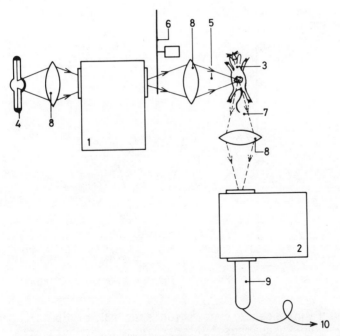

Fig. 2.   Schematic of the used spectro fluorimeter: 1, 2. monochro-
          mators; 3. rat with tumor containing HpD; 4. Xe-arc lamp;
          5. excitation light; 6. chopper; 7. fluorescence light;
          8. lensen; 9. photomultipliertube; 10. to lock-in amplifier
          and recorder.

        Monochromator 2 (see fig. 2) was fixed at a detection wavelength
of 620 nm ($\Delta\lambda$ = 3nm) which lies in the first emission band of HpD.
The sample was excited with light from a 500 W Xe arc lamp filtered.
through monochromator 1. The Xe lamp has a nearly continuous spectrum
between 350 nm and 600 nm, which is suitable to excite the HpD.

        The relative intensity of the 620 nm emission light was measured
as a function of the excitation wavelength, by scanning monochromator 1. The thus obtained spectra (e.g. fig. 1) were corrected for the
intensity distribution of the Xe lamp plus monochromator 1.

RESULTS

        Fig. 3 presents a typical example of a fluorescence excitation
spectrum of HpD in the previous mentioned squamous cell carcinoma.
It is taken 24 hours after injection of the HpD. For comparison the
excitation spectrum of HpD solved in saline is also given.

        A comparison of the two spectra indicates, apart from a broa-
dening of the band around 400 nm, a relative increase of the three

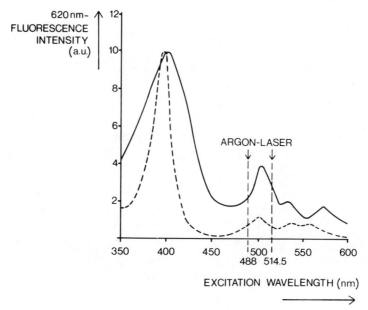

Fig. 3. —— : Fluorescence excitation spectrum of HpD in living
             RUC-2 squamous cell carcinoma, 24 hours after injec-
             tion of 20 mg/kg HpD
        ---- : Fluorescence excitation spectrum of HpD solved in
             saline, as in fig. 1.

small bands above 460 nm in the in vivo spectrum. This explains
why also an argon ion laser can effectively be used to excite HpD.

    It is suggested that the change of the in vivo spectrum with
respect to the in vitro spectrum, is due to the presence of blood
in the tumor tissue.

    The effective light distribution as a function of wavelength
(i.e. both for excitation and fluorescence light) in tissue containing blood can be computed using the optical parameters of HbO_2 and
tissue scattering and transmission as given in fig. 4. A method to
compute the effective yield of emission light at the surface of the
tissue was developed by Van der Putten and Van Gemert[2], applying the
Kubelka-Munk theory.

    Following this computation method, the in vitro spectrum as
given in fig. 2 and fig. 3, is corrected by assuming the presence
of 1.2% of HbO_2 in the tissue. The result is presented by the dashed
curve in fig. 5.

    With this amount of HbO_2 the computed spectrum is more or less
fitted with the measured excitation spectrum in vivo. From this we

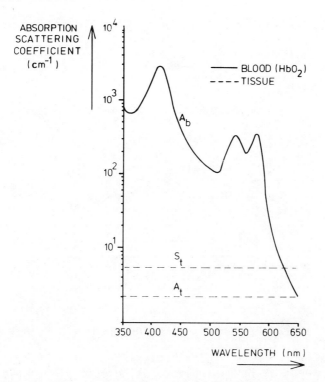

Fig. 4. Absorption coefficient of $HbO_2(A_b)$ and the estimated
coefficients of absorption (A_t) and scattering (S_t) of tissue.

see that the relative increase of the three small bands in vivo can
indeed be explained by taking into account the optical behaviour
of blood in the tumor.

The fitting of the computed spectrum with the excitation spectrum in vivo is not fully satisfactory. The same computations have
been performed on the excitation spectrum of HpD solved in saline
with 10% of human serum. This corrected spectrum for the presence
of 1% HbO_2 and tissue is shown in fig. 6, as the dashed curve
together with the excitation spectrum in vivo.

In this case the fitting is nearly perfect.

DISCUSSION AND CONCLUSION

From the presented results it is concluded that fluorescence
emission of HpD in vivo can be observed by excitation with light
of a wavelength greater than 400 nm, especially around 500 nm. The
observed ratio of the fluorescence excitation in vivo at 400 nm
and 514.5 nm is only a factor 2.5, while in vitro this ratio is
about 10.

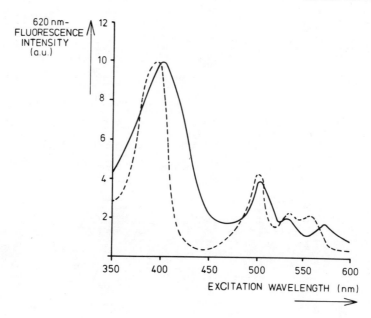

Fig. 5. ——— : Fluorescence excitation spectrum of HpD in vivo,
               as in fig. 3.
         --- : Fluorescence excitation spectrum of HpD computed from
               spectrum HpD in saline, using optical behaviour of
               tissue containing 1.2% of HbO_2.

        This leads us to the conclusion that to localize small tumors
an argon ion laser can be used, which may have advantages over the
use of a Hg-arc lamp or a krypton ion laser[3]. The argon laser begins
to be a common instrument in a hospital.

        In conclusion, the presence of blood in tumor tissue has been
predicted to be responsible for changes in the fluorescence excitation spectrum in vivo with respect to the spectrum in vitro.

ACKNOWLEDGEMENTS

        We are indepted to Cees Verlaan for handling the rats and to
Willem Star for supplying the HpD.

REFERENCES

    1. D.R. Doiron, Fluorescence bronchoscopy for the early locali-
       zation of lung cancer, Ph.D. Dissertation, University of
       California, Santa Barbara (1982).

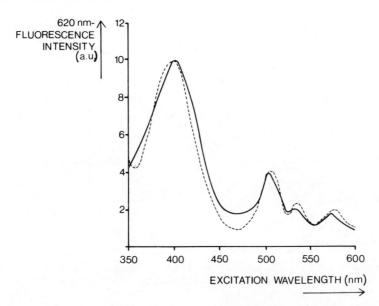

Fig. 6. ————: Fluorescence excitation spectrum of HpD in vivo, as
in fig. 3
- - - - -: Fluorescence excitation spectrum of HpD, computed
from the spectrum of HpD in saline with 10% of human
serum using the optical behaviour of tissue containing
1% of HbO_2.

2. W.J.M. van der Putten and M.J.C. van Gemert, A modelling
approach to the detection of sub-cutaneous tumors by
Hematoporphyrin-Derivative Fluorescence, Phys.Med.Biol.
28: 639-645 (1983).
3. W.J.M. van der Putten and M.J.C. van Gemert, Hematoporphyrin-
derivative Fluorescence in vitro and in an animal tumor,
Phys.Med.Biol., 28: 633-638 (1983).
4. J. Langelaar, G.A. de Vries and D. Bebelaar, Sensitivity
improvements in spectrofluorimetry, J.Sci.Instrum. 46:
149 (1969).

IN VIVO OBSERVATIONS OF PORPHYRINS AND OF THE LIGHT ACTION

R. Plus

Auxil-Fatima, 40140 Magescq (France)

SUMMARY

We have registered the fluorescence spectra of IN SITU porphyrins on alive anaesthetized and even awaked animals. These works
permitted us to evidence (i) a natural compound, (ii) the light
action on porphyrins, and (iii) to study the relation which exists
between natural porphyrins and cancer. The Natural General Action
of porphyrins is considered.

An important difficulty in Phototherapy is to evidence the
photosensible compound in the studied tissues. So we have develop-
ped in Paris a technic permitting to obtain the registered fluorescence spectra of the studied tissus.

MATERIAL AND TECHNIC

We excite the fluorescence of the tissues by light in the visible range (1a, b, c). We use an Argon Laser and generally the exciting wavelength is λ exc = 501,7nm, in the range of the band IV
of the absorption spectrum of porphyrins that we have studied previously by Raman Spectroscopy (1d, e).
We have used a very feeble laser power and we have even worked
with 0,02mw only. The tissues or the animals are lighted and placed
in front of the entering slits of a spectrometer, a Coderg Raman
spectrometer was used, which permits an analysis of the diffused
light.
The spectrum is then registered to determine the fluorescence
wavelength. This method allows us to work not only on different
tissues but also on alive and even on awaked animals that it needs
only to place in the laser beam.

SPECTROSCOPIC STUDIES

The figure 1 shows the spectra of tumours extracted from animals who had received 1 or 1,5 mg of hematoporphyrin (HP): A-mammary tumour, B-subcutaneous solid Ehrlich Ascit, C-liquid Ehrlich Ascit.

For all these spectra, the 2 bands observed centered at 625nm and at 690nm are typically porphyrins and they correspond with what is waiting for HP.

The figure 2 shows the spectrum of the light diffused by the cutaneous area of mammary tumour of an awaked mouse 19 hours after the intraperitoneal injection of 1mg of HP. We recognize again the HP spectra.

All these spectra show that it is possible to characterize HP IN SITU and IN VIVO. This method can be used for the observation and the identification of IN SITU compounds, for their comparative proportion between diverse tissues or different organs and equally for the follow of their evolution in function of various parameters as injected doses of HP, time of lighting and so on...

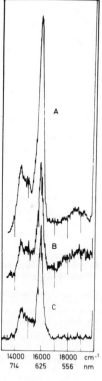

Fig. 1.

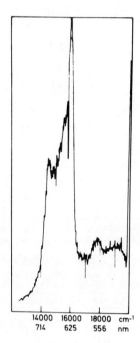

Fig. 2.

NATURAL COMPOUND

    We have evidenced an unexpected phenomenon : it is the pre-
sence of a fluorescence toward 560nm. This new fluorescence that
we can see with a faint intensity on the figure 2 is easier
observed when the doses of injected HP are more feeble and when
the exciting wavelength is different (λexc=514,5nm) (1c).
    The figure 3 shows the spectrum of this natural compound re-
gistered from mice with mammary tumours and which have received
0,05mg of HP only : A-awaked animal, B-extracted tumour.
    We can ascertain that these spectra are composed of 2 bands.
They correspond with what we are waiting for porphyrins.
    We have attributed this spectrum to a natural porphyrin and
more precisely to a metalloporphyrin.
    It is interesting to note here that we agree with others re-
search workers that have mentionned the presence of a typical cancer porphyrin (2) and effectively we have ourselves established that
this natural porphyrin is present in all animals carrying adenocarcinomas that we have studied (9 mice) that they had received HP
(from 0,05 to 1 mg) or not. On the other hand, it is not observed
on healthy animals even if they have received HP.

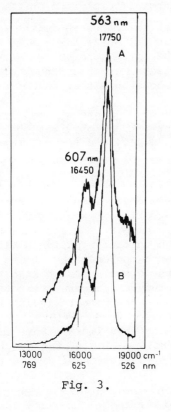

Fig. 3.   Fig. 4.

EVOLUTION WITH LIGHT

We are going to study the evolution of the natural porphyrin
and of HP when the animals are lighted.

The figure 4 evidences the action of light on the porphyrins
IN SITU on an awaked animal with a mammary tumour which received
0,5 mg HP. We observe the cutaneous area above the tumour.

- The A spectrum is registered 26 hours after the injection
of HP. We see the fluorescences of injected HP and of the natural
compound called F_{17750}.

The B spectrum is registered after 30 minutes of the lighting
of the animal and the C spectrum after again 30 minutes. We observe
that the fluorescence of HP reduces when the second one grows up.

These unexpected results suggest that light favors the production of natural porphyrins and it is remarkable that other research workers have reach the same conclusion in studying the porphyrin metabolism on Human Beings or on animals (3-4).

Now, let us say that it appears that if we have to consider
the injected porphyrins, it is also necessary to study the natural
porphyrins present in the organisms carrying tumours, the metabolism of which is affected by light and by injected porphyrins and
so, some teams claim the incidence of Natural Porphyrins on cancer:

1°- The first category is dealing with the cases where there
is a concentration of natural porphyrin in malignant tissues to
certain levels of tumoral development. The first observation was
made in 1924 by Policard about the rat's sarcomas (5). Since, other
research workers have signalized this phenomenon either on Men or
on animals (6 to 11).

2°- The second category concerns the cases where a cutaneous
porphyria is observed among cancer patients. These observations are
associated with a lot of various tumours (4- 12) and for the team
of Goulon, Gadjos et al (13) this high level of porphyrin and cancer cannot be fortuitous.

3°- The third category is dealing with the cases where there
is a high level of natural porphyrin observed in blood, urines and
faeces of cancer patients. Once more, the various tumours studied
(14) and the number of observations had to come to the conclusion
that the porphyrin rate is abnormally high on cancer patients (15).

4°- The fourth category is dealing with the endurance to the
cancer. Some authors have observed that the organisms rich in natural porphyrins are more resistant to the induced cancer. It is the
case of the Harder's glands of the rat which are more resistant that
the salivary glands or that the subcutaneous tissues (9-10).

5°- The fifth category concerns the observed improvements :
diminished weight of tumours (16) and a prolongation of the survival time of animals has been observed after injection of HP (16 to
19-9).

6°- The last category is dealing with resorption of tumours,
because effectively, it has been observed a spontaneous resorption

of tumours when the production of natural porphyrins lasts to a
superior rate above the normal. These observations were made on
Brown-Pearce's tumours inserted on rabbits (20).

All these observations brought some authors to consider the
light action on organisms by cutaneaous porphyrins which may act
either directly or by electromagnetic radiations on a target
cell enhancing organic defences (16-17-4).

All these works have brought ourselves to consider that the
natural porphyrins may intervene in the defence system of the organisms, for example, by tranforming and diffusing the energy is-
sued from photonic energy by the mean of transference chain of
Szent Gyorgyi.

Here we can recall that these transformations are naturally
realized by the chorophylls, which are found in the porphyrins family, in the photosynthesis where the conversion of photonic energy
initiates a transfer of electrons by way of a transporting chain.
Then, the fact is that it has been established that the chloro-
phylls have an inhibitive effect on tumoral growth induced in the
mice and in the rat (21-22-9)

We have called this porphyrin action the "NATURAL GENERAL AC-
TION".

THE NATURAL GENERAL ACTION

So, actually, the researches on porphyrins and light actions on organisms are purchased according to two principal directions (23).

In the Local Action, that you know very well,
- We try at first to enrich selectively in porphyrin a tissue
or an organ,
- Light is localized to the treated zones,
- We want to provoke a local necrosis,
- We think that this action occurs by means of the photo-dynamic
properties of porphyrins (mediated through the formation of singlet
oxygen that is to say a short lived excited electronic state).
In the local action, the porphyrins are used in the same way
as other already tested chemical substances, as crange acridine or
fluorescein for example, and the association porphyrin-light is used
as a tool assigned to provoke a local cellular destruction confined
to the undergone zone.

In the Natural General Action,

- The whole deficient organism is enriched in porphyrin,
- The whole body is softly lighted (the daylight is well adapted),
- We want to help the conversion and the transference of the
photonic energy,

-We want to produce an exaltation of the defence system of the organism.

In the Natural General Action, the association porphyrin-light is a part of the defence system of the organism.

Works are currently purchased to study the Natural General Action of porphyrins. This action which has to exalt the natural defence of the organism must intervene in cancerology and in virology and so very cheerful results are obtained particularly with leukaemia and Viral Hepatitis and we propose to test this action on herpetic virus who make so damages in the USA where 20 millions persons are already affected and on AIDS syndrom: Retrovirus HTRV and Gallo's virus HTLV.

Finally, to complete what we said before, let us add that others teams in USA have tested HP in other ways, as in parasitology, by treating Trypanosoma of the sleeping sickness and in pleomorphic infection in rabbits (24-25).

REMARKS

Concerning with the Natural General Action, we have to precise that a solution is drunk (0,75mg/kg/dayly) and the whole body is exposed to natural light by small sessions.

The purpose of this treatment is to enrich in porphyrin the deficient organism. We must feed more to cure according to the process that Nature provides by remedying the defect of the alimentation and of the transmission of energy and, consequently, of the inter-cells and inter-organs informations.

We can note that our observations dealing with sain or ill patients show that porphyrin can have an incidence on the neuro-encephalic system and we can find, for example, a kind of excitation. The family has to pay attention for because not only the good tendancies can be exalted.

This neuro-encephalic incidence can be understood when we recall that the neuro-physiologists claim that the brain is the first organ alimented.

This stimulation of the brain by the porphyrin brings us to the question of the influence of the encephalon on the development of illness such as cancer, the persons the cerebral functions of whom are overloaded being a favourable ground.

We can note that this tie permets to understand why there is pratically no cancer in Psychiatric Hospitals by the incurable that the Hospital keeps all life long (26). In connection with this idea it would be interesting to verify that generally the brain is not subject to primar cancers but rather to metastasis.

As a conclusion, we think that the neuro-encephalic incidence of the porphyrins can be the symptom of a reinforced cerebral activity rather a neurotoxicity as it has been sometimes putted forward by practitioner.

REFERENCES

1. a- R. Plus, Rapports du Commissariat à l'Energie Atomique,
        DRA/SRIRMA 76/39 et 76/40 (1976).
    b- R. Plus, Spec, Sc. Tech 5:3 (1982).
    c- R. Plus, Comptes-rendus Congrès Laser Médical, Paris (1983),
        to be published.
    d- R. Plus, Thèse Doctorat d'Etat, Paris, A.O.12204 (1976).
    e- R. Plus, M. Lutz, Spec. Lett. 7:133 (1974), 7:73 (1974),
        8:119 (1975).
2. B. Zawirska, Path Europ. 7:67 (1972).
3. I. Magnus, V. Jonousek, K. Jones, Nature 250:504 (1974).
4. H. Perrot, "La porphyrie cutanée tardive", Simep., ed., (1968).
5. A. Policard, Compt. Rend. Soc. Biol. :1423 (1924).
6. J. Schultz, H. Shay, S. Gruenstein, Cancer Res. 3:157 (1954).
7. K. Medras, J. Nal. Cancer Inst. 25:465 (1960).
8. G. Rubino, L. Rasetti, Panm. Med. 8:290 (1966).
9. B. Zawirska, Arch. Imm. Ther. Exp. 13:238 (1965).
10. B. Zawirska, Neoplasma 14:622 (1966).
11. B. Zawirska, Neoplasma 26:223 (1979).
12. R. Thomson, B. Nicholson, T. Farman, D. Whitmore, and R. Wil-
        liams, Gastroenter. 59:779 (1970).
13. M. Goulon, A. Gadjos, J. Lougovoy-Visconti, and F. Nouilhat,
        Rev. Neurol. 121:423 (1969).
14. P. Carricaburu, Bull. alg. Carcin. 5:210 (1952).
15. H. Rabinowitz, Cancer Res. 9:672 (1949).
16. W. et H. Amsallem, Bull. alg. Carcin. 6:135 (1953).
17. E. Albertini, and R. Della Volpe, Arch. Ital. Patol. Clin.
        Tumori 2:167 (1958), 2:962 (1958), 2:183 (1958), 3:1334
        (1959).
18. Y. Tazaki, H. Furue, Cancer Chem. Rep. 13:41 (1961).
19. N. Lijima, K. Matsura, A. Ueno, K. Fujita, T. Aiba, H. Ukishi-
        ma, F. Nohara, Q. Ikehara, T. Koshizuka, and S. Mori, Cancer
        Chem. Rep. 13:47 (1961).
20. S. Gulieva, A. Kubatiev, Vop. Onkol. 16:85 (1970).
21. S. Burgi, Zeitschr. Ges. Exp. Med. 110:259 (1942).
22. H. Kurten, Zeitschr. Inn. Med. 11:531 (1956).
23. M. D. de la Monneraye, Thèse "l'hématoporphyrine dérivée",
        Nantes (France) (1983).
24. S. Meshnick, R. Grady, S. Blubstein, and A. Cerami, J. Phar.
        Exp. Ther. :1041 (1978).
25. A. Fairlamb, Trends Biochem. Sc. 7:249 (1982).
26. Y. Salles, and P. Greig, Private Communication, Ste Anne Ho-
        spital, Mont de Marsan (1975).

MONITORING OF HEMATOPORPHYRIN INJECTED IN HUMANS AND CLINICAL

PROSPECTS OF ITS USE IN GYNECOLOGIC ONCOLOGY

Piero Fioretti, Virgilio Facchini,
Angiolo Gadducci and Ivo Cozzani

Istituto di Clinica Ostetrica e Ginecologica and
Istituto di Biochimica, Biofisica e Genetica
University of Pisa, 56100 Pisa, Italy

INTRODUCTION

The use of hematoporphyrin (HP) and its water soluble derivatives (HPD) as tumor localizers[1] and sensitizers for phototherapy of
neoplasias[2] is well documented and receiving rapidly increasing interest.

Gynecologic oncology is an important area of application of
porphyrins in association with visible light for both early diagnosis and phototreatment, owing to the large occurrence and the wide
variety of tumors easily accessible to coherent or non-coherent
light sources, eventually coupled to fiber optic endoscopes. Ready
to start a plan of clinical experiments of diagnosis and phototreatment of gynecologic tumors with hematoporphyrin - visible light, we
have studied, in some selected patients undergoing surgical ablation
of the tumor masses, the location of administered HP in the neoplastic and surrounding tissues and the whole processes of clearance
of the dye from the patients bodies. Actually the present extension
of the method to different oncologic fields and to different stages
of neoplastic growth and invasion requires a precise knowledge of
the rates and extents of distribution of the sensitizers in different normal and malignant tissues, to optimize phototreatment and
diagnostic procedures. Moreover the clearance rates and features of
the dye from the body are essential parameters to control and prevent side effects.

Finally these clinical studies may provide essential contributions to the elucidation of the mechanisms of photodinamic effects
of porphyrins in vivo.

PROCEDURES AND RESULTS

Administration and monitoring of HP

HP for clinical use was prepared from a lot of hematoporphyrin
IX hydrochloride (Porphyrin Products, Logan, Utah, U.S.A.), estimated 95-97% pure by high pressure liquid chromatography. The product,
dissolved with sterile isotonic saline and filtered through milli-
pore under nitrogen pressure, was administered by intravenous injection at the dose of either 2.5 or 5 mg/Kg of body weight.

For the first set of clinical experiments, two patients with
primary vulvar tumors, undergoing total vulvectomy, were selected.
Previous clinical examination and laboratory tests excluded alterations of liver and kidneys functions. Since the time of HP injection the patients were kept 10 days in a room with darkened lights,
the eyes being protected by sunglasses. The patients were then
warned not to expose to direct sunlight for the additional two
weeks. At regular intervals from HP injection the monitoring of HP
concentrations in serum, faeces and urine was performed throughout
24 days. The HP concentrations in tumor and normal surrounding
tissues were also determined, following dissection under a magni-
fier and separated extrations of fresh samples obtained from
bioptic or surgical specimens.

The concentrations of HP in solid tissues and body fluids were
measured spectrophotofluorometrically[3], following extraction or dilution with buffered 1% sodium dodecylsulfate.

Preferential distribution of injected HP in malignant tissue, and
in vivo detection of HP fluorescence

The comparative distribution of injected HP in tumor and in the
normal surrounding tissues confirmed that the preferential affinity
of malignant cells for porphyrins observed in isolated cells and in
animal tissues in vivo[3,4,5], can be demonstrated also in humans.
Fig.1 shows a typical spectrophotofluorometric assay of HP content
in a surgical specimen of a vulvar squamous cell carcinoma, in comparison with the control normal skin tissue. The differential HP
concentrations in vulvar tumor masses with respect to the surrounding tissues allowed us to observe and photograph the characteristic

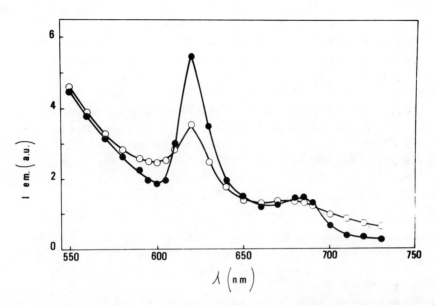

Fig. 1. Comparative spectrophotofluorometric determination of HP
         in malignant (●) and normal surrounding tissue (○) in
         a surgical specimen, 48 hours after intravenous injection
         of 2.5 mg of HP / Kg of body weight. Other details are
         reported in the text.

pink-red fluorescence emission of HP on illumination of the tumor
areas with a mercury vapor lamp. Both the tumor-to-normal HP concentration ratios and the HP fluorescence observed in vivo increased
during the first 48 hours after HP infusion.

Monitoring of HP concentrations in serum and kinetics of its clearance.

     Fig.2 shows the variations of HP concentrations in the serum
of two patients following the intravenous injections of 2.5 or 5
mg of HP / Kg of body weight. The patterns of HP concentrations in
serum are very similar (as are the kinetics of HP clearance through
the intestine and the kidneys), the differences being accounted for
by the different dose injected. In particular it was observed that

all the injected HP was removed from serum within 24-48 hours, according to the dose (Fig.2). During this interval HP bound to specific protein carrier is vehiculated to liver and other body organs.
Experimental evidences indicated that HP administered parenterally
in acqueous solutions to normal rats or to animals bearing solid or
ascites hepatomas was cleared off from normal and malignant cells
at different rates[3,4], thus providing tumor-to-normal HP concentration ratios suitable for phototreatment or diagnostic investigations. Our preliminary data in humans are in agreement with this
view. As shown in Fig.2, a second lower peak of HP bound to serum
proteins was observed at considerable delay from the drug's administration. The specific protein carrier of HP was isolated and purified from one patient's serum and its structural and functional

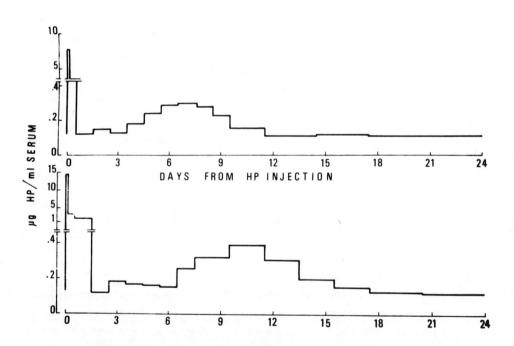

Fig. 2.   Time-course of HP concentrations in serum of gynecologic
          patients, following intravenous injection of 2.5 mg of
          HP / Kg of body weight (upper diagram) or the double dose
          of HP (lower diagram).

properties are presently under investigation.

The patterns of HP elimination through faeces and urines (Fig.3) closely match the variations of serum HP levels, although with appreciable delay. Our results indicate that an important fraction of HP injected in humans is eliminated through the intestine without degradation of the tetrapyrrole macrocycle, in agreement with recent observations in animals[6]. The urinary excretion is also quantitatively important, although the peak concentrations are lower.

The limit of three weeks reported for risk of skin photosensitization is in fairly good agreement with the kinetics of HP elimination we have observed.

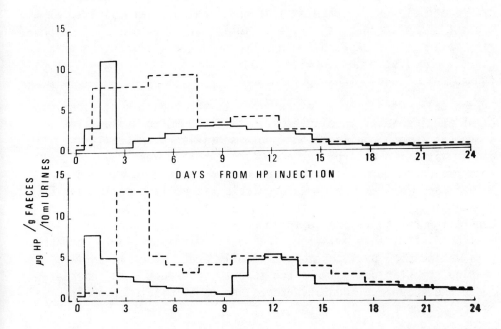

Fig. 3.   Kinetics of HP clearance through intestine (continuous lines) and kidneys (broken lines) in gynecologic patients, following intravenous injection of 2.5 mg of HP / Kg of body weight (upper diagram) or the double dose of HP (lower diagram).

DISCUSSION AND CLINICAL PROSPECTS

Although the reported clinical experience is very limited, we estimate that it has focussed some crucial points to be considered in the future applications of porphyrins and visible light in clinical oncology. The monitoring of HP distribution in normal and malignant tissues as well as in body fluids appears to be essential to determine the times and features of the therapeutic and diagnostic procedures. This choice appears to be critical in the present clinical practice, since the differential binding of HP or HPD in acqueous solution to the tumor tissue probably occurs within a limited interval from HP injection. Our observation of a delayed peak of bound HP in serum after complete removal of the drug originally injected, besides its own mechanistic significant, may have interesting clinical implications.

Additional important informations can be obtained by systematic investigation of the kinetics of HP accumulation in neoplasias as a function of the time and dose injected, tumor type, location, grades and stages. Such investigations, that are very limited at the present moment, can be extended by monitoring the uptake of porphyrins by tumor tissues, following diagnostic or therapeutic administration in vivo or by in vitro studies on slices of fresh tissues from bioptic or surgical specimens.

Finally we attach great interest to the possible clinical use of HP and its water insoluble derivatives bound to unilamellar liposomes, as tumor localizers and photo sensitizers. Actually in vitro and in vivo studies from our and other laboratories indicate that liposome-bound porphyrins are accumulated at high levels and retained for considerable times by neoplastic cells and tissues, thus substantially increasing both the time interval and porphyrin concentration ratios favorable for phototherapy and diagnostic exploitment of fluorescence emission. The local administration of porphyrins vehiculated by liposomes, presently under study in animals bearing subcutaneously implanted tumors, is expected to enhance again the above outlined advantages and to eliminate or greatly reduce the risk of side effects.

REFERENCES

1. D. A. Cortese, J. H. Kinsey, L. B. Woolner, W. S. Payne, D. R. Sanderson, and R. S. Fontana, Clinical application of a new endoscopic technique for detection of in situ bronchial car-

cinoma, Mayo Clin. Proc. 54: 635 (1979).

2. T. G. Dougherty, Hematoporphyrin derivative for detection and
    treatment of cancer, J. Surg. Oncol. 15: 209 (1980).

3. G. Jori, G. B. Pizzi, E. Reddi, L. Tomio, B. Salvato, P. L.
    Zorat, and F. Calzavara, Time-course of hematoporphyrin
    distribution in selected tissues of normal rats and in ascites
    hepatoma, Tumori 65: 43 (1979).

4. I. Cozzani, G. Jori, E. Reddi, A. Fortunato, B. Granati, M.
    Felice, L. Tomio, and P. L. Zorat, Distribution of endogenous
    and injected porphyrins at the subcellular level in rat hepa-
    tocytes and in ascites hepatoma, Chem. Biol. Interactions
    37: 67 (1981).

5. I. Cozzani and J. D. Spikes, Photodamage and photokilling of
    malignant human cells in vitro by hematoporphyrin-visible
    light: molecular basis and possible mechanisms of photocyto-
    toxicity, Med. Biol. Environ. 10: 271 (1982).

6. L. Tomio, P. L. Zorat, G. Jori, E. Reddi, B. Salvato, L. Corti,
    and F. Calzavara, Elimination pathway of hematoporphyrin
    from normal and tumor-bearing rats, Tumori 68: 283 (1982).

Chapter 5

Clinical Applications of HpD Phototherapy

HEMATOPORPHYRIN DERIVATIVE PHOTORADIATION THERAPY,

IN THEORY AND IN PRACTICE

J.C. Kennedy and K. Oswald

Department of Radiation Oncology
Queen's University
Kingston, Ontario K7L 2V7

INTRODUCTION

A patient has been referred to you for possible photoradiation therapy. She has breast cancer, treated in the past by bilateral mastectomy, radiotherapy, hormone therapy, and chemotherapy. It is now recurrent to the anterior, lateral, and posterior chest wall in the form of several hundred subcutaneous and cutaneous nodules ranging in diameter from 1 to 10 mm. We face two basis questions: (1) What is the goal of treatment? (2) What type of light source and light delivery system will best help us to reach that goal?

Our goal presumably is palliation. There is now no hope of cure, but there is hope that we can destroy the cutaneous and subcutaneous nodules, and thus prevent the skin of the thorax from becoming a very unpleasant mess. However, since prevention of skin breakdown is the goal of our treatment, whatever we do must not itself lead to skin breakdown, or add to the problems of the patient.

Interstitial photoradiation therapy via implanted optical fibres clearly is not the optimal approach in this situation, since there must be many more nodules present than the several hundred that we can see or palpate. What we need is a technique that will allow us to destroy both the detectable and the undetectable nodules in a field that covers most of the thorax. The purpose of this paper is to outline several useful approaches to the treatment of fields that involve large areas of the body. In all such clinical situations, some form of external beam therapy is necessary for optimal results.

365

EXTERNAL BEAM PHOTORADIATION THERAPY

The goal of external beam photoradiation therapy is to give a lethal dose of photoactivating light to malignant tissue that lies in or beneath an accessible body surface, but to do so without causing unacceptable damage to overlying or adjacent non-malignant tissues. We know that non-malignant tissues can be destroyed if the dose of photoactivating light is too large. It follows that the upper limit to the dose is determined by two characteristics of the non-malignant tissues within the treatment field: (1) their ability to survive the planned treatment, and (2) their value to the patient. We know also that the intensity (or dose) of photoactivating light will decrease as the depth of penetration increases, and that the intensity at any given depth will be proportional to the intensity (or dose) at the surface. Consequently, to produce maximum depth of kill of malignant tissue, we need to use the maximum dose that can be tolerated by the overlying or adjacent non-malignant tissues. When trying to treat just below this limit of tolerance, it is very important that the dose to non-malignant tissues and made as uniform as possible, in order to avoid the production of localized areas of overdose and consequent tissue necrosis.

TREATMENT PLANNING GOALS

One major goal is to work out techniques that will result in a uniform dose of light to every part of the surface of the treatment field. Since dose = intensity x duration of exposure, we can simplify our treatment planning by keeping the duration of exposure constant. Our planning goal then becomes "the uniform illumination of all parts of the surface of the treatment field".

Two factors dominate treatment planning when we have such a goal: (1) the geometry of the surface being treated, and (2) the optical characteristics of the treatment beam. For example, restricted areas on the anterior and posterior aspects of the thorax of our hypothetical breast cancer patient will approximate a plane surface. If we consider the whole of the thorax from the clavicles to the waist, it resembles a somewhat deformed cylinder or a truncated cone. Approaches to treatment that have been worked out using geometric solids as models often can be adapted for use with parts of the body that approximate the geometric solids in question. Several examples of such are described below.

UNIFORM ILLUMINATION OF PLANE SURFACES

The ideal light source for this purpose is one that can produce a collimated beam with a diameter larger than the largest dimension of the treatment field, and with a radiant energy density that is uniform across the whole diameter. With such a beam, changing the distance between the treatment field and the source will not change the intensity of illumination. Changes in the angle at which the axis of the beam meets the surface will change the intensity of illumination at all points on that surface (cosine correction for angle of incidence), but since all of the changes will be equal, the surface will continue to be illuminated uniformly.

The sun is a simple and inexpensive source for such a beam. As viewed from the earth, the sun subtends a half-angle of 0.25°. However, forward scattering within the atmosphere increases this angle to an effective value of approximately 3.5°. Solar radiation has a peak normal irradiance of approximately 1 kW/m at the surface of the earth, and a spectrum that varies with the angle at which the light passes through the atmosphere, but approximates that of a black body of appropriate colour temperature. We use a large second-surface mirror of aluminized glass to direct a broad beam into the treatment room, where several smaller mirrors intercept this beam and redirect the resultant smaller beams to appropriate treatment fields. Superimposing several of the smaller beams on the same treatment field can lead to very high intensities and correspondingly short treatment times. Since the angle the sun makes with the first (large) mirror changes with time, it is necessary to make that mirror adjustable. We tried mounting this mirror on a motorized stand that adjusted the beam direction automatically whenever the sun strayed from the original configuration, but this is not really necessary. However, it certainly is necessary to use a power meter than can integrate dose of light with time, since wisps of cloud than can not be detected visually can cause substantial although unsuspected variation in the intensity of the treatment beam.

Most of the UV and much of the far IR is removed as the beam passes through the glass of the two second-surface mirrors and the window. Water-absorption bands in the IR can be removed by passing the beam from the first mirror through a water filter of suitably large dimensions. To remove most of the visible wavelengths below 600 nm, we generally cover the lab window with Rubylith masking film (Ulano), or with some other red plastic film of suitable transmission spectrum. Although it would require less filter material to cover the small mirrors instead of the window, it should be noted that with such an arrangement the light will pass through each filter twice, with a consequent change in the transmission spectrum and a large decrease in intensity. In either case, care should be taken to cover or remove the filter when it is not in use, since the film fades badly if exposed to continuous sunlight. The addition of 2×10^{-4} gm/ml of Rhodamine B to the water filter will remove much of the radiation below 600 nm, and thus extend the lifetime of the colour filter. All filtrations are best carried out before the light has been concentrated by the second mirrors, since the power of an unfiltered but concentrated beam is capable for cracking glass and melting plastic.

In most northern countries, the sun is not very dependable as a source of photoactivating light. A much more expensive but also much more dependable source of a "nearly collimated" beam with an appropriate spectrum and a reasonably uniform radiant energy density can be made from a power ful arc lamp that is manufactured by Vortek Industries, Vancouver, Canada. This lamp can produce a spectrum similar to the "air mass 2" solar spectrum, with an average irradiance of 1.1 kW/m^2 at a distance of 10.5 m. Since our largest treatment fields usually do not exceed 50 cm in their largest dimension, the half-angle subtended by a treatment field at 10.5 m will rarely be more than 3°. Under such conditions, the uniformity of illumination of a plane surface is quite adequate. As with sunlight, mirrors and filters can be used to amplify and modify the treatment beam. The main problem with this system is its cost (close to $ 100,000 U.S.A.) and high power requirements (125 kilowatts).

Although a broad collimated beam of uniform radiant energy density, suitable emission spectrum, and adequate intensity would be ideal for treating plane surfaces, a large diffuse source of photoactivating light can be a useful substitute. In principle, the best such source would be a very large plane surface that was capable of emitting light with uniform radiant intensity from every point on its surface. With a such a source, the illumination at any point on the treatment field (also a plane surface) would not be affected by moderate variations in the orientation of the target with respect to the source, or in the distance between them. However, a black-body source of this size, operating at the required colour temperature, would require a substantial amount of power and produce a correspondingly large amount of waste heat.

High-pressure sodium lamps produce a useful amount of energy between 600 and 640 nm, with relatively little output in the IR. Accordingly, as an approximation to a diffuse source, we arranged four 1000 watt high-pressure sodium lamps (General Electric Lucalox) with the light-emitting elements parallel to each other and in the same plane. The elements of these lamps are 23.5 cm long and 8.8 mm in diameter. When four elements are arranged so that the inner two are each 9.7 cm from the midline while the outer two are an additional 9.0 cm distant, they can produce relatively uniform illumination (3.5% variation about the mean) of a flat surface approximately 24 cm long x 14 cm wide when it is placed parallel to the plane of the lamps and 24 cm from it.

Increasing the distance between the plane of the lamps and a flat surface placed parallel to that plane causes a decrease in the intensity of illumination. When both the original and the new distance are within our usual working range, then the decrease is approximately proportional to (original distance/new distance). Any change in the spacing between the lamps changes (1) the intensity of illumination of a field, (2) the optimal distance for producing

uniform illumination of a given size of field, and (3) the maximum
size of field that can be illuminated uniformly. To calculate the
optimal spacing for fields of various sizes located at various
distances from the plane of the lamps, we may consider the lamp
elements to be a linear array of point sources that radiate uniformly in all direction. Each point source in the rod will obey the
inverse square law that relates the radiance at a given point in
space and the distance between that point and the source. In addition, since we are interested in calculating the power per unit area
at various points on a flat surface (rather than the power passing
through the equivalent points in space), it is necessary to make a
correction for the angle of incidente of the rays arising from each
hypothetical point source. Since the isointensity curves produced
by computer are a good fit for similar curves that we obtained experimentally, it appears reasonable to use the computer to work out
the optimal positions for the lamps when facing a situation that
involves a new geometrical relationship.

The output of the high-pressure sodium lamps must be filtered
to remove wavelengths below 600 nm. Our primary filter consists of
two parallel sheets of Pyrex glass (42 x 24 cm), separated by a gap
of 12 mm through which flows an aqueous solution of Rhodamine B at
a concentration of 2×10^{-4} gm/ml. The solution enters at the bottom of the filter, is pushed out at the top, and then drains by gravity to a water-cooled heat exchanger. From there it is pumped to a
reservoir that is open to the atmosphere (to relieve the pressure
that builds up with an increase in temperature), and fastened above
the filter in such a way that the average hydrostatic head between
the filter and the reservoir is constant, no matter what the position of the filter. Gravity drainage then returns the solution to
the filter. Such an arrangement prevents dangerous changes in pressure that may burst the filter. The final filter is a red acetate
sheet (Transilwrap) that is placed over the glass plate nearest the
patient. Care must be taken in selecting the plastic filter, since
transmission spectra may vary significantly from one sample to another.

We use this light source routinely for treating large, relatively flat areas such as the anterior or posterior chest wall. Our standard approach is to give a dose of 25 mWhr/cm^2 in the morning, and
then an additional 5 or 10 mWhr/cm^2 in the afternoon if the skin reaction is about as strong as expected. At our standard treatment
distance of 15 cm from the outer surface of the filter, the dose
rate is such that approximately 0.43 minutes are required to give a
dose of 1.0 mWhr/cm^2. Note that it is essential to use a cosine-
corrected power meter when calibrating this, or any other, source
of diffuse light.

Both the sun and our array of high-pressure sodium lamps produce beams whose behaviour can be predicted mathematically. In con-

trast, projectors produce beams whose radiant energy density distribution measured across a diameter does not follow any simple or constant pattern. Consequently, we have found it best to be completely empirical when planning a treatment for which projectors are to be the source of photoactivating light. We use to methods. First, we may use a model, a figure that has been painted flat white in order to simulate the mixture of specular and non-specular reflectance of dry human skin. Second, we may remove the Hoya R-60 filter that we use during treatment, replace it by a R-66, and then use the patient as our model, since the wavelengths passed by the R-66 filter will not active HpD. If the surface of the treatment field shows significant variation in either texture or colour, it is best to place material of uniform reflectivity (white cloth) on the surface of the field at the points at which measurements are to be taken. In either case, we measure the light scattered from various points on the surface, and then adjust the projectors by trial-and-error until the intensities at each point are similar. Intensity measurements usually are made by means of a meter that has been modified to accept only a very limited cone of light. This allows us to make measurements at sufficient distance to prevent shadowing of the field by intrusion of the light meter. An attempt to digitize the output of a video camera and use it as a light meter that would be capable of simultaneous measurement of the intensity at every point on the surface was not a complete success, since we could not obtain adequate linearity.

A 500 watt slide projector equipped with a Hoya R-60 filter and a f/2.8 or f/2.5 lens produces much less light than does our array of high-pressure sodium lamps. In the past we attempted to overcome this problem by using up to 5 projectors when it was necessary to treat large flat areas such as the anterior chest wall, but this occasionally produced localized areas of second degree burn when our treatment planning was not adequate. At present, we never use more than one projector, and then for small areas only. We minimize the non-uniformity of the beam by using only the central third, where the degree of non-uniformity is acceptable if the projection lens is focussed properly. It is best to use a lens with as long a focal length as possible, provided the f-number is at least 2.8 (preferably 2.5). Attempts to make the beam more uniform by using a neutral density filter that absorbed more in the centre of the beam than at the edges were successful, but there was too great a loss of intensity for this technique to be very useful.

A Kodak slide projector equipped with a 500 watt tungsten or halogen lamp, a Hoya R-60 filter, and a 130 cm f/2.8 lens, focussed so that the central third of the beam covers an area 5 cm square, will require about 8.6 minutes to deliver 1.0 mWhr/cm^2 of photoactivating light. Obviously, a dose of 25 to 35 mWhr/cm^2 will require a long exposure. The system should be calibrated immediately before

each use, since the output of the tungsten lamp will decrease sig-
ificantly with time.

UNIFORM ILLUMINATION OF SOLID CYLINDERS OR CONES

The thorax of our hypothetical cancer patient resembles a somewhat flattened cylinder or truncated cone. As was the case for a
plane surface, the ideal treatment beam is collimated, with a diameter larger than the largest dimension of the treatment field, and
a uniform radiant energy density across the whole of that diameter.
As discussed above, the sun or a solar simulator of adequate intensity are suitable sources for such a beam.

Several different techniques may be used to give a uniform dose
of photoactivating light to the external surface of a cylinder or
cone when such a beam is available. First, the treatment beam may
be rotated with constant angular velocity about the axis of the cylinder or cone. Secon, the beam may be fixed, and the cylinder or
cone rotated about its own axis with constant angular velocity.
Third, the cylinder or cone may be exposed to multiple beams of equal
intensity that are distributed radially in a plane at right angles
to the axis of the target. It should be noted that there may be a
difference in the biological effect if the beams are applied in sequence rather than simultaneously, even though the dose of photoactivating light may be identical in both cases.

Table 1. Relationship Between the Uniformity With Which the Surface
of a Cylinder or Cone Is Illuminated by Broad Collimated
Beams of Uniform Radiant Energy Density, and the Number
and Radial Distribution of Those Beams in a Plane Perpendicular to the Axis of the Cylinder or Cone.

Number of beams	Angle (degree) between adjacent beams	Number of maxima	Number of minima	Maximum variation in intensity (minimum intensity = 100%)
1	360	1	1	100%
2	180	2	2	100%
3	120	6	6	15.5%
4	90	4	4	41.4%
5	72	10	10	5.1%
6	60	6	6	15.4%
7	51.4	14	14	2.6%
8	45	8	8	8.2%
9	40	18	18	1.6%
10	36	10	10	5.2%

Table 1 summarizes the variation in intensity of illumination
to be expected when different numbers of beams are evenly spaced
radially about a cylinder or cone. It should be noted that an odd
number of beams is to be preferred. Since the beams are collimated,
the intensity of illumination will not change when the source-to-
-target distance is changed, and consequently the calculations apply
even when a cylinder has been somewhat flattened. Flattened cones
present a more complex dosimetry problem.

As noted previously, broad collimated treatment beams of uniform
radiant energy density are either unreliable (sunlight) or expensive (Vortek lamp solar simulator). Consequently, we generally use
our array of high-pressure sodium lamps when treating cylindrical
surfaces such as the thorax or leg. Unfortunately, the mathematics
of dosimetry for a continuously convex curve illuminated by a pseudo-
-diffuse source is not as simple as it is when a plane surface is
involved. Since our source contains four lamps, the surface of a
cylinder or cone will have one area that is illuminated by all four
lamps, plus semi-shadowed areas on each side that are illuminated in
turn by either one, two, or three lamps. We are now in the process
of developing a computer programme for determining how best to place
the lamps when treating cylindrical or conical surfaces, but a present we must use empirical methods. For example, when treating the
entire thorax, we usually start by giving the planned dose to the
anterior chest wall, but do not attempt to shield the sides of the
thorax from the edges of the treatment beam. We then rotate the
patient and/or the source approximately 110° about the axis of the
thorax, and give another full exposure, this time allowing the edges
of the beam to spill over onto the anterior chest wall. With our
particular arrangement of lamps, the area of overlap between the
treatment fields receives a dose that is reasonably close to that
given to the field directly beneath the lamps. The best source-to-
-target distance and the angle between the adjacent treatment beams
must be determined empirically for each patient. It must be admit-
ted that, as a result of inadequate dosimetry, we occasionally come
very close to producing a second degree burn in the area of the
thorax where the edges of the beams overlap.

Another way in which the diffuse beam produced by an array of
high-pressure sodium lamps can be used to treat a cylindrical surface into treatment fields that approximate plane surfaces. These
are then patched together. As with all such techniques, the junction line is often given either too much or too little radiation.
However, up to the present we have not caused any actual skin breakdown.

The diverging beams of non-uniform cross-section that are produced by slide projectors are not suitable for the uniform illumination of cylinders or cones. A single projector is not powerful
enough to treat a large area unless a very long exposure time is

used, and it is very difficult to blend beams from several projectors
to produce illumination that is uniform enough to be safe.

HAZARDS OF TREATING LARGE AREAS OF THE THORAX

Pain is a common problem, even when the dosimetry has been
exact. The "sunburn" response of normal skin is not usually a
source of much more than mild discomfort unless very large areas
have been treated. Serious pain seems to be caused by the stretching a dermis by edematous tissue or fluid. It is noterworthy that
a patient who has multiple percutaneous and cutaneous nodules of
malignant tissue of approximately equal size will usually feel pain
after treatment only in relationship to the cutaneous nodules.
thick-walled vesicles may develop in the skin over the cutaneous nodules, but the serum that oozes freely from the percutaneous nodules
is never confined sufficiently to stretch the adjacent or underlying skin. Cutaneous nodules smaller than 3 mm in diameter rarely
cause pain following treatment, presumably because they are too
small to cause much intradermal edema. Larger nodules that are
located in any confined space that is bounded by relatively inelas-
tic tissues such as fascia may be a source of serious pain.

Necrosis of normal skin can result from unexpectedly strong
reactions to a dose of photoactivating light that ordinary would
cause no problem. We have seen such skin damage under two conditions: (1) when the patient has been given multiple injections of
HpD within what we now know (by hindsight) was too short a period
of time for that particular patient to have excreted residual drug
before the next injection; (2) when the patient has taken doxo-
rubicin. The severity of such unexpected phototoxicity can be reduced if each patient is instructed prior to treatment to let you
know as soon as itching, tingling, or burning sensations are noted
in the area number treatment. A burning sensation indicates serious
tissue damage, and treatment should be stopped instantly. Itching
or tingling sensations are common after at least two-thirds of the
planned dose has been given, but they indicate unusual skin reactivity if reported during the first third of the treatment.

An accidental overdose of photoactivating light also can cause
necrosis of skin. The usual causes are either inadequate treatment
planning, or inaccurate dosimetry. We have produced small areas of
overdose (and subsequently of necrosis) within a treatment field
when attempting to use treatment beams that were not suitable for
the surface configuration of the field in question. Surfaces that
are made up of compound convex curves, or of a mixture of convex
and concave curves, are especially difficult to illuminate uniformly.

SUMMARY OF CLINICAL RESULTS FOR CYLINDERS AND CONES

We have used photoradiation therapy to treat 19 thoraces (all with subcutaneous, intradermal, and/or percutaneous recurrences of breast carcinoma), and 3 legs (two with Kaposi's sarcoma and one with a soft tissue sarcoma whose histological classification was ambiguous). The clinical results may be summarized in the following sentences.

With one exception, all of the nodules were damaged semi-selectively by the treatment. The exception was a single nodule of breast carcinoma whose histology was indistinguishable from that of adjacent nodules, but whose doubling time was much less. This nodule showed what must be considered an absolute resistance to HpD photoradiation therapy. Repeated injections of HpD directly into this nodule were followed by huge doses of photoactivating light, with no effect. The other nodules in the same patient showed the expected response to treatment, and all of the nodules had approximately equal HpD fluorescence.

As expected, the best responses in all cases were obtained with the smaller and more superficial nodules. A good illustration of this rule was provided by several patients who had inflammatory breast carcinoma involving the anterior, lateral, and posterior surfaces of the thorax. The areas of inflammation in which no nodules could be palpated responded very well; the itching stopped immediately, and the red rash changed to a brown colour that did not blanch readily under pressure. The areas containing nodules that were less than 5 mm in diameter also responded well; in many cases the nodules were completely destroyed by a single treatment, and those that were not were badly damaged. As the size of the nodules increased, the proportion that was completely destroyed decreased. Nodules larger than approximately 10 mm in diameter were damaged but not destroyed by doses of light large enough to cause significant phototoxic damage to the normal skin. We found that even these larger nodules sometimes could be destroyed without causing significant harm to the normal skin, if we gave repeated treatments at intervals long enough to permit the skin to repair the phototoxic damage caused by the previous treatment. This procedure was effective only when the doubling time of the nodules was long enough that they did not show significant regrowth before the next treatment.

In summary, large field external beam photoradiation therapy is appropriate for flat, cylindrical, or conical treatment fields containing multiple small nodules.

EVALUATION OF PHOTORADIATION THERAPY (PRT) IN 20 CASES OF CANCERS

Guo Zhonghe, Huang Yingcai, and Wen Zangmin

Chinese PLA General Hospital

Beijing, China

INTRODUCTION

The application of HpD-laser photoradiation in the diagnosis and treatment of malignancies is now under investigation in a few countries [1]. In China, Hematoporphyrin Derivative (HpD) has been prepared from the blood of cattle by Beijing Pharmaceutical Institute and used in animal experiment since August 1980. The laser apparatus used in this study is also made in China, its clinical application having started in 1981. Using this apparatus, 20 cases of malignancy have been studied in our hospital.

MATERIAL AND METHODS

The Use of HpD

Skin test for hypersensitiveness was done first. In case of no reaction HpD, 2.5-5 mg/kg body weight, was injected slowly intravenously, or that diluted with 250 ml nomal saline injected by intravenous drip. To avoid generalized photosensitivity lasting about 30 days, all patients were informed to avoid exposure to direct or strong sunlight during this period. Both diagnosis and treatment were started 48-72 hours after HpD injection.

Laser Apparatus

For diagnosis: Argon ion laser with a wavelength of 4888 Å and power output of more than 50 mW was used. For treatment: Argon-dye laser with a wavelength of 6300 Å and output of 400 mW was used. The light was irradiated through a quartz fiber.

Table 1. Laser-HpD Fluorescence Observed with Naked Eye.

	No. of cases	DIAGNOSTIC RESULTS		
		Positive reaction	Doubtful reaction	Comformity
MALIGNANCIES:				
surface cancer	10	10	–	10
gastric cancer	5	5	–	5
urinary bladder cancer	2	2	–	2
BENIGN LESIONS:				
ulcer of mouth	2	–	1	1
leukoplakia of oral mucosa	1	–	–	1
richen of oral mucosa	3	–	1	2
Total	23	17	2	21

Irradiation for Treatment

The cancer was irradiated with 80–250 mW/cm^2 of an Argon dye laser beam at a distance of 1–3 cm from the lesion via a quartz fiber for 20 minutes on each irradiated point. In the treatment of visceral tumors, such as gastric cancer, the laser beam was transmitted via the quartz fiber inserted through the instrumentation channel of the endoscope.

Diagnosis of Malignancies

The diagnosis was finally confirmed by histopathological examination both in surface tumors and in visceral ones [6,7].

Criteria for Therapeutic Effectiveness

Because no international criteria for PRT therapeutic effectiveness have been laid down, the criteria used in this study were formulated by modifying international criteria for chemotherapy. They were divided into 4 grades: (1) Complete remission (CR), the tumor disappears and the result maintains for at least one month. (2) Partial remission (PR), the volume (estimated by the product of two greatest vertical lines in the tumor outline) of tumor decreases by 50–99% and maintains in such size for at least one month. In case of gastric cancer PR means extensive necrosis of the tumor and slough off of the necrotic tissue; (3) Mild remission (MR), the tumor volume reduces by more than 50%. In case of gastric cancer MR means superficial necrosis of tumor. MR cases usually are added to the PR group to estimate the total effect rate. (4) No remission (NR), there is no obvious necrosis, or only necrosis without reduction of the tumor volume. In case of gastric cancer NR means no response.

RESULTS

Fluorescence of Malignant Tumors and Other Diseases

See Table 1.

Clinical Data of Malignancies Treated by Laser HpD Technique

The 20 patients were 12 males and 8 females. Their ages are reported in Table 2, while the type of malignancies and the therapeutic effects are shown in Table 3 and Table 4, respectively.

Table 2. Age Distribution

Age	21-30	31-40	41-50	51-60	61	Total
No. of cases	2	3	4	5	6	20

Table 3. Clinical Type of Tumors

Type*	Cancer of Skin	Cancer of Cervix	Cancer of Stomach	Cancer of Urinary Bladder
No. of cases	7	1	10	2

*The localization of all visceral cancers was done by endoscopy.

Table 4.   Therapeutic Effect

Type	CR	PR and MR	NR
Skin cancer	3	3	2
Gastric cancer	1	8	1
Urinary bladder cancer	1	1	-
Total	5	12	3

Side Effect

The main side effect of this type of therapy was allergic der-
matitis, which occurred in 3 cases after HpD injection and subsequent exposure to sunlight, manifesting as mild or moderate swelling
of the sites exposed to sunlight, which usually subsided within 2-3
weaks, provided that there was no further exposure to sunlight in a
dim room. Blood and urine examinations, hepatic and renal function
test were normal before and after treatment. In the gastric cancer
group, there were 3 cases which showed melanorrhagia lasting for 3
days.

DISCUSSION

According to reports in the literature and the result in this
study, it appears that PRT exerts some lethal action to the tumor
cells [1-5]. Even in the NR group of this series, slight necrosis has
been observed. Because of the requirement of HpD itself, the laser
light used should be red at a wavelength of 6300 Å and the output
low. The effect of the laser on the tumor is superficial, usually
deep about 1 cm or less.

These factors greatly limit its usefulness and jeopardize its
clinical applications.

Further investigation on photosensitizer and the increase of
depth of the killing action is in an urgent need in the development
of this technique. From the data of this series, it may be seen
that laser-HpD technique is effective on various kinds of tumor in
different sites. It is also effective on recurrent neoplasms which
have been treated by surgery, irradiation or chemotherapy. This
fact indicates that this method provides an opportunity of therapy
for those cases in which the tumor cells have developed resistance
to chemotherapy.

A selective action seems to happen with this method. This means, that the tumor cells are killed, leaving normal tissues undamaged or less damaged. There is no harmful effect on the heart, liver, kidneys or bone marrow. This may be particularly useful in those cases in which damage to some important organs have occurred and other therapeutic measures have deteriorated patient's conditions as for example, in patients with coronary disease, liver cirrhosis, hypersplenoses or spleen hyperfunction. For the malignant tumors of some sites such as the face, the hand, or the foot, while operation may cause a diminished function or an esthetic damage, this technique is certainly a method of choice and may be easily accepted by the patients. In case with dysphogia due to obstruction by cancer of the stomach the patients usually suffer greatly and this method can provide an alleviative effect.

As mentioned before, the most apparent drawback of PRT is its superficial penetration. Solid tumors of considerable size can be radically treated by this method. The problem of tumor metastasis also can not be solved with this method. In PRT performed via endoscope, the equipment and technology needs further improvement.

CONCLUSIONS

This paper reports the use of HpD and laser in the diagnosis and treatment of various malignant neoplasms. Fluorescence observation for diagnosis was performed in 17 cases of malignancies with positive reaction in all cases, and in 6 cases of benign lesions with suspicious reaction in 2. Twenty cases of malignancy were treated by PRT, and the results are CR in 5, PR in 12, and NR in 3.

The advantages and disadvantages of this method have been discussed. It is effective on various kinds of neoplasms located in different sites and is usable according to different clinical requirements.

The penetrating power of the laser is shallow. This disadvantage limit its effect and application. The finding of new photosensitizing drugs and the way to increase the penetrating power of the laser irradiation is now in urgent need for the further development of this technique. The equipment and technology for PRT in the treatment of visceral tumors also require further improvement.

REFERENCES

1. T. J. Dougherty, J. Surg. Oncol. 15:209 (1980).
2. T. J. Dougherty, R. E. Thoma, D. G. Boyle, and K. R. Weishaupt, Interstitial photoradiation therapy for primary solid tumors in pet cats and dogs, Cancer Res. 41:401 (1981).
3. T. J. Forbes, P. A. Cowled, A. S. Y. Leong, A. D. Ward, R. B. Black, A. J. Blake, and F. J. Jacka, Phototherapy of human

tumors using Hematoporphyrin Derivative, <u>Med. J. Aust</u>. 2:489 (1980).

4. Y. Hayata, H. Kato, C. Konaka, J. Ono, and N. Takizawa, Hemato-porphyrin Derivative and laser photoradiation in the treatment of lung cancer, <u>Chest</u>. 81:269 (1982).
5. Y. Hayata, <u>Med. Imaging Inf</u>. 14:19 (1982).
6. R. L. Lipson, E. J. Baldes, and M. J. Gray, <u>Cancer</u> 20:2255 (1967).
7. R. W. Henderson, <u>Br. J. Exp. Path</u>. 61:345 (1980).

HEMATOPORPHYRIN PHOTOTHERAPY OF MALIGNANT TUMORS

P.L. Zorat, L. Tomio, L. Corti, F. Calzavara,
G. Sotti, G. Jori*, E. Reddi* and G. Mandoliti

Division of Radiotherapy, Civil Hospital
*Institute of Animal Biology, University of Padova

INTRODUCTION

More than ten years have elapsed since Diamond et al. demonstrated[1] the possibility of using the photodynamic properties of hematoporphyrin (Hp) to cure malignant tumors in vivo. At present, the so-called photoradiation therapy (PRT) is under clinical investigation as a new technique to treat a wide variety of solid tumors. Up to now about 2000 patients have been treated with PRT in several different countries[2]. Generally, PRT is performed by using the hematoporphyrin derivative (HpD) as the photosensitizing agent. HpD is intravenously injected; after 2-5 days, the malignant lesions are exposed to visible light of wavelengths between 620 and 640 nm.

Recently, we demonstrated[3] that Hp is a powerful photosensitizer which can selective destroy malignant tumors in patients exposed to red light. In this report, we outline our initial experience with Hp-phototherapy and technical guidelines for future use in the clinical field.

MATERIALS AND METHODS

Hematoporphyrin

Hp was obtained from Porphyrin Products (Logan, Utah) and prepared in a sterile injectable form by Monico Pharmaceutical Company (Venice, Italy) according to the procedure previously described[3]. Typically, 5 mg of Hp per kg of body weight were injected intravenously 24 h prior to PRT.

Light Sources and Procedure

Two light sources were used in this study. A 4,000 W Xenon arc-lamp was employed for treating single or multiple lesions of external diameter larger than 2 cm, as well as areas up to approximately 20 cm^2 containing multiple lesions of small diameter. A red beam (590-690 nm) was isolated by filtering the emitted light with a combination of a chemical filter and a heat-reflecting glass filter. The total intensity delivered at the level of the patient was 25 mW/cm^2 over a circular light spot with an overall diameter of 5 cm. In practice, since the red absorption band of Hp encompasses the all cases, the total delivered light dose was 22.5 J/cm^2 in each session of the phototreatment.

The second light source was a He/Ne laser (Valfivre, Florence, Italy) generating a monochromatic (632.8 nm) light beam focused on the proximal end of a single quartz optical fiber of 1,100 um diameter by means of an alignment device. Output power at the distal end of the optical fiber was 20 mW. By coupling five sources a maximal intensity of 100 mW could be obtained. We used the latter modality for treating single superficial lesions whose diameter approached 1 cm and, less often, single infiltrating lesions up to 2 cm in diameter or areas smaller than 7 cm^2 containing multiple lesions. If one neglects the light scattering by tissue and eventual inhomogenities of the tumor surfaces, the total intensity ranged between 100 and 15 mW/cm^2 depending on the distance between the lesion and the distal end of the optical fiber. Lesions were also treated with various total light doses (17-72 J/cm^2) depending on exposure time. Occasionally, 180 J/cm^2 were used; however, skin necrosis was observed. Usually, the phototreatment was performed at 24 h and 48 h after Hp administration. The exposure time was 60 min. in each session with the Xenon lamp, and varied within 10-30 min. with the He/Ne laser.

Clinical Cases

Fourteen patients affected by a variety of primary and metastatic or recurrent malignant lesions of the skin were treated. One patient presented a lesion from Kaposi's sarcoma on the oral pharynx. The main characteristics of the patients are given in table 1. All patients had biopsy-proven malignancy. Fully informed consent for phototreatment was obtained in all cases and the patients were cautioned to avoid direct sun exposure during the two weeks immediately following Hp injection. A total number of 32 lesions were treated. Six patients received a second dose of Hp at 15-20 days after the first phototreatment and were reexposed to light according to the above outlined protocol. Assessment of tumor response and results are given as previously described[3]. Before treatment and during the follow-up period, blood and urine samples were taken for Hp analysis by a spectrophotofluorimetric procedure[4].

RESULTS

The responses observed for various phototreated patients are summarized in tables 2 and 3. Five lesions are not considered owing to the short post-irradiation follow-up. Out of the 27 evaluable lesions, we observed 13 complete and 5 partial (below 50 percent) responses. Specifically, 10 complete responses were obtained by phototreating small lesions (5 basal cell carcinoma, 4 Kaposi's sarcoma and 1 squamous cell carcinoma) which were 5 mm-thick and were treated with the He/Ne laser (total light doses ranged between 57 and 180 J/cm^2). The other complete responses consisted of three large exophytic and ulcerated nodules from Kaposi's sarcoma treated with Xenon arc-lamp and total light doses of 22.5 J/cm^2. We wish to outline the optimal response obtained in a basal cell carcinoma of the external auditory duct previously treated by surgery and topical chemotherapy; the only alternative modality of tumor treatment would have been represented by high doses of radiation therapy with important side effects.

The phototreatment was unsuccessful in 2 lesions from pigmented melanoma in agreement with previous reports[5] and in single or multiple lesions from breast cancer. In the latter case both the Xenon arc-lamp and the He/Ne laser were ineffective probably owing to the infiltrating characteristics of the lesions and the low light doses used.

The time-dependence of Hp concentration in blood and urines from several patients subjected to PRT (Fig. 1) indicated a rapid accumulation of the porphyrin, followed by a slow clearance. In most cases, the serum porphyrin levels returned to those typical of endogenous porphyrins only after some weeks. This observation may explain the reported persistence of photosensitivity in humans injected with Hp[6]. Only a small fraction of Hp undergoes elimination in the urines, in agreement with previous findings[7] indicating that the main route for Hp elimination involves the gut.

DISCUSSION

Our initial data show that free base Hp is taken up by different kinds of tumors which can be photosensitized to the action of red light, thus leading to a massive necrosis of the neoplastic lesion.

The quality of the tumor response is strongly dependent on the total light dose. Our optimal results were obtained in the case of small superficial lesions exposed to light doses higher than 50 J/cm^2. Dougherty et al.[7] showed that in PRT using HpD the response of the normal skin to the activating light is the major factor limiting the light dose so that the light should be delivered 3 or 4 days after HpD administration to avoid skin necrosis. On the contrary,

Table 1. Cases and physical data

Case no.	Age	Sex	Histology	Site	Number of Lesions	Dimension (cm)	Total dose (J/cm^2)
1	35	F	Malignant Melanoma	Shoulder	2	2	22.5
2	72	M	Squamous Carcinoma	Anus	1	6	22.5
3	79	F	Kaposi's Sarcoma	Foot	3	0,6-3	22.5
					4*	0,6-0,3	180-68
4	61	F	Breast Carcinoma	Chest Wall	2	0,5 (mult.)	22.5
5	62	F	Breast Carcinoma	Chest Wall	1	5	22.5
					2*	2	38
6	48	F	Breast Carcinoma	Chest Wall	1*	2	38
					3*	1	26
7	54	M	Squamous Carcinoma	Neck	1	5	22.5
8	49	M	Kaposi's Sarcoma	Arm	3*	0,5 (mult.)	35
				Oral ph.	1*	0,6	60
9	61	M	Basal Cell Carcinoma	Face	1*	1,5	26
10	75	F	Basal Cell Carcinoma	Face	2*	1	57
11	82	M	Basal Cell Carcinoma	Ear	1*	1	57
12	72	M	Basal Cell Carcinoma	Head	2*	1	57
13	80	F	Squamous Carcinoma	Head	1*	1	68
14	71	F	Malignant Melanoma	Foot	1	6	22.5

* Lesions treated by He/Ne laser. Other lesions treated by Xenon lamp.

we did not observe necrosis of the overlying or surrounding skin even when the phototreatment has been performed only 24 h after Hp administration. Finally we want to outline that, when the power output is small, good results can be obtained by fractionating the

Table 2. Results obtained with patients treated with hematoporphyrin and red light

Histology		Number of sites	CR	PR	R	S	NV
Basal Cell Carcinoma		6	5			1	
Squamous Cell Carcinoma		3	1		1		1
Breast Carcinoma		9			3	6	
Melanoma	Pigmented	2				2	
	Unpigmented	1			1		
Kaposi's	Skin	10	7				3
	Oral pharynx						1
TOTAL		32	13		5	9	5

CR= complete response; PR= partial response; R= regression; S= stable, no change; NV= not valuable

Table 3. Summary of patients treated with hematoporphyrin and red light

Light Source	CR or PR/Total	S/Total*
Xenon	5/10	5/10
He/Ne	13/17	4/17

*Symbols as in Table 2

light dose, thus avoiding long exposure times which may be inconve= nient for the patients.

ACKNOWLEDGMENT

This work was partially supported by C.N.R.(Italy) under the Progetto Finalizzato "Controllo della crescita tumorale maligna", contract No. 82.00252.96

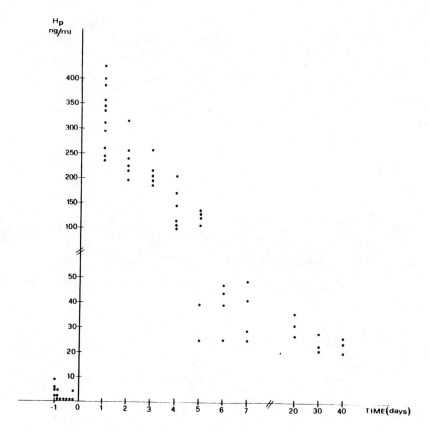

Fig. 1.   Recovery of HP from biological fluids of patients subje-
          cted to photoradiation therapy.

REFERENCES

1. I. Diamond, A. F. McDonagh, C. B. Wilson, S. G. Granelli,
       S. Nielsen, and R. Jaenicke, Photodynamic therapy of mali-
       gnant tumors, Lancet 1175 (1972).
2. T. J. Dougherty, An overview of the status of photoradiation
       therapy, in:"Porphyrin localization and treatment of tumors,"
       D. Doiron, ed., Alan R. Liss Inc., New York (1983).
3. L. Tomio, F. Calzavara, P. L. Zorat, E. Rossi, E. Reddi, and
       G. Jori, Photoradiation therapy for cutaneous and subcuta-
       neous tumors using hematoporphyrin, in:"Porphyrin localiza-
       tion and treatment of tumors," D. Doiron, ed., Alan R. Liss
       Inc., New York (1983).
4. G. Jori, E. Reddi, L. Tomio, B. Salvato, P. L. Zorat, and
       F. Calzavara, Time-course of hematoporphyrin distribution in
       selected tissues of normal rats and in ascites hepatoma,
       Tumori 65:43 (1979).

T. J. Dougherty, Photoradiation therapy for cutaneous and subcutaneous malignancies, J. Invest. Dermatol. 77:122 (1981)

6. G. L. Zalar, M. Poh-Fitzpatrik, D. L. Krohn, R. Jacobs, and L. C. Harber, Induction of drug photosensitization in man after parenteral exposure to hematoporphyrin, Arch. Dermatol. 113:1397 (1977).

7. L. Tomio, P. L. Zorat, G. Jori, E. Reddi, L. Corti, and F. Calzavara, Elimination pathway of hematoporphyrin from normal and tumor-bearing rats, Tumori 68:283 (1982).

HEMATOPORPHYRIN-DERIVATIVE AND PHOTOTHERAPY IN EXTENSIVE BASAL-CELL CARCINOMA OF THE DORSAL SKIN

G. Bandieramonte, R. Marchesini, F. Zunino, E. Melloni,
S. Andreola, C. Andreoli, S. Di Pietro, P. Spinelli,
G. Fava and H. Emanuelli

National Cancer Institute, Via Venezian, 1
20133 Milano, Italy

SUMMARY

A 75 year old male patient was diagnosed of multiple basal cell carcinoma in a surface area of 18 x 21 cm^2 of the dorsal skin. Contraindications for surgery and radiation therapy made the patient eligible for phototherapy. After hematoporphyrin-derivative (HpD) administration at the dose of 3 mg/kg, body weight, the entire area of lesions was treated 2 times and in 12 fractionated areas, by using Argon or Dye lasers and different exposure times. Five of the 12 fractions were treated with Argon-ion laser at 100 mW/cm^2 average irradiance for 20 min, whereas 7 fractions were treated at the same irradiance with Dye laser for 10 min in one, 15 min in 3 and 20 min for the remaining 3. Energy dose of 60 J/cm^2 with Dye laser irradiation and 120 J/cm^2 with Argon-ion laser irradiation resulted in similar effectiveness from clinical and histologic standpoints for the studied surface epitheliomas.

INTRODUCTION

In the framework of an Oriented National Research Project, the "Biomedical Applications of Lasers" phototherapeutic procedures with HpD and visible light have been developed at the National Cancer Institute of Milan, both for intracavitary and surface neoplastic lesions. Crucial problems in that method of treatment were recognized to be light dosimetry[1]. For a given wavelength, penetration depth in tissue and total energy density delivered are the most critical parameters to evaluate the therapeutic effectiveness[2,3] and to avoid adverse effects[4]. Thus, in a pilot study, extensive neoplastic lesions at the surface level were treated after photosensitization, by using Argon or Dye laser at different energies,

389

and the clinical and histologic effects were evaluated on the treated areas.

PATIENT AND METHODS

A 75 year old male patient was diagnosed of multiple basal cell
carcinoma in a surface area of 18 by 21 square centimeters of the
dorsal skin. The tumors had arisen 17 years after local radiation
therapy for spondylitis ankylosans. (Fig. 1). The maximum depth
of tumor infiltration was 1.7 mm, measured on several biopsy sites.
Since the patient was considered as a poor condidate for surgery
as a consequence of his general conditions and age, moreover being
questionable the success of plastic reconstructive surgery because
of the extension of the lesion area and of the previous radiation
treatment, the phototherapy was the treatment of choice. Because of

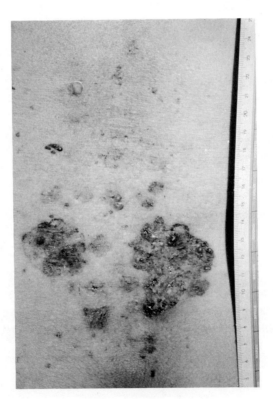

Fig. 1. Extensive dorsal skin epitheliomas in a 75 year old patient.

the large extension of the lesions – which required many irradiation fields and consequently long irradiation time – the treatment
was performed in two times, with and interval of two months. Before
and after each treatment, biopsy samples were taken for histologic
examination. HpD was administered at a dose of 3 mg/kg, body weight,
48 hours before laser irradiations.

The treatments were performed either with Argon-ion laser (all
lines) or with the Dye laser emitting at 630 nm wavelength as
checked with a monochromator (Mod. 7240 Oriel). The delivered powers
were measured with a power meter (Mod. 201 Coheerent) and an average
irradiance was defined as ratio between power and illuminated area.
In the first series of treatments the laser beam, enlarged by lens
was directed on the lesions by means of mirrors. Conversely, in the
second series of treatments the output of the laser (Argon or Dye)
was coupled into the proximal end of an optical fiber 400 μm in
diameter. A mechanical support allowed us to direct and fix the
optical fiber in the direction orthogonal to the treated area.
Fig. 2 shows the map of the 12 fractions of the entire treatment.
Since the average irradiace of laser light were kept constant at
100 mW/cm^2 for each fraction, the energies varied only for Dye laser,
ranging from 120 J/cm^2 to 60 J/cm^2, depending on exposure time.

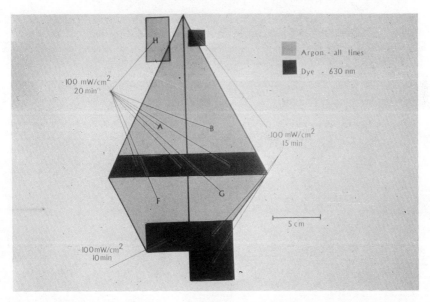

Fig. 2. Schematic drawing of the 12 fractionated areas for photo-
        therapy.

The first treatment was done on the areas A and B with Argon laser
and C-D-E with Dye laser at the same dose (120 J/cm^2). Masks of
white papers were used for covering the surrounding areas during
each fraction of treatment.

RESULTS

The macroscopic appearance of the irradiated area after 2 weeks
showed evident necrosis in the Dye laser treated sites. After 2
months, ulcerations of 5 mm depth were still persistent and painful
(Fig. 3). Multiple biopsy samples 2 months after the first treatment
demonstrated no residual disease in area B, previously treated with
Argon laser and in area C, previously treated with Dye laser. But,
at the left upper border of area A, a persistence of a small pigmented lesion was found and histologically confirmed.

The second treatment was performed on day 61 in 7 fractions.
This time the same irradiance for both laser was used, whereas the
energies for Dye laser were reduced. 90 J/cm^2 were used in areas

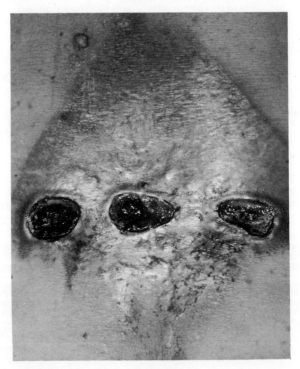

Fig. 3. Clinical aspect of the lesions 2 months after the first
        treatment.

L-M-N, and 60 J/cm^2 in area I, in order to avoid the strong side
effects previously noted. Moreover, for the same reason, Argon laser
irradiation was used on the areas immediately below the Dye-produ-
ced ulcerations. The temperature measurements were done by means
of thermocouples and thermographic maps. It was found a maximum
temperature increase of 7°C at the surface level. The gross appearance of the lesions, after the second treatment did not show deep
ulcerations present in the previously treated sites. Also bullous
edema and pain were minor than that of the first treatment. The
aspect of the dorsal skin 2 months after the second treatment
(Fig. 4) demonstrated the completion of the healing process in all
fractions. In the lower right part of the treated sites, persisten-
ces of small pigmented lesions midway between two Dye-treated sites
horizontally, and at the border between Dye and Argon-treated sites
vertically were histologically demonstrated.

CONCLUSIONS

    Dougherty previously reported the effectiveness of phototherapy
in the treatment of primary skin epitheliomas[5]. First purpose of

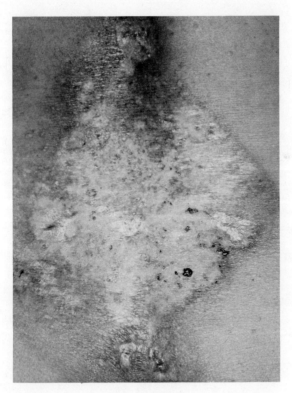

Fig. 4. Final aspect of the lesions, 2 months after the second
        treatment.

this study was to evaluate the effectiveness at different energies of Dye system in phototherapy of basal cell carcinoma of the skin; second, it was useful to compare the two laser systems as regards, to the cure capability and side effects. Based on this pilot study we may conclude that:

1. Residual disease appeared to be related either to the border effects or to the pigmentation of the lesions, rather than the laser system used.
2. The lowest energy used (60 J/cm^2) for Dye laser system resulted in sufficient effectiveness for the cure of the lesions.
3. The side effects (ulcerations) after the highest dose (120 J/cm^2) of Dye laser irradiation for shallow lesions, indicated a light overdose.

Thus, proper energies of Dye and Argon laser resulted in similar effectiveness in phototherapy of the studied surface epitheliomas. Finally, hematoporphyrin-derivative and laser irradiation demonstrated to be an encouraging alternative treatment modality for selected surface lesions, especially when conventional therapeutic methods are poorly indicated or contraindicated.

REFERENCES

1. A.E. Profio, D.R. Doiron, Dosimetry consideration in phototherapy, Med. Phys.8: 190 (1981).
2. T.J. Dougherty, J.E. Kaufman, A. Goldfarb, K.R. Weishaupt, D. Boyle, and A. Mittleman, Photoradiation therapy for the treatment of malignant tumors. Cancer Res.38: 2628, (1978).
3. A. Dahlman, A.G. Wile, R.G. Burns, G.R. Mason, F.M. Johnson, M.W. Berns, Laser photoradiation therapy of cancer. Cancer Res. 43: 430 (1983).
4. D.A. Cortese, G.H. Kinsey, Endoscopic management of lung cancer with hematoporphyrin-derivative phototherapy. Mayo Clin. Proc. 57: 543 (1982).
5. T.J. Dougherty, K.R. Weishaupt, D.G. Boyle, Photosensitizers, in: "Cancer principles & practice of oncology". V. De Vita Jr., S. Hellman, S.A. Rosenberg, eds. Lippincott, Philadelphia, (1982).

HEMATOPORPHYRIN DERIVATIVE PHOTORADIATION THERAPY OF ENDOBRONCHIAL LUNG CANCER

Daniel R. Doiron and Oscar J. Balchum

University of Southern California, School of Medicine, Los Angeles, CA 90033

INTRODUCTION

Hematoporphyrin derivative (HpD) photoradiation therapy (PRT) has been reported as an effective treatment for a variety of tumors (1,2). This technique relys on the tumor localizing and photosensitization potential of HpD to selectively destroy tumors.

When injected, HpD distributes throughout the tissue, but clears preferentially faster from most normal tissue. Waiting 24 to 72 hours post injection in humans has been found best for obtaining preferential HpD distribution in the tumor and therefore a more selective photosensitization response. The principle cytotoxic agent is thought to be singlet oxygen generated by an energy transfer from the excited triplet state of the HpD (3). This highly reactive form of oxygen readily oxidizes biological components. Oxidation of these components leads to disruption of vasculature and tissue structures and cell membrane function, thereby causing cell death. Since the HpD is preferentially retained in and around the tumor tissue the reaction can be very specific to the tumor if the light dosimetry is properly done. Cell death and tissue necrosis may be seen within 24 hours of the light application.

We have applied HpD-PRT to over 60 patients with endobronchial tumors. This report outlines the methods and results in the last 22 patients employing a fairly well standardized protocol based on the experience gained in the earlier trials.

METHODS

HpD

Hematoporphyrin derivative was obtained in a sterile
injectable solution from Oncology Research and Development,
Inc., Cheektowaga, New York. This material is given the trade
name of Photofrin and is provided at a concentration of 5
mg/ml. It is used in humans under T.J. Dougherty's
investigative new drug (IND) permit #12678, with O.J. Balchum
listed as a co-investigator.

Standardized HpD dosage is 3 mg/kg body weight. Delivery
is by a single intravenous injection in a free flowing saline
drip at 72 hours prior to PRT treatment.

Light Application

Wavelength of the light used to activate the HpD was 630
nm $\pm$ 1 nm. It was generated from an continous argon pumped dye
laser containing rhodamine-B (Spectra Physics Model 375 dye
laser and Model 164 argon laser). Delivery of the light to the
tumor was via single step index quartz fibers (Quartz product
QSF-125, QSF-200 and QSF-400) inserted into the biopsy channel
of a flexible bronchoscope (Olympus Model BF-2T or BF-4B2).
Exposure to the tumor was either by surface illumination or by
interstitial implantation of the fiber.

Surface illumination was either by the forward directed
output from the fiber or by use of a scattering matrix applied
to the fiber tip. The forward directed exposure is termed
forward surface (FS). The effective numerical aperature of the
fiber was increased to 0.40 by physically pinching the fiber.
Full illumination of the lesion was obtained by sweeping of the
output over its surface. The scattering matrix was applied to
the core of the fiber to give an isotropic distribution around
the fiber circumference and along its length. This is termed
cylindrical surface (CS) illumination when the fiber is placed
in an open bronchus. Typical cylinder lengths used were 0.5
cm, 1.0 cm and 1.5 cm.

Interstitial illumination was provided by inserting the
optical fiber directly into the tumor. If a flat cut fiber was
used it was termed point insertion (PI) while if a isotropic
cylindrical fiber was used it was termed cylindrical insertion
(CI). If a tumor tissue was too firm to allow direct insertion
of a fiber a 22 guage 1.0 cm long flexible-sheath endoscopic
needle was used with a 125 micron core fiber. This was termed
PIN.

A visual examination through the bronchoscope was made throughout the treatment to assess that adequate delivery and light diffusion was maintained.

Bronchoscopic Procedure

Bronchoscopic procedures were done under topical anesthesia (1% Lidocaine) through a bronchoscopic endotracheal tube attached to a ventilator utilizing 100% oxygen. Prior to each treatment a fluorescence examination of the tumor area was done using an intensified fluorescence endoscope system (4).

Patients were re-bronchoscoped two to four days post PRT to assess response and clean out necrotic tissue and exudate if present. Removal was by endoscopic forceps and suction. Specimens from the clean up bronchoscopy were studied cytopathologically. If further PRT treatment was deemed necessary at this time, patients were given another series of treatments using 3.0 mg/kg at 72 hours prior to red light applications.

Patient Selection and Workup

The 22 patients reported here included 4 women and 18 men ranging from 40 to 71 years of age. Tumor locations included those from the lower trachea to the sub-segmental bronchi. Twelve had squamous carcinoma, one large cell carcinoma, five adenocarcinoma, one carcinoid, one metastatic thyroid cancer, one malignant fibrous histiocytoma and one local fibrous mass (See Table 1).

Patients were evaluated by complete history, particularly for shortness of breath, and for debility in the form of weight loss, weakness, poor apetite and food intake. Chest x-rays in four views and CT scans of the chest were taken and evaluated along with pulmonary function, lung volume and blood gas analysis. Perfusion scans using $^{99}T_c$ and ^{81}Kr were also obtained. Care was takin in evaluating these test results in determining possible risk due to impairment of ventilation that may occur after PRT.

Light Doses

Planned total light dose were 100 ± 20 J/cm^2 for FS or CS, 200 ± 20 J for PI or PIN and 200 ± 20 J/cm for CI. These values were adjusted when multiple treatments in closely

related areas were deemed necessary, when light diffusion in
the tissue was visually poor and when limitations on the length
of the procedure did occur.

RESULTS

     The twenty-two patients were treated as outlined in Table
1.   Twenty were deemed to have a complete response (no
endobronchial tumor).   Nineteen had partial obstructing masses
(40-90%) and one had carcinoma in-situ (CIS).

     Patient No. 18 had a firm mass obstructing 50% of the
right main stem with what appeared to be normal mucosa covering
it.   The histological status of this mass was of questionable
origin after two previous biopsies.   PRT was performed to
assess its ability in removing such an obstruction.   No
fluorescence was visualized in the lesion prior to the
application of the red light and no siginificant response was
obtained.   A post rigid bronchoscopy and large forcep biopsy
showed fibrous tissue and no tumor cells.

     Patient No. 17 had a partial response with a hard tumor
mass remaining which did not permit insertion of the fiber or
needle and exhibited poor light diffusion.   Further treatment
was deemed not possible.   Fifteen of the 21 patients with tumor
required only one treatment while the remaining 7 received two.
The second treatment were given due to either multiply tumor
sites or extention beyond the area of prior treatment that was
previously not accessable.

     All of the tumor masses showed true positive fluorescence.
The carcinoid and thyroid cancer showed low level fluorescence
and poor red light diffusion but did respond to PRT.

Complications

     No deaths or complications occured during the PRT or
clean-up bronchoscopies.   Three patients developed
staphylococcal pneumonia 7 to 10 days after PRT that responded
to antibiotic therapy.   Two patients (No. 7 and 13) had a left
pneunothorax 5 and 1 day post PRT respectively.   These were
thought to be due to coughing and not due to the PRT treatment
directly since both occured distantly from the PRT application
site.   Both patients acheived full lung expansion with the
insertion of chest tubes which were removed at 7 days without
complications.

Table 1. Photoradiation Therapy in Twenty-two Patients with Obstructing Endobronchial Cancer

Patient No., Sex, Age	Location	Histol. Type	Light Applicators Length in cm.	Light Dosages
1. M, 55	MC, RMS, LMS	SC Ca.	CI - 0.5, CI - 0.5	200J/cm, 255 J/cm
2. M, 54	RUL	SC Ca.	CI - 0.5	202 J/cm^2
3. M. 53	RMS (CIS)	SC Ca.	CS - 1	129 J/cm
4. M, 54	MC, RMS	Carcinoid	CI - 0.5, CI - 0.75	200 J/cm
5. F, 41	RMS, BI	Adenoca	CI - 1, Submucosal	202 J/cm, 198 J/cm
6. M, 60	BI, RMS	SC Ca.	CI - 1; PI; Submuc.	200 J/cm; 202 J/cm, 182 J
7. M, 44	LMS	Adeno-large cell	CI - 1	200 J/cm
8. M, 67	RLL-6	Adenoca	CI - 0.5	200 J/cm
9. M, 59	RMS, RUL	SC Ca.	CI - 0.5	200 J/cm
10. M, 49	LMS	SC Ca.	CS - 1; CI - 1	50 J/cm^2, 200 J/cm
11. M, 68	MC, LMS, RMS	SC Ca.	CI - 0.75	264 J/cm
12. M, 57	LMS, MC, RMS, RLL	SC Ca.	CI - 0.5	418 J/cm (Poor Diffusion)
13. M, 68	BI, LUL	SC Ca.	CI - 1.5	225 J/cm
14. F, 53	LMS, MC, Trachea	SC Ca.	CS - 1.5, CS - 1.5, FS; CS - 1.5; CI - 0.5; CS - 1.5, CS - 1.5	55 J/cm^2, 89 J/cm^2, 94 J/cm; 200 J/cm^2, 216 J/cm^2; 60 J/cm^2, 80 J/cm
15. F, 53	LUL, LMS	Adenoca	PI. CI - 0.5; CI - 1; CI - 0.5	55 J, 330 J/cm; 144 J/cm, 144 J/cm
16. M, 71	Lingula, LLL	Adenoca	CI - 0.5; CI - 0.5; CS - 0.5; FS	296 J/cm^2, 270 J/cm^2; 86 J/cm^2, 5] J/cm^2
17. M, 69	LUL	SC Ca.	PI	202 J
18. M, 45	RMS	Benign	PI	243 J
19. M, 52	LMS, MC, BI	SC Ca.	PI; PI; PI	220 J, 210 J, 126 J
20. M, 51	LMS	SC Ca.	CS - 1.0	126 J/cm^2
21. M, 36	LLL	Met. Thyroid Ca.	CS - 1.0	76 J/cm^2
22. F, 64	LUL	Malig. Fibrous Histiocytoma	PI, PI	147 J, 149 J

MC-Main Carina
RMS-Right Main Bronchus
LMS-Left Main Bronchus
BI-Bronchus Intermedius
RUL-Right Upper Lobe Bronchus
RLL-Right Lower Lobe Bronchus
RLL-6 Sup Seg RLL
LUL - Left Upper Lobe
LLL - Left Lower Lobe
SC Ca - Squamous Cell Ca.

Patient Followup

Fifteen of the 22 patients remain alive at the time of
this writing. The longest followup is one year. Of the seven
deceased, 3 died of local extension and/or metastasis of the
tumor. Two of those were at 3 months (No. 14 and 22) and one
at one year (No. 20). Patient No. 13 died of pneumonia having
severe COPD at 3 months after PRT. Patient No. 17 died of
pulmonary and cardiac failure 3 weeks after COPD. He was
receiving radiation therapy at that time. Patient No. 12 was
found dead at 3 - 5 weeks post PRT of unknown causes even after
autopsy. The treated LMS bronchus was still found to be 50%
open. Patient No. 11 took an overdose of sedatives 3 weeks
after discharge.

DISCUSSION

This report outlines the successful palliative treatment
of extensive and large obstructing endobronchial cancers by
photoradiation therapy (PRT), employing the photodynamic action
of HpD activated by red light (630 nm). The purpose of these
clinical trials was to abolish endobronchial tumor, control its
growth and extension, to open up bronchi for ventilation in
order to decrease shortness of breath and to prevent the
retention of secretions and bacteria that may lead to
pneumonia.

Patients were selected whose lung cancer was stable by
chest x-rays, and who were in reasonable physical condition,
ambulatory and carrying on activities of daily living.

The light dosages and techniques of illumination used
(Table 1) resulted in very little bronchial inflammation
(erythema, edema). There was no significant bleeding during
interstitial PRT. Occasionally, a slight amount of blood
accumulated around the insertion site but posed no problem.
Withdrawal of the fiber after PRT showed no coatings of
carbonaceous or other material. Fibers were clean with only
occasionally adherence of a small clot of blood. No
complications of accidents occured such as ignition of fiber
tips nor damage to the bronchoscope in the presence of PRT on
100% oxygen. This was attributed to the technique used. Only
a small amount of light was applied to the fiber before
insertion. After placement, the power was turned up to the
desired level and then turned off completely before fiber
withdrawal.

Treated endobronchial tumor at the time of rebronchoscopy
usually appeared intact, very similar to its appearance before

PRT. However, removal by forceps showed that it was debris.
Removal resulted in no bleeding indicating that it was necrotic
(and by microscopic examination).   Tumor debris was removed
only down to the level of the bronchial mucosa. Bleeding was a
signal of unaffected tumor remaining and need for repeat PRT.

A reaction that did commonly occur in the bronchus
following PRT and observed during clean-up bronchoscopy was the
accumulation of thick mucus. At times, this was loose but at
other times firm, to the point of forming a membrane over the
surface, or even a plug. This response was generally only seen
in patients receiving higher light doses, and occured from
stimulation of bronchial and mucosal mucus glands.

Our criterion for complete response was the visual absence
of endobronchial tumor at the time of clean-up bronchoscopy,
within one week following PRT.   In eight instances,
bronchoscopic washings and biopsies at cleanup were negative
for cancer cells, including the one patient with CIS. In all
instances a bronchial lumen of 6 mm or more was acheived, and
the bronchus was opened up to its full extent.

The techniques of light application varied with the size,
extent and location of the lesions. Cylinder light application
methods (CS, CI) were used for illumination of endobronchial
tumor extending along a considerable length of bronchus, or
having a large volume. Insertion methods (PI, CI) were used
for large tumor masses. FS illumination was used to treat
discrete areas and small tumor sites. The light dosage applied
was selected on the basis of the light diffusion
characteristics of the tumor tissue, and the degree of
anticipated bronchial exudate accumulation.

In the previous 40 patients receiving PRT in our studies,
various dosages of HpD were used (2.5 - 5.0 mg/kg) with only PI
and FS types of illumination. Light dosage were also higer
than for the 22 cases present in this report. Typically, they
were 200 J/cm^2 and 400 J for FS and PI illumination
respectively. Clean-up bronchoscopy within a few days after
PRT was not consistently done in these previous 40 cases. With
the development of more effective light applicators a more
uniform light dose could be easily obtained. As a result, long
lengths of endobronchial tumor could be treated with only one
PRT treatment. In addition, the light dosage was reduced to
decrease bronchial inflammation around the tumor site. This
has led to a decrease in thick mucus, tenacious exudate and
membrane formation.

Light dosage delivery was aimed to achieve about 200 J/cm for CI, 200 J for PI, and 100 J/cm^2 for FS or CS. The amount of light applied to a given tumor mass was determined by estimating the light penetration in the tissue and the extent of the tumor mass. There were no visible heat effects, such as charring and coagulation of the tissue around the fiber or on the tumor surface. Visualization during clean-up bronchoscopy several days after PRT showed minimal redness, inflammation and edema in the surrounding bronchial tissues.

The more distal the obstructing lesion, the safer is PRT in that occlusion of the lumen by loose exudate or firmer membrane in the several days after PRT had little or no noticeable effect in terms of causing breathing difficulty. In the central airways, the trachea and/or main bronchus, this is not the case. Breathing difficulty may become increased within a day or two after PRT, indicating the need for clean-up bronchoscopy. No specific test or method of assessment has been found to give information needed to predict an increase of dyspnea after PRT. Symptoms and chest auscultation were closely and sequentially assessed, as was the pulse rate, to determine whether clean-up bronchoscopy should be done. These patients all had decreased lung function from COPD, previous radiation, lung resection, extent of the lung cancer, and many were elderly.

Radiographic atelectasis was infrequent, and probably was prevented by prompt clean-up bronchoscopy within two or three days. It was repeated when required. The lower light doses in these trials reported here were associated with a significant decrease in mucus, preventing consequent respiratory distress, compared to our experience in the previous 40 patients. This was not a significant problem in these 22 patients, with the exception of No. 12 which occurred after radiation therapy.

We judged from our follow-up contacts that our patients have benefitted from PRT symptomatically. Many who had been working returned to work, and others maintained reasonably good activity and living. Presumably this was assisted by the successful abolishing and local control of endobronchial tumors, opening up of airways, decreased dyspnea, decreased retention of secretions and bacteria, and potentially prevention of pneumonia. The ultimate effect on life span will depend upon the rapidity of endobronchial recurrence, local spread in the lung and mediastinum, and distant metastasis. Longer follow-up with re-bronchoscopies are planned to depict the real value of palliative PRT to patients with obstructing endobronchail cancer.

ACKNOWLEDGMENTS

      The technical assistance of Nick Razum and Leon Chaput, our
laser technicians, are greatly appreciated, as was the assistance
of Joyce Portugal in records and specimen handling. We thank Albert
Castorena for assistance in the preparation of this manuscript.

REFERENCES

1.   T. J. Dougherty, J. B. Kaufman, A. Goldfarb, K. R. Weishaupt,
         D. G. Boyle, and A. Mittleman, Photoradiation therapy for
         the treatment of malignant tumors, Cancer Res. 38:2628 (1978).
2.   D. Kessel and T. J. Dougherty, Advances in Experimental Medicine
         and Biology, in: "Porphyrin Sensitization", D. Kessel and
         T.H. Dougherty, eds., Plenum Press, New York (1983).
3.   K. R. Weishaupt, C. J. Gomer, and T. J. Dougherty, Identifica-
         tion of singlet oxygen as the cytotoxic agent in photo-inac-
         tivation of a murine tumor, Cancer Res. 36:2326 (1976).
4.   A. E. Profio, D. R. Doiron, O. J. Balchum, and G. C. Huth,
         Fluorescence bronchoscopy for localization of carcinoma in
         situ, Med. Phys. 10:35 (1983).

PHOTORADIATION THERAPY IN EARLY STAGE CANCER CASES OF THE LUNG,
ESOPHAGUS AND STOMACH

Yoshihiro Hayata, Harubumi Kato, Chimori Konaka,
Jutaro Ono, Makoto Saito, Hidenobu Takahashi and
Takahisa Tomono
Department of Surgery, Tokyo Medical College
Tokyo, Japan 160

INTRODUCTION

Photoradiation therapy (PRT) was performed in clinical cancer
cases ascertaining the therapeutic effectiveness and safety of
this new modality in experimentally induced canine central type
lung cancer. In the canine experiments, weekly submucosal injections
of the carcinogen 20-methylcholanthrene were made at the bifurcation
of the right apical and cardiac lobe bronchi in beagles and mongrel
dogs[1]. This is one of only a very few successful dog lung cancer
models in the world.

While much work in this method has been performed over the
past few years by several researchers, most notably by Dr. Dougherty[2,3,4,5], its role in the treatment of early stage cancer cases
was not clearly defined. In 1978 Dr. Dougherty's work was introduced to us by Dr. E. Carmack Holmes of U.C.L.A.. Dr. Holmes suggested that our dog lung cancer model could be used to evaluate the
effectiveness of the diagnostic and therapeutic applications of
this method in large animals. The results of a study using our
dog lung cancer model and made feasible by Dr. Dougherty's cooperation in providing not only hematoporphyrin derivative (HpD) but
also much helpful advice established for the first time the applicability of these methods in early stage lung cancer lesions.

Since 1980 we have been performing laser photoradiation therapy
after administration of HpD in the treatment of cancer at Tokyo
Medical College Hospital[6,7,8]. One hundred and eighty cancer cases
of various organs, consisting of 73 cases of lung cancer, 11 cases
of esophageal cancer, 25 cases of gastric cancer, 18 cases of
bladder cancer, skin metastases from 16 cases of breast cancer and

37 others were treated with PRT plus HpD.

This paper describes the therapeutic results of PRT in 31 cases of early stage cancer, consisting of 13 cases of central type lung cancer, 4 cases of esophageal cancer and 14 cases of gastric cancer.

MATERIAL and METHODS

HpD was provided initially by Dr. Dougherty of Roswell Park Memorial Institute, Buffalo, and subsequently by Oncology Research and Development Inc., (Photofrin, Cheektowaga, NY). The lesion was photoradiated via a 400 micron quartz fiber (Quartz Products, Plainfield, NJ) inserted through the instrumentation channel of a fiberoptic endoscope. PRT was performed with the tip of the fiber at a distance of 1-3 cm from the tumor or else inserted intra-tumorally, with a power of 90-600mW for 10-40 minutes (120-240 Joules/cm^2) 48 hours or more after i.v. injection of 2.5-5.0mg/kg body weight HpD.

As a light source we used an argon dye laser system. An argon laser (model 171-08, wavelength 457.9-514.4nm, 15W power, Spectra-Physics) pumped a dye laser (model 375-01, wavelength 630-640nm, Spectra-Physics) using rhodamin B dye to obtain a red light beam of 630nm. In some cases we used a Cooper 770 argon dye laser system that provides a beam of similar wavelength. We used red light as it has the best tissue penetration characteristics. The procedure was performed under local anesthesia. Atropin sulfate (0.5mg) was administrated 15-30 minutes prior to the procedure and in particu-larly nervous cases 35-70mg meperdine or 25-50mg hydroxyzine (Ata-raz-P) was also injected intramuscularly.

Diagnosis of early stage cases was perfformed endoscopically, roentgenologically, cytologically or histologically.

Evaluation of therapeutic effects was divided into 4 grades as follows; complete tumor remission (CR) meaning that no tumor was evident endoscopically, cytologically or histologically, signi-ficant remission (SR) meaning that 60% or more of the original tumor volume disappeared, partial remission (PR) meaning that more than 20% but less than 60% of the original tumor volume disappeared and no remission (NR) meaning that less than 20% of the original tumor volume disappeared.

RESULTS

Table 1 shows the therapeutic results of PRT in early stage cancer cases of the lung, esophagus and stomach. CR was obtained in 58%, SR in 32.2% and PR in 3.2%.

Table 1. Therapeutic results of PRT in early stage
cancer cases

	No. of cases	CR	SR	PR	NR
Lung cancer	13	10	3	0	0
Esophageal cancer	4	2	1	0	1
Gastric cancer	14	7	6	1	0
Total	31	19	10	1	1

Lung cancer:

Eight of the 13 central type lung cancer cases were either inoperable due to poor pulmonary function or they refused surgery. CR was obtained in all and they are disease free from 8-36 months after PRT (Table 2).

These cases are being followed up endoscopically, cytologically and histologically. In 5 cases resected after PRT, CR was obtained in 2 and SR in 3. All 13 cases were squamous cell carcinoma. The reasons for SR were limited penetration of the leaser beam due to the location of the tumor (2 cases) and insufficient power of the argon dye laser beam due to mechanical problems (one case).

Case No. 2 of the non-resected group was a 59-year-old female with negative chest X-ray but positive sputum cytology. A superficially invaded tumor and thickening of the bifurcation of the right upper lobe bronchus was observed endoscopically.
The patient was inoperable due to poor pulmonary function and asthma, therefore PRT was performed 72 hours after intravenous injection of 5.0mg/kg body weight HpD, with a power of 600mW for 40 minutes. This was equivalent to 360Joules/cm^2. The tumor disappeared after PRT and at present she is disease free 25 months after PRT (Fig. 1).

Table 2. Therapeutic results of PRT in non-resected
early stage central type lung cancer cases

Case no.	Age	Sex	Location of tumor	Histologic type	Reason for PRT	Result	Survival	Recurrence
1.	74	M	R. B2b	Sq. ca.	Refused surgery	CR	36 months	–
2.	76	M	L. B10ai	"	Poor pulm. func.	CR	26 "	–
3.	59	F	R. u. lobe br.	"	"	CR	25 "	–
4.	70	M	R. u. lobe br.	"	"	CR	19 "	–
5.	62	M	L. B1+2ab	"	"	CR	14 "	–
6.	70	M	R. u. lobe br.	"	"	CR	12 "	–
7.	62	M	L. B1+2	"	Refused surgery	CR	11 "	–
8.	71	M	L. B3	"	"	CR	8 "	–

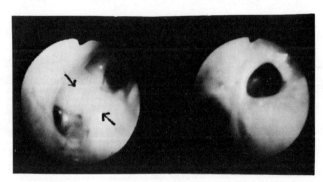

Fig. 1. PRT in case No. 2 of the non-resected group
The tumor in the right upper lobe bronchus (left)
disappeared after PRT (right).

Esophageal cancer:

     Of the 4 cases of early stage esophageal cancer two CR cases
were not resected due to refusal of surgery and recurrence after
reconstruction. They are disease free at 15 and 25 months after
PRT at present. The other two cases were resected after PRT and
the results were SR and NR respectively. The reasons for only
SR and NR were technical failure in the former and an unsuitable
wavelength due to decomposition of rhodamin B dye in the latter.
Case report. A 64-year-old male noted a burning sensation behind
his chest wall in October 1978. In March 1979 superficial cancer
of the esophagus was recognized. In April 1979, total gastrectomy
(due to lymph node metastasis to the gastric angle), total resection
of the esophagus and right hemicolectomy with antethoratic reconstruction were performed. In the resected specimen 2 early stage
lesions were observed. In June 1979 superficial esophageal cancer
was recognized in the residual cervical esophagus. 70 Gy radiotherapy was performed, however, biopsy subsequently showed cancer
cells. Therefore additional course of 74Gy was performed in June.
Biopsy in December of that year was again positive. In February
1981 PRT was performed with a power of 400mW for 15 minutes (420
Jouls/cm^2) after intravenous injection of 2.5mg/kg HpD and after
a further 24 hours PRT was again performed for 20 minutes at the
same power level (244Joules/cm^2). The tumor disappeared after
PRT and no recurrence has been recognized as of 1983 (Fig. 2).

Gastric cancer:

     Of the 14 early stage gastric cancer cases, 3 cases were not
resected due to poor general condition or refusal of surgery and
CR was obtained in all. They are apparently disease free from
16-29 months after PRT. Eleven cases were resected after PRT

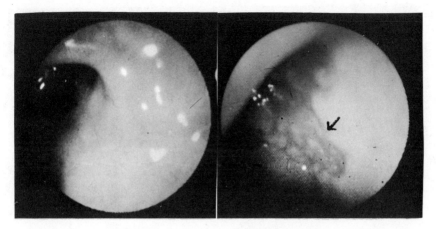

Fig. 2. PRT in early stage esophageal cancer case
A superficial invading tumor can be seen in the cervical
esophagus (left) and the tumor disappeared after PRT (right).

and CR was obtained in 4, SR in 6 and PR in one (Table 3). The
reasons for not obtaining complete remission were due to difficult
photoradiation angles because of the location of the tumor
(3 cases), overlooking of an accessory lesion (one case), technical
failure (one case), submucosal growth (one case) and light obstruction by gastric folds (one case).

Case report: Well differentiated tubular adenocarcinoma was diagnosed in the antrum. Endoscopic findings showed irregular mucosa
and thickened plica accompanied by ulcer formation. Since this
patient, a 54-year-old male, addamantly refused surgery, PRT was
performed three times, 100mW for 30 minutes, 48 hours after intravenous injection of 2.3mg/kg HpD, 300mW for 20 minutes 24 hours
after the first PRT and 200mW for 20 minutes 24 hours after the
second PRT (total 244Joules/cm^2). The tumor disappeared after
PRT, the mucosa become smooth and biopsy failed to reveal tumor
cells. He is apparently disease free 18 months after PRT at present (Fig. 3).

Table 3. Therapeutic results of PRT in 14 early stage
gastric cancer cases

Surgery	No. of cases	CR	SR	PR	NR
Non-resected	3	3	0	0	0
Resected	11	4	6	1	0
Total	14	7	6	1	0

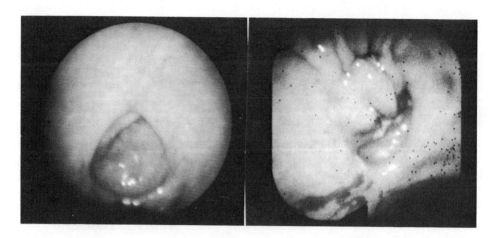

Fig. 3. PRT in early stage gastric cancer case
Superficial tumor can be seen in the antrum (left) and
the tumor disappeared after PRT (right).

DISCUSSION

The principal purpose of PRT in cancer cases is to treat the
lesion curatively. However, this method is not indicated in advanced cancer because there are limitations to the penetration of
the argon dye laser beam and there is also danger of perforation
in canalicular organs with extensive invasion. Therefore, curative
PRT is limited to early stage cancer cases. Since 1980 we have
performed PRT with HpD in over 180 cancer cases of various organs
after ascertaining the therapeutic effectiveness of experimental
PRT in canine central type lung cancer induced in dogs exerimenta-
lly.

Excellent therapeutic results of PRT were obtained in 31 early
stage cases of cancer of the lung, esophagus and stomach especially
in lung cancer. Our clinical experience suggests that the indications of PRT are as follows; prophylactic treatment of precancerous
lesions (although we have no case of gastric mucosal atypia, 3
cases of severely atypical squamous cell metaplasia of the bromchial
epithelium were treated with PRT and the atypia disappeared), and
treatment of inoperable early stage cancer. Further indications
for PRT in advanced cancer include preoperative PRT for reduction
of the extent of resection and widening of the indications of surgery, pretreatment for radiation therapy to decrease the required
focal dose and in combination with chemotherapy. PRT for recurrent
lesions and intratumor PRT in inoperable tumors using multiple
quartz fibers are also promising.

Although excellent therapeutic results were obtained in early stage cancer cases with PRT. The fact that in some cases complete tumor remission was not obtained is a very important problem. The reasons why CR was not obtained in all early stage cancer cases can be considered due to the laser beam not penetrating the entire lesion due to the angle of the beam or location of the tumor, technical failure or obstruction of the laser beam by gastric folds. We have been using a quartz fiber with a divergence angle of 22-53°. In order to obtain complete tumor remission in all early stage cancer cases with PRT improvement of the quartz fiber is necessary. A new fiber which provides a 360° field has been developed by Dr. Dougherty and his colleagues, and this holds considerable province. Also improvement of technique is necessary in organs with conspicuous folds or peristaltic movement such as the esophagus and stomach.

Another important problem in PRT in early stage cancer is how to definitively diagnose the case as early stage. We decide the clinical stage of lung cancer, esophageal cancer and gastric cancer on the basis of endoscopic and roentgenological findings. However, histological examination is also necessary to determine the depth of tumor invasion in the mucosa of the bronchus, esophagus and stomach.

In some non-resected cases with PRT, chemotherapy, radiation therapy or immunotherapy were performed after PRT. Such combined therapeutic approach with PRT should be considered to prevent recurrence or metastasis. On the other hand the optimal doses of HpD and laser beam power have not yet been definitively decided. In our series both doses were decided according to the extent of invasion and location of the tumor and on the basis of experimental experience in animals.
In case No. 2 of the non-resected group, stenosis of the right upper lobe bronchus ocurred after PRT (Fig. 1). This was probably due to the high dose of HpD and high power of argon dye laser. Therefore problems should be also studied.

This series of early stage cancer cases has clearly demonstrated the effectiveness of HpD and PRT in the treatment of certain cases of cancer in a wide variety of organs.

ACKNOWLEDGEMENTS

The authors would like to express their appriciation to Drs. T. J. Dougherty and E.C. Holmes and Mr. J.P. Barron for their co-operation. Supported in part by a Grant-in-Aid for Scientific Research from the Ministry of Education and a Cancer Research Grant from the Ministry of Welfare, Japan.

REFERENCES

1. Y. Hayata, H. Kato, C. Konaka, M. Hayashi, M. Tahara, T. Saito,
    and J. Ono, Fiberoptic bronchoscopic photoradiation in expe-
    rimentally induced canine lung cancer, Cancer 51:50 (1983).
2. T.J. Dougherty, G.B. Grindey, K.R. Weishaupt, and D.G. Boyle,
    Photoradiation therapy II. Cure of animal tumors with Hema-
    toporphyrin and light, J. Natl. Cancer Inst. 55:115 (1975).
3. T.J. Dougherty, J.E. Kaufman, A. Goldfarb, K.R. Weishaupt, D.G.
    Boyle, and A. Mittleman, Photoradiation therapy for the
    treatment of malignant tumors, Cancer Res. 38:2628 (1978).
4. T.J. Dougherty, G. Lawrence, J.E. Kaufman, D.G. Boyle, K.R. Wei-
    shaupt, and A. Goldfarb, Photoradiation in the treatment of
    recurrent breast carcinoma, J. Natl. Cancer Inst., 62:231
    (1979).
5. T.J. Dougherty, R.E. Thoma, D.G. Boyle, and K.R. Weishaupt,
    Photoradiation therapy for treatment of tumors in pet and
    dogs, Cancer Res. 41:401 (1981).
6. Y. Hayata, H. Kato, C. Konaka, J. Ono and N. Takizawa, Hemato-
    porphyrin Derivative and laser photoradiation in the treat-
    ment of lung cancer, Chest. 81:269 (1981).
7. Y. Hayata, H. Kato, C. Konaka, J. Ono, Y. Matsushima, T. Yone-
    yama, and K. Nishimiya, Fiberoptic bronchoscopic laser pho-
    toradiation for tumor localization in lung cancer, Chest.
    81:10 (1982).
8. Y. Hayata, H. Kato, C. Konaka, M. Aida, J. Ono, and K. Nishimi-
    ya, Hematoporphyrin Derivative and photoradiation for tumor
    localization and treatment of lung cancer, in: "Lung Cancer
    1982", S. Ishikawa et al., ed., Excerpta Medica, Amsterdam-
    -Oxford-Princeton (1982).

EXPERIMENTAL AND CLINICAL STUDIES ON HPD-PHOTORADIATION THERAPY

FOR UPPER GASTROINTESTINAL CANCER

Shigeru Okuda, Seishiro Mimura, Toru Otani,
Makoto Ichii and Masaharu Tatsuta
Department of Gastroenterology, The Center for Adult
Diseases, Osaka
3-3, Nakamichi 1-chome, Higashinari-ku, Osaka 537,
Japan

INTRODUCTION

There have been reports of the use of photosensitizing agents and conventional light source in experimental tumor destruction. In 1972, Diamonds et al. showed that hematoporphyrin was effective as a photosensitizing dye in treatment of animal tumor in vivo. In 1974, Tomson reported the use of acridine orange and aron laser in treatment of mouse epithelial tumors. Recently, Dougherty and Hayata reported success in the clinical treatment of human tumors by using hematoporphyrin derivative and dye laser. In the present paper, we first investigated the phototoxic effect of acridine orange (AO) and hematoporphyrin derivative (HPD) on implanted rat stomach tumor and then reported the clinical results of HPD-photoradiation therapy of the upper gastrointestinal cancers.

METHODS

Experimental studies: Tumor cells from Walker 256 carcinosarcoma tumors were implanted into the gastric mucosa of Wistar strain rats as described by Brøyn. Between 5 to 10 days after tumor implantation, gastric tumors had become tumors of 4-6 mm in diameter. Then tumor-bearing rats were devided into 6 groups and treated as follows: Group 1 was injected i.p. with 40 mg per kg of AO 2 hr. before laser irradiation as described by Tomson. The abdomen was opened and the forestomach was opend along the greater curvature. Then the gastric tumors were exposed to argon laser at 488 nm at an intensity of 15 mW per sq cm. After irradiation, the stomach and then the abdomen was closed. Group 2 was injected i.p. with AO in the same way as Group 1, but without irradiation with argon laser. Group 3 was treated with argon laser, but with-

out pretreatment with AO. Group 4 was injected i.v. with 5 mg per
kg of HPD 24 hr. before laser irradiation. The gastric tumors
were exposed to dye laser at 630 nm at an intensity of 15 mW per
sq cm. Group 5 was injected i.v. with HPD in the same way as
described as Group 4, but without irradiation with dye laser.
Group 6 was treated with dye laser, but without pretreatment with
HPD. Rats were killed 5, 10, and 20 min. after laser irradiation
and on experimental day 7, and the gastric tumors and adjacent
gastric mucosa were examined to determine the response of stomach
tumors and adjacent mucosa by phase-contrast, and electron microscopy, and histological examination. The surface temperatures of
the gastric tumor and adjacent gastric mucosa were measured with
thermister thermometer.

The effect of a singlet oxygen-trapping agent, 1,3-diphenyli-
sobenzofuran, on the phototoxic effects of AO and HPD was examined.
Tumor-bearing rats were given AO or HPD as described in Groups 1
or 4. One hour before irradiation, 1 ml of 5 X 10^{-4} M diphenylisobenzofuran was injected i.p., and then gastric tumors were treated
with laser irradiation.

Clinical studies: Two patients with early esophageal cancer, 5
patients with early gastric cancer and one patient with advanced
gastric cancer with poor risk were given 3 mg per kg body weight
of HPD intravenously by the method of Dougherty and Hayata. Two
or three days later, a gastrofiberscope was inserted and the
lesion was irradiated with a dye laser beam of 300 mW power at
the fiber tip. As a light source, a continuous tunable dye laser,
model 375, from Spectra Physics, Inc. with rhodamine 6G dye to
obtain a spectral output centered at 630 nm. A 500 μm quartz
fiber was inserted through the forceps channel of a gastrofiberscope to transmit the laser beam to the stomach or esophagus.
After insertion of the gastrofiberscope, the tip of the quartz
fiber was placed about 3.5 cm from the lesion, giving a light spot
of 1 cm^2. When the lesion was more than 1 cm^2, the fiber was
moved so that the light covered the entire lesions. Irradiation
at 300 mW at the fiber tip for 5 minutes gave 90 joules per cm^2
at the lesion.

RESULTS

Experimental studies: Measurement of the surface temperature of
the gastric tumors and adjacent gastric mucosa showed that the
temperature did not increase more than $3^{\circ}C$ during irradiation with
laser.

By phase-contrast microscopy, the first signs of degeneration
of the tumor treated with AO were seen as early as 5 min. after
irradiation. As shown in Fig. 1, 20 min after the beginning of
irradiation the nucleus had become markedly pyknotic and the
nuclear menbranes thicker and irregular; dense chromatin aggregates were seen in the nucleus. Electron microscopy (Fig. 2)

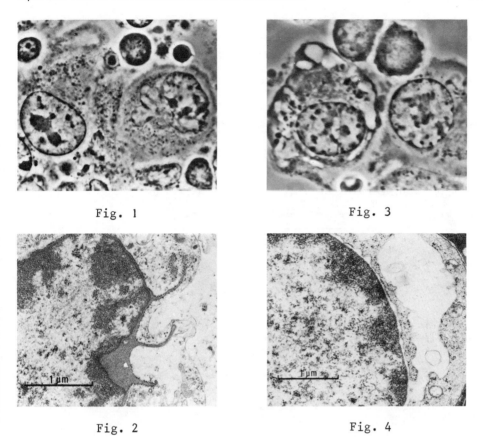

Fig. 1

Fig. 3

Fig. 2

Fig. 4

Table 1. Response of Gastric Tumors to Photoradiation Therapy

Group No. & Treatment	Response of gastric tumors			Total
	CR	PR	NR	
1. AO+Argon laser	8	7	0	15
2. AO alone	0	0	6	6
3. Argon laser alone	0	0	8	8
4. HPD+Dye laser	10	5	0	15
5. HPD alone	0	0	5	5
6. Dye laser alone	0	0	5	5

Table 2 . Effect of 1,3-Diphenylisobenzofuran on Phototoxic Effects of AO and HpD

Treatment	Incidence of degenerative tumor cells
AO+Argon laser	80.0%
AO+Furan+Argon laser	45.6%
HPD+Dye laser	60.0%
HPD+Furan+Dye laser	40.2%

Table 3 . Digestive Cancer Cases Treated with HpD-Photoradiation Therapy

No.	Patient	Gross Type (Location)	Depth of Invasion	Histology of Biopsy	Size of Lesion	Irradiated Area	Output (Time)	Dose* (Joule/cm²)	Response (Follow up)
Esophagus									
1	Y.S. 76 ♂	I + IIc (Im)	m	Squamous cell ca.	3 cm²	8 cm²	400 mW (68 min.)	204	CR (1Y2M)
2	K.F. 79 ♂	IIc (Im~EI)	sm	Squamous cell ca.	14 cm²	30 cm²	300 mW (75 min.)	45	PR (1Y2M)
Stomach									
3	K.M. 78 ♂	IIc+III (Angle~Antrum)	sm	well diff. adeno-ca.	10 cm²	15 cm²	300 mW (60 min.)	72	CR (6M)
4	S.Y. 74 ♂	IIc conv.(−) (Angele)	m	mod. diff. adeno-ca.	1 cm²	3 cm²	300 mW (15 min.)	90	CR (5M)
5	S.K. 85 ♂	IIa+IIb (Corpus)	sm	well diff. adeno-ca.	32 cm²	30 cm²	300 mW (90 min.)	54	PR (5M)
6	I.O. 57 ♂	IIc conv.(−) (Antrum)	sm	Signet.	2 cm²	4 cm²	260 mW (30 min.)	117	CR (3M)
7	K.K. 79 ♂	Bor. 1 (Angle)	pm	well diff. adeno-ca.	25 cm²	27 cm² / 25 cm²	200 mW (90 min.) / 200 mW (109 min.)	40 / 52	MR (3M)
8	S.T. 76 ♂	IIa (Antrum)	m	well diff. adeno-ca.	0.5 cm²	1 cm²	100 mW (10 min.)	60	CR (2M)

* Dose=Joule/cm² ÷ mW × min. × 60 × 10⁻³/cm²

CENTER FOR ADULT DISEASES
Osaka, 1983. 2.

showed that at this time the two layers of nuclear envelope were
separated by irregular shaped gaps and that the karyoplasm had
been released into the nuclear envelope, sometimes forming
expanded cavities with a dense matrix. On the contrary, in rats
treated with HPD and then dye laser, the first signs of degeneration of the tumor cells were seen after 10 min after irradiation by phase-contrast microscopy. Laser irradiation produced
progressively more damage of the tumor cells, but the degenerative
changes were seen more remarkably in the cytoplasm than in the
nucleus. As shown in Fig. 3, 30 min after the beginning of irradiation, many vacuoles of various size were seen near the nucleus.
Electron microscopy (Fig. 4) showed that at this time the outer
layer of the nuclear envelope remarkable expanded into the cytoplasm, forming large vacuous cavities. Treatment with AO or HPD
without irradiation or laser irradiation without AO or HPD treatment had little or no influence on tumor cells.

The histological changes of gastric tumors 7 days after AO or
HPD treatment and/or laser irradiation are summarized in Table 1.
Tumor irradiation with argon or dye laser caused extensive
necrosis of all tumors in Groups 1 and 4 treated with AO or HPD.
Eight of 15 rats in Group 1 and 10 of 15 rats in Group 4 had no
microscopically detectable tumor cells, but normal adjacent
gastric mucosa.

The effects of 1,3-diphenylisobenzofuran on the phototoxic
effect of AO and HPD are summarized in Table 2. Degenerations of
tumors treated with AO or HPD were protected by this treatment.
This indicates that singlet oxyngen is the cytotoxic agent in both
experimental system.

Clinical studies: Table 3 summarizes results of 8 treatments of
esophageal and gastric cancer with poor risk. All the lesions
treated were responded to photoradiation therapy. Five responses
were complete, 2 were partial and one was slight in follow-ups
for 2 to 14 months. Case No. 1, with squamous cell carcinoma of
the esophagus, has survived 14 months without recurrence, and so
can be considered to have been cured. This treatment had no side
effect.

Figure 5 shows in a patient with superficial wide esophageal
cancer treated with HPD and then dye laser irradiation. Figure
5A and B show the endoscopic appearance of the esophageal cancer
before irradiation. A wide superficial cancer with a small flat
elevated lesion was seen. Figure 5C shows extensive necrosis of
the tumor. Figure 5D taken one month later shows complete epithe-
lization of the necrotic area. No recurrence was seen 14 months
after photoradiation therapy. Figure 6 shows X-ray findings of
the same patient before and after HPD-photoradiation therapy. In
Figure 6A, a wide superficial cancer with an elevated lesion was
seen in the middle portion of the esophagus. Figure 6B and 6C
are X-ray findings 6 weeks and 12 weeks after HPD-photoradiation
therapy, showing no abnormally in the esophagus.

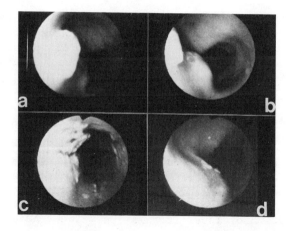

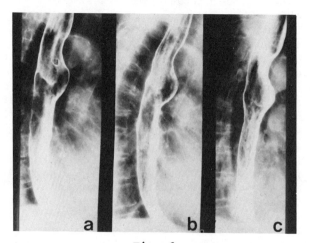

Fig. 6

Stage of cancer	CR	PR	MR	Total
Early cancer	○○○ ○●	○●		7
Advanced cancer			○	1
Total	5	2	1	8

CR: Complete response, PR: Partial response
MR: Minor response, ○: Gastric cancer, ●: Esophageal cancer

Fig. 7. Tumor responses to HpD-photoradiation
        therapy in relation to the stage of
        the lesion.

Figure 7 summarizes the tumor responses to HPD-photoradiation therapy in relation to the stage of esophageal and gastric cancers. The response was complete in 5 of 7 early cancers of the stomach or esophagus. After photoradiation therapy, multiple biopsy specimens from the lesions revealed no tumor cells histologically and cytologically. In contrast, only a slight response was obtained in a patient with an advanced elevated gastric cancer.

Figure 8 summarizes the tumor responses to HPD-photoradiation therapy in relation to the dose of irradiation. Complete responses were obtained in patients with early gastric and esophageal cancer when the dose of laser irradiation was more than 60 joules/cm^2, while no complete response was obtained in any patients with early cancer when the dose was less than 60 joules/cm^2.

Figure 9 shows results in a patient with a minute early gastric cancer treated with HPD and then dye laser irradiation. Figure 9A shows a minute depression on the lesser curvature of the angulus. Figure 9B shows the endoscopic appearance immediately after dye laser irradiation. The swelling and discoloration of the lesion and its surrounding gastric mucosa were seen. Figure 9C taken 7 days after irradiation shows a wide extensive necrosis of the lesion and of normal gastric mucosa. But, in Figure 9D taken 70 days after irradiation, ulcer appears completely healed with converging folds. In this patient, the wide extensive necrosis of the normal surrounding mucosa corresponded well with the discolored area immediately after laser irradiation.

DISCUSSION

Dougherty et al. identified singlet oxygen, a metastable state of normal oxygen, as a cytotoxic agent that was probably responsible for inactivation of carcinoma cells after incorporation of HPD and exposure to red light. In the present work, we obtained the same results. Moreover, we showed that singlet oxygen was the agent responsible for toxicity in the phototoxic system using AO and argon laser. Electron and phase-contrast microscopy showed that cytotoxicity was mediated by the nuclear and cell membrane, and intracytoplasmic organellae. But the phototoxic process of AO and HPD seemed to act at different site in the cell due to the different distribution of the sensitizing agent in the cells.

Phototoxic system using HPD and dye laser is useful for treating early esophageal and gastric cancer. Complete responses were obtained in patients with early gastric and esophageal cancer when the dose of dye laser irradiation was more than 60 jouels/cm^2. However, extensive necrosis of the normal gastric mucosa was seen all patients by our method. This suggested that besides a phototoxic effect of HPD there may be a heat effect in our system.

CONCLUSION

Phototoxic system using HPD and dye laser is useful for

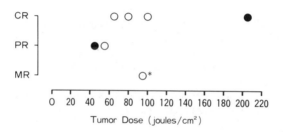

CR: Complete response, PR: Partial response, MR: Minor response,
○: Gastric cancer, ∗: Advanced cancer, ●: Esophageal cancer

Fig. 8. Cancer responses to HpD-photoradiation therapy in relation
to tumor or dose of laser irradiation.

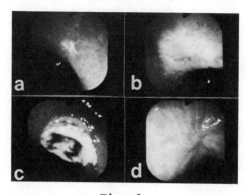

Fig. 9

treating gastrointestinal cancer, and this cytotoxicity is mediated
chiefly by changes in the nuclear membrane and intracytoplasmic
organellae.

This work was supported in part by a Grand-in-Aid for Cancer Research (56-5) from the Ministry of Health and Welfare.

REFERENCES

1.   T. J. Dougherty, J. E. Kaufman, A. Goldfarb, K. R. Weishaupt,
D. G. Boyle, and A. Mittleman, Photoradiation therapy for

the treatment of malignant tumors, Cancer Res. 28:2628 (1978).

2. Y. Hayata, H. Kato, C. Komaka, J. Ono, and N. Takizawa, Hematoporphyrin Derivative and laser photoradiation in the treatment of lung cancer, Chest 81:269 (1982).

3. S. Okuda, T. Otani, S. Mimura, M. Tatsuda, M. Ichii, H. Mishima,
   and S. Ishiguro, Application of dye laser to gastroendoscopy,
   in: "Laser Tokyo '81", K. Atsumi and N. Nimsakul, eds., Inter
   Group Corp., Tokyo (1981).

4. M. Tatsuta, M. Yamamura, R. Yamamoto, M. Ichii, H. Mishima, T.
   Hattori, and S. Okuda, Photodestruction of rat gastric tumors
   after acridine orange and argon laser, in: "Laser Tyokyo '81",
   K. Atsumi and N. Mimsakul, eds., Inter Group Corp., Tokyo
   (1981).

ENDOSCOPIC HpD—LASER PHOTORADIATION THERAPY (PRT) OF CANCER

P. Spinelli, S. Andreola, R. Marchesini, E. Melloni,
V. Mirabile, P. Pizzetti, and F. Zunino

Istituto Nazionale Tumori, Milano, Italy

INTRODUCTION

Efforts are being made all over the world to improve the survival rate and the quality of life of cancer patients. These are
the main reasons why new methods of treatment are developed and
find their place in the management of the disease. It has been demonstrated for many years that malignant tissue as well as embryonic
and traumatized tissues possess selective affinity for porphyrins [1,2]
and particularly for an acetic-acid-sulfuric-acid derivative of
Hematoporphyrin (HpD) [3]. At the same time, endoscopic application
possibilities have been identified [4]. More recently, after a large
experimental study, Dougherty et al. [5] reported to succeed in the
treatment of malignant tumors in humans, and Cortese and Kinsey [6]
and Hayata et al. [7] reported clinical endoscopic applications.

The purpose of our work is to test the HpD—laser system in its
various possible applications.

MATERIALS AND METHODS

HpD was supplied by Dr. T. J. Dougherty of Roswell Park Memorial
Institute, Buffalo, N.Y., USA, and after, as "Photofrin", from Oncology Research and Development Inc., Cheektowaga, N.Y., USA. The
drug was kept away from light, at a temperature of 4°C.

The laser light source was a Rhodamine B dye laser (Spectra
Physics, model 375) pumped by an argon laser (Spectra Physics, model 171): the dye laser produces a red radiation of 630 nm wavelength.
Red light is focused at one end of a 400 micron quartz fiber light
guide. The fiber can be passed through the channel of a rigid or
a fiberoptic endoscope.

Patients are selected as follows: 1) primary advanced carcinomas obstructing respiratory (trachea, main or lobar bronchus) or digestive (esophagus, stomach, large intestine) tract; 2) recurrent carcinomas after traditional therapeutic possibilities have been exploited; same locations; 3) early carcinomas in high-risk patients; same locations.

Steps of treatment are: intravenous administration of HpD (Photofrin) 3 mg x kg body weight (patients are then kept away from sunlight for at least 3 weeks); 48 hours after the injection, irradiation with Rhodamine B dye laser (wavelength 630 nm) is delivered to the lesion for 10 to 30 min.; the power ranges between 250 mW and 600 mW, with an irradiance of 200-270 mW/cm^2.

RESULTS

The results are presented in Table 1. In case of partial response the results are given in terms of percentage of tumor mass destruction. We treated 3 rectal carcinomas of the circumferential stenosing type; case 1 was a recurrence after surgery and radio-

Table 1.   Results of Endoscopic HpD-Laser Treatment.

Case	Age	Sex	T.S.[*]	Site	Spread	F-u[**]	Results
1	33	F	1	Rectum (recur)	adv.M+	2	60%
2	73	M	2	Sigm.-rect junct.	adv.M+	13	40%
3	51	M	5	Right main bronchus	adv.N.	5	50%
4	53	M	2	Left upper bronchus	early?	8	CR
5	67	M	2	Stomach antrum	early?	9	CR
6	75	M	2	Rectum	adv.M+	6	70%

[*]T.S. Treatment sessions

[**]Follow-up in months.

therapy; case 2 and 6 were poor-risk patients with intermittent intestinal obstruction; case 1 died 2 months after photoradiation therapy (PRT) for cancer cachexia, cases 2 and 6 are still alive with no symptomus of obstruction. Case 3 had a right main bronchus carcinoma that covered the main carina and grew into the trachea, causing obstructive respiratory symptoms: after PRT it was reduced to the right system up to disclosure of the right main bronchus. Case 4 was a small carcinoma (1.4 cm) of the left upper brochus supposed to be "early", in a patient operated for light inferior bilobectomy; complete remission (CR) has been obtained in this case. Case 5, a patients with stomach antral carcinoma supposed to be "early" and measuring 6 cm in diameter, had a CR and is disease free, like to former, at the last control.

The therapeutic effect was evaluated on both endoscopic and radiologic basis.

DISCUSSION

This report confirms previous results and gives preliminary information on the possibility of treating large stenosing intestinal tumors: in these cases, PRT treatment allows maintence of a sufficient intestinal passage, thus avoiding surgical palliation. The treatment can be repeated two or more times by reinjection of HpD and reexposure to laser light.

In cases of "early cancer", in the respiratory as well as in the digestive tract, CR has been obtained. It appears to be related to light penetration in the tumor framework, which in cases of "early cancer" is generally not very thick and can be completely destroyed. In cases of advanced intra- and extra-cavitary tumors, the double (endoscopic and radiologic) evaluation has allowed a more definite estimate of the eventual modifications in the tumor mass.

In our experience, PRT has produced a constant response of tumor necrosis, with the only complication of hemorrhage, of the oozing type in rectal cancers and of spurting type in gastric cancer. Hemorrhage required blood transfusions (4 fresh blood units) in the gastric tumor case, but was not clinically important in rectal cancers. No complications were observed in bronchial carcinoma treatments. No damage to the normal tissues surrounding the tumor was detected by common histologic methods, which confirms the extreme selectivity of the necrotizing action of PRT in cancer tissue.

The authors thank the Istituto Ricerche Onde Elettromagnetiche for supplying the special fiberoptics.

REFERENCES

1. F. H. J. Figge, G. S. Weiland, and L. O. J. Manganiello, Cancer
    detection and therapy. Affinity of neoplastic embryonic and
    traumatized regenerating tissues for porphyrins and metallo-
    porphyrins, Proc. Soc. Exptl. Biol. Med. 68:640 (1948).
2. F. H. J. Figge, and G. S. Weiland, Studies on cancer detection
    and therapy: the affinity of neoplastic embryonic and trau-
    matized tissue for porphyrins and metalloporphyrins, Cancer
    Res. 9:549 (1949).
3. R. L. Lipson, F. J. Baldes, and A. M. Olsen, The use of a deriv-
    ative of Hematoporphyrin in tumor detection, J. Natl. Cancer
    Inst. 26:1 (1961).
4. R. L. Lipson, E. J. Baldes, and A. M. Olsen, Hematoporphyrin
    Derivative: A new aid to endoscopic detection of malignant
    disease, J. Thorac. Cardiovasc. Surg. 42:623 (1961).
5. T. J. Dougherty, J. E. Kaufman, A. Goldfarb, K. R. Weishaupt,
    D. G. Boyle, and A. Mittleman, Photoradiation therapy for
    the treatment of malignant tumors, Cancer Res. 38:2628 (1978).
6. D. A. Cortese, and J. H. Kinsey, Endoscopic management of lung
    cancer with Hematoporphyrin Derivative phototherapy, Mayo
    Clinic Proc. 57:543 (1982).
7. Y. Hayata, H. Kato, C. Konaka, J. Ono, and N. Takizawa, Hemato-
    porphyrin Derivative and laser photoradiation in the treat-
    ment of lung cancer, Chest. 81:269 (1982).

DYE-LASER-PHOTORADIATION-THERAPY OF BLADDER CANCER AFTER PHOTO-SENSITIZATION WITH HEMATOPORPHYRIN DERIVATIVE (HpD)-BASIS FOR AN INTEGRAL IRRADIATION

D. Jocham, G. Staehler, E. Unsöld*, Ch. Chaussy, and
U. Löhrs
Urologische Klinik und Poliklinik, Pathologisches
Institut, Ludwig-Maximilians-Universität,
D-8000 München, W. Germany

* Gesellschaft für Strahlen- und Umweltforschung mbH
Abteilung für Angewandte Optik, Zentrales Laser-Labor
D-8042 Neuherberg, W. Germany

Bladder carcinoma is the second most common type of tumor within the urinary tract. Single bladder tumors can be treated and successfully destroyed by conventional methods such as transurethral electroresection of tumor or laser induced heat coagulation using, for example, a neodym.-YAG laser beam. However, for at least 60% of all bladder carcinomas we are confronted with a multifocal growing tumor. In addition to the major tumor areas, which can be recognized easily macroscopically, the bladder very often contains widely distributed carcinoma in situ. It is not possible to treat these minute tumor foci sufficiently by means of conventional methods, including topical cytostatics treatment.

Frequently a tumor cell positive urinary cytology shows that despite the lack of visible tumor, and even after removing all macroscopically recognisible tumor foci, carcinomas still exist in the bladder. Such foci are at least in part responsible for the high rate of tumor recurrence of up to 80% during the first 24 months after surgical treatment. At present it is often not possible to spare the patient the ultimate treatment of cystectomy in order to halt the course of the disease.

The development of flexible light fibers has opened up the possibility of PRT by means of endoscopy. Since 1979 our own efforts have been aimed at developing a method for the photoradiotherapy (PRT) of HpD-photosensitized bladder tumors.

427

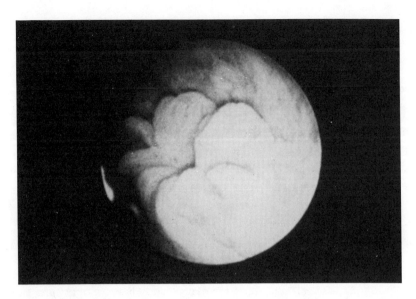

Fig. 1.   Endoscopic view of a Brown-Pearce-carcinoma transplanted
          transurethrally to the urinary bladder of a rabbit
          4 days earlier.

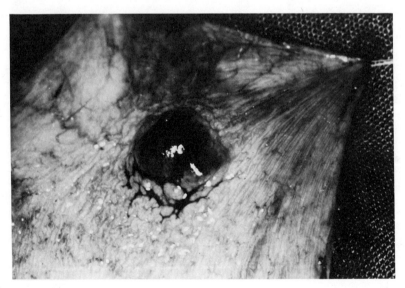

Fig. 2.   Transplanted Brown-Pearce-tumor in the opened urinary
          bladder (rabbit) .

Kelly and coworkers reported as early as 1976, that HpD was selectively stored by human bladder carcinoma. More recent investigations, for example those of Benson and coworkers, have both confirmed these results and shown that carcinoma in situ also stores HpD selectively.

These results suggest theoretically that by means of PRT one may destroy selectively not only the macroscopic major tumor areas, but also the very minute areas which are distributed in a diffuse manner, and in addition, the invisible carcinoma in situ.

This paper describes the step by step development of a new method for homogeneous integral irradiation of hollow organs such as the urinary bladder.

For the photosensitization we initially used HpD, which we prepared ourselves according to the method of Lipson. Later we switched to photofrin I^R. A dye laser pumped by an argon laser, was used as a light source in all investigations. The maximum output power of the red laser light (630 $\pm$ 10 nm) at the end of the flexible fiber was 3,5 W. Originally the fiber was introduced into the bladder through a cystoscope and the light was directed onto the transplanted tumor. The first experiments were carried out using Brown-Pearce-transplant-tumors. The tumor transplantation was carried out using an endoscopically controlled injection by means of which the tumor cell suspension was directed into the bladder wall of rabbits.

Within 4 days, rabbits showed pea-sized tumors endoscopical-ly (Fig. 1). A convincing therapeutic effect was seen for all 25 photosensitized transplanted tumors after irradiation with 200 to 400 J/cm^2. However in all but 4 cases some remaining acti-ve tumor material was found.

Laser irradiation of tumors in open bladders (Fig. 2) did not enhance the effect of the therapy significantly even when we tried scanning the bladder wall.

Fig. 3 shows a large bladder tumor mass on the left after dye laser treatment without HpD-photosensitization in comparison with an almost totally destroyed tumor after photosensitization and PRT shown on the right.

We have to assume that besides insufficient photosensitiza-tion of individual transplant tumors, not all tumor areas were sufficiently exposed to the laser irradiation when using the con-ditions described above.

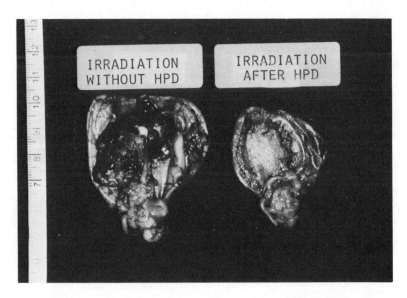

Fig. 3. Therapeutic effect of laser-irradiation:
        left: large tumor mass after treatment without HpD
        right: almost totally destroyed tumor after irradiation
               following HpD-photosensitization.

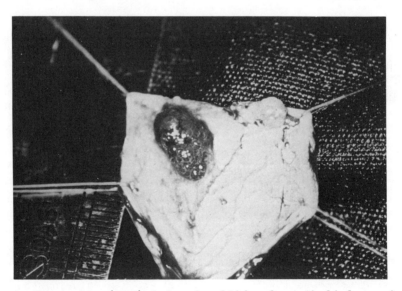

Fig. 4. Chemically (BBN) induced multifocal urothelial carcinoma
        in rat-bladder.

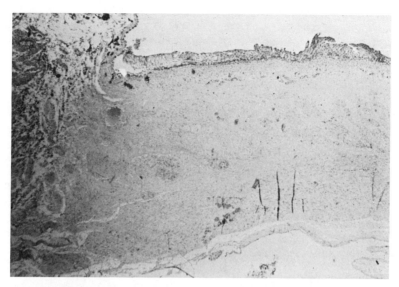

Fig. 5. Circumscribed heat-coagulation of the full depth of the
bladder wall after Neodym-YAG laser treatment.

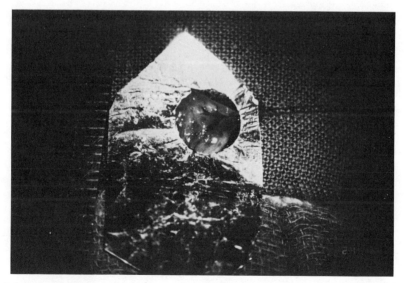

Fig. 6. Rat bladder covered in part by a mask to give an internal
standard.

Similar results were obtained for direct, and line by line, irradiation of urothelial bladder tumors in rats which were chemically induced using BBN, a nitrosamine (Fig. 4). Despite photosensitization with 10 mg HpD/kg BW, and despite an irradiation dosis of up to 400 J/cm^2, 35% of all photosensitized tumor-bearing rats showed some unaffected remainders of tumors. On the other hand tumor bladders which had <u>not</u> been photosensitized were completely unaffected by the laser irradiation.

In summary these experimental data suggested that satisfactory therapeutic results could not be expected in the case of multifocal human bladder using the technique as described above, even when applying the technically rather difficult method of line by line irradiation of all wall areas. On the other hand there is little justification for using PRT, with the related side effects of transient photosensitization for treatment of single tumors as long as there are other efficient methods of treatment. Tumors which can be recognized macroscopically can be destroyed safely by means of conventional methods as described in the introduction (Fig. 5).

Because of the unsatisfactory results using directed or line by line PRT we decided to test the effect of diffusely scattered laser light in a series of experiments using opened rat bladder. A clearly defined area of the rat bladder was covered by a mask and thus excluded from the irradiation (Fig. 6). In this way every experiment on a particular bladder was self calibrated. The first experiments in this series were performed on normal tumor free rat bladders.

Fig. 7 shows the effect of PRT following laser irradiation of mucosa membrane inside the normal bladder 6 hours after supplying 10 mg HpD/kg BW intravenously. There is clear evidence of significant necrosis of the normal bladder mucosa within the irradiated area. On the other hand if the low energy laser irradiation is performed more than 24 hours after supplying HpD, no damage of the normal bladder mucosa is observed (Fig. 8). At this time no differences were observed between rat bladder mucosa irradiated with the dye laser, rat bladder mucosa photosensitized and subsequently irradiated, and normal rat bladder.
However, when the photoradiotherapy was carried out on tumor affected bladders 24 or even 60 hours after supplying HpD intravenously, the diffuse irradiation resulted in complete destruction of the tumors. Fig. 9 shows the total necrosis of a tumor. Complete destruction of the tumors was achieved in 13 out of 14 cases using an irradiation dosis of 60 J/cm^2 over a time period of 20 minutes. Tumor areas which were not exposed to light remained unaffected after receiving HpD (Fig. 10).

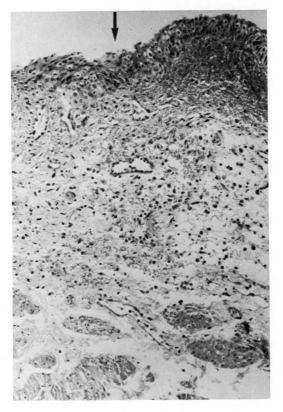

Fig. 7.   Irradiation of normal bladder wall: 6 hours after i.v.
          HpD-injection,
          left: partial necrosis of the urothelium
          right: intact mucosa in the masked area.

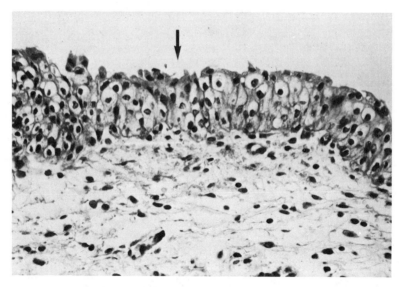

Fig. 8. Irradiation of normal bladder wall: 24 hours after i.v. HpD-injection no damage seen in laser exposed area (to the left of the arrow).

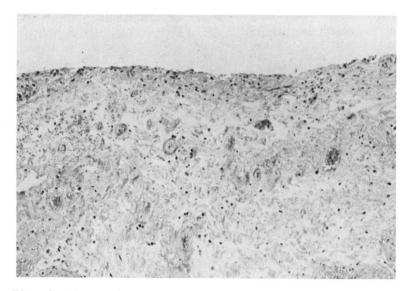

Fig. 9. Laser irradiation of tumor bearing rat bladder. 24 to 60 hours after i.v. HpD-injection causes total necrosis of the tumorous material.

These results – when compared with the results of the earlier experiments – show clearly that the requirement for successful therapy is a homogeneous irradiation of the tumor area. By
carefully selecting the time after HpD application for irradiation, the PRT therapy can have an effect sufficient for complete
destruction of tumor whilst at the same time sparing the normal
bladder areas. This is an essential prerequisite to the clinical
application of integral irradiation of the total bladder wall.

Initially we considered achieving homogeneous irradiation
by means of a rotating light fiber, along the same lines as the
clinically routinely used rotating transurethral ultrasonic
probe. This method however is rather extravagant. Furthermore
it is known to be difficult to achieve sufficient irradiation
of the bladder front wall and bladder neck.

We then proceeded to look for other methods for homogeneously scattering the red light of the dye laser by modifying the
fiber end to a bulb shape inside the bladder. A considerable expansion of the light zone was achieved. However, this procedure
still gave insufficient retrograde illumination. We therefore
explored a third possibility in which we scattered the beam
using a clinically harmless light scattering medium. In order
to keep this method as simple as possible, it was necessary to
find a medium which would have no harmful side effects if it came
into contact with the mucosa or accidentally entered the vascular
system. Such a medium could be used for irrigation of the bladder. Tests of light scattering were performed using different
glass models. The light dosage was measured by a photocell which
was moved mechanically around the sphere.

Fig. 11 shows the relative distribution of irradiation at
different positions on the glass sphere. The upper curve shows
the scattering properties of laser light entering a physiological
saline solution through a flat cut fiber. The laser beam has been
only moderately expanded. The lower curve shows the scattering
properties of a special fat emulsion which is suitable for clinical use. An almost completely homogeneous light distribution can
be achieved using even a flat fiber top. The particles inside
the solution gave rise to absorption losses of the laser energy
of typically 10 to 60% at the wall of the hollow organ. This has
to be taken into account in the therapeutical irradiation dosimetry. The scattering characteristics of the solution depend on
a number of factors including the concentration of the scattering
medium i.e. the number of scattering particles in it. An optimum
concentration of the scattering medium can be determined for a
given volume. The solution is not significantly heated by the
incident irradiation energy and this effect can be neglected clinically.

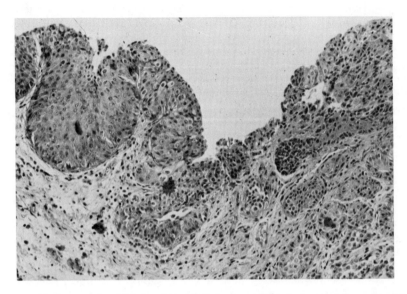

Fig. 10. Tumor treated with HpD but without laser irradiation remains unaffected.

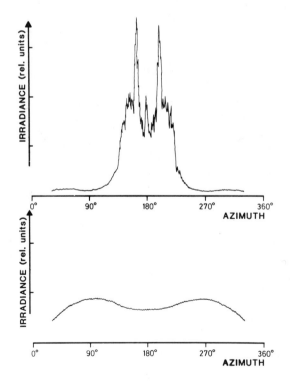

Fig. 11.
Light distribution using
a flat laser fiber
without (top)
and
with (bottom)
a light scattering
medium.

Possible contamination of the solution by impurities arising from
the influence of the laser light or as a result of mixing with
urine or blood, can be avoided by a permanent exchange of the
solution during the irradiation. The light diffusing medium did
not cause any wavelength shifts in the therapeutic red light.

Solutions with good light scattering properties were investigated in animal experiments. A fat emulsion was used for treatment of rabbits bearing (Brown-Pearce) bladder tumor. The photosensitization was performed with 5 mg HpD per kg body weight.
The integral irradiation was carried out 60 hours after supplying
HpD. At this time practically no HpD is present in the normal
bladder tissue. As already mentioned this is extremly important
for protecting normal tissue areas from damage due to the integral irradiation. The light fiber was introduced transurethrally
into the bladder and was directed into the centre of the bladder
past the tumor located at the bladder neck.

This ensured that there was no direct irradiation of the
tumor. The bladder was irrigated with light diffusion medium to
a volume such that the total wall was irradiated with a dose of
50-60 J/cm^2 .The average length of irradiation was 25 minutes.
Applying this method of integral dye laser therapy to the photosensitized tumors we were able to completely destroy tumor tissue
in 19 of the 22 rabbits tested.

Tumors in a control group without HpD showed a tumor growth
which was unaffected by the irradiation.

In conclusion, integral photoradiotherapy of hollow organs
(e.g. bladder) can be successfully performed using a light scattering medium.
- The light scattering medium is clinically well-tolerated,
  even when injected intraveneously.
- The application of integral irradiation is simple. There are
  no mechanical moving parts. Successful effects on tumor tissue
  can be achieved even in areas of the bladder which are difficult to reach.
- Normal bladder wall is unaffected by low dose laser irradiation, if the irradiation is performed at the right time.

Integral irradiation in combination with a scattering medium
offers a genuine possibility for the successful therapy of multifocal bladder carcinoma and especially carcinoma in situ.
The method promises to be superior to all other existing methods
of urological treatment for tumors of this type. We are in the
process of developing a special bladder catheter which will further simplify the described method and will make the procedure
easy and comfortable for doctor and patient, as well as solving
laser security problems.

REFERENCES

1. R. C. Benson, G. M. Farrow, J. H. Kinsey, D. A. Cortese, H.
    Zincke, and D. C. Utz, Detection and localization of in situ
    carcinoma of the bladder with Hematoporphyrin Derivative,
    Mayo Clin. Proc. 37:548 (1982)
2. R. C. Benson, The use of Hematoporphyrin Derivative (HpD) in the
    localization and treatment of transitional cell carcinoma
    (TCC) of the bladder, in: "The Clayton Foundation Symposium
    on Porphyrin Localization and Treatment of Tumors", Alan R.
    Liss Inc., ed., New York (in press).
3. D. Jocham, G. Staehler, Ch. Chaussy, C. Hammer, and U. Loehrs,
    Dye laser therapy of bladder tumors after photosensitization
    with Hematoporphyrin Derivative (HpD), in: "Laser Tokyo '81",
    K. Atsumi and N. Mimsakul, eds., Inter Group Corp., Tokyo
    (1981).
4. D. Jocham, C. Hammer, U. Loehrs, G. Staehler, Ch. Chaussy, and
    R. Dietrich, Farblasertherapie photosensiblilisierter Blasen-
    tumoren, in: "Chir. Forum '82 f. experim. und klinishe For-
    schung", Hrsg. S. Weller, ed., Springer Berlin, Heidelberg,
    New York (1982).
5. D. Jocham, E. Unsöld, G. Staehler, and Ch. Chaussy, Use of a
    light dispersion medium for an integral dye laser therapy of
    bladder tumors after photosensitization with Hematoporphyrin
    Derivative (HpD), in: "The Clayton Foundation Symposium on
    Porphyrin Localization and Treatment of Tumors, Alan R. Liss
    Inc., New York (in press).
6. J. F. Kelly, and M. E. Snell, Hematoporphyrin Derivative: a pos-
    sible aid in the diagnosis and therapy of carcinoma of the
    bladder, J. Urol. 115:150 (1976).

PHOTORADIATION THERAPY WITH HEMATOPORPHYRIN DERIVATIVE AND AN ARGON DYE LASER OF BLADDER CARCINOMA

Tetsutaro Ohi*, Harubumi Kato**, Akira Tsuchiya*,
Nobuo Obara*, Koichi Imamura*, Katsuo Aizawa***,
Chimori Konaka*, Jutaro Ono**, Norihiko Kawate**,
Kazuo Yoneyama**, Makoto Saito**, Hidenobu Takahashi**,
Sumiyaki Tsukimura**, Hideki Shinohara**,
Johnson Lay**, and Yoshihiro Hayata**

*Department of Urology, Tokyo Medical College, 6-7-1
 Nishishinjuku, Shinjuku-ku, Tokyo 160, Japan
**Department of Surgery, Tokyo Medical College, 6-7-1
 Nishishinujuku, Shinjuku-ku, Tokyo 160, Japan
***Department of Physiology, Tokyo Medical College, 6-7-1
 Shinjuku, Shinjuku-ku, Tokyo 160, Japan

INTRODUCTION

Hematoporphyrin Derivative (HpD) which has an affinity for malignant tumors is excited by light exposure and reacts photodynamically in tumor tissue. Therefore it is possible to treat malignant tumor selectively without any damage to surrounding normal tissues. HpD is excited by a light in the spectrum from ultraviolet to visible red. Previously arc lamps and slide projectors were used for excitation of HpD but laser beams which facilitate photoradiation via endoscopes has been used recently. Much of the early basic and clinical studies on HpD and light photoradiation therapy was performed by Dougherty and his coworkers[1]. Hayata et al. investigated photoradiation therapy using an argon dye laser following an intravenous HpD administration in mice, and on cultured human lung cancer cells[2], and in experimentally induced canine lung cancer and demonstrated its therapeutic effectiveness[3]. Malignant bladder tumor were treated by this new technique in this study.

MATERIALS AND METHODS

Hematoporphyrin Derivative

HpD and Photofrin were used in this study. HpD was provided
by Dr. Dougherty, Department of Radiation Biology, Roswell Park
Memorial Institute, Buffalo, New York, who prepared it by means of
a modification of Lipson's method[4] and Photofrin, a commercial name
for HpD, was provided by Oncology Research and Development Co., Ltd.
Cheektowaga, New York. They were both stored in darkness until used.

Laser equipment

An argon laser system was used as a light source in this study.
This system consists of an argon laser, model 171-08, 15 W, 457.9-
-514.9 nm (Spectra Physics, Co., Mountain View, CA) and a dye laser,
model 375-01, using Rhodamine B dye. The whole line wavelength of
the argon dye laser beam was converted to approximately 630 nm wavelength beam by a dye laser. A quartz fiber (400 micron, Quartz Products Co., Plainfield, N.Y. and Fujikura-Muto Co., Tokyo) was used
for the transmission of laser beam. The maximum laser output power
at the quartz fiber tip was 600 mW. A flexible cytoscope (Takei
Ikakoki Co., Ltd., Tokio) was used (Fig. 1).

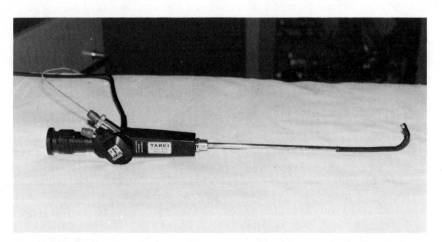

Fig. 1.   Flexible cytoscope (Takei Ikakoki Co. Ltd, Tokyo). A quartz
          fiber is inserted through a instrumentation channel of cy-
          toscope.

Procedures

2.5 mg/kg body weight HpD or Photofrin was injected intravenously 72 hours prior ro laser photoradiation. Photoradiation therapy (PRT) was performed for 20 minutes with the dose rate of approximately 100 mW/cm^2 which approximates 120 Joules/cm^2 with the bladder inflated by air after aspiration of urine. Because of a slight amount of systemic photosensitivity to sunlight, lasting approximately 30 days, all patients were cautioned to avoid sunlight during this period.

Patients

11 patients with superficial bladder carcinoma were selected for the PRT (Table 1). 10 cases were male and 1 case was female, and the age distribution was from 36 to 75, averaging 59.2. Of these 3 were primary cases and 8 cases were recurrent or recurrent cases with histories of partial bladder resection, or transurethral resection (TUR). All except cases 2 and 5 had undergone radiotherapy. The lesions were all less than 1 cm in size. 4 cases out of 11 were solitary tumors and the other 7 cases had multiple tumors. Histologically all cases were transitional cell carcinoma and they were T_a-T_1 according to the UICC classification, except 2 cases which showed invasion of the muscular layer (T_2).

Table 1. Results of HpD and laser photoradiation in bladder carcinoma.

Case	Age	Sex	Condition	Site	Grade	Period After PRT	Results
1	69	M	sol	sup lt ureter	GI	22 m	CR
2	71	M	sol	lt post	GII	22 m	CR
3	36	M	mult	rt post	GI	19 m	t cystectomy
4	69	M	mult	rt post lat	GI	22 m	CR
5	55	M	mult	rt lat	GII	10 m	p cystectomy
				post lat	GII		
6	43	M	mult	rt lat	GI	20 m	CR
				post lat	GI		
7	54	M	mult	rt post	GII	19 m	CR
8	55	M	mult	lt ureter	GII	14 m	t cystectomy
9	67	M	sol	lt lat	GII	10 m	CR
10	57	F	mult	lt lat	GII	10 m	CR
11	75	M	solt	rt lat	GII	10 m	CR

All cases were transitional cell carcinoma. M:male, F:female, m:month, t:total, p:partial, G:grade, lt:left, rt:right, sol:solitary, mult: multiple, sup:superior, lat:lateral, post:posterior, CR:complete remission of tumor.

Results

11 patients were treated by HpD administration and argon dye laser photoradiation therapy. The results are shown in Table 1. All cases were T_a-T_1 by the UICC classification, but cases 3 and 5 showed invasion of the muscular layer (T_2) by biopsy before the treatment. Figs. 2 and 3 show the endoscopic and histological findings before treatment.

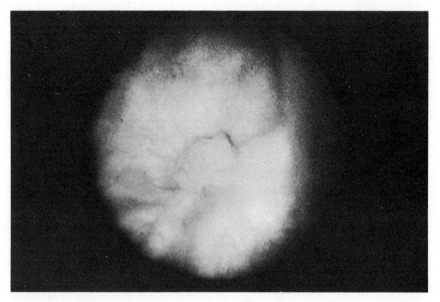

Fig. 2.   Endoscopic findings before treatment show a solitary poly-
          poid tumor above the left ureter in the case 1.

Follow-up endoscopic examinations of the lesion were performed after treatment. Swelling and edema were observed endoscopically after the 20 minutes PRT and biopsy at this time revealed remarkable interstitial and tumorous edema. Necrosis of the irradiated site was seen as a whitish mass the day following PRT (Fig. 4). Complete covering of the lesion by a whitish mass was recognized 7-14 days after photoradiation therapy. A chronological series of biopsies showed a regressive changes (Fig. 5). Complete remission of the tumors in 8 out of 11 cases was obtained (Table 1, Fig. 6). However 3 cases showed tumor recurrence 2, 5 and 6 months following photoradiation. Surgery was performed in these cases. In one of these cases, the tumor focus was located in the right lateral site where there is a blind spot. This prevented sufficient photoradiation, resulting in tumor recurrence after photoradiation therapy.

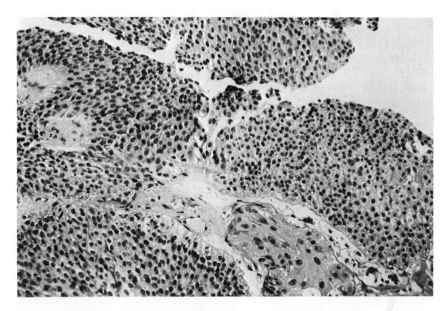

Fig. 3. Histological findings before treatment show transitional
cell carcinoma. H.E. X100

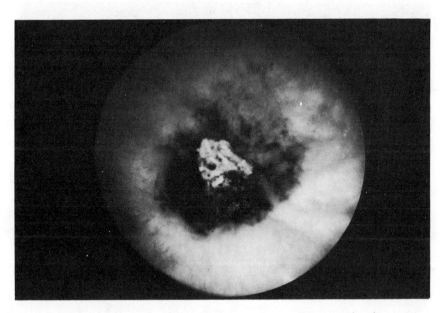

Fig. 4. Endoscopic findings 3 days after photoradiation therapy
show necrosis of the tumor.

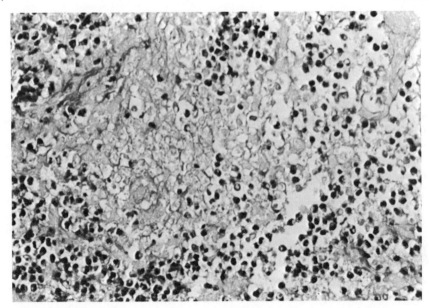

Fig. 5. Histologic findings 4 weeks after photoradiation therapy show complete destruction of tumor cells and infiltration of inflammatory cells. H.E. X100

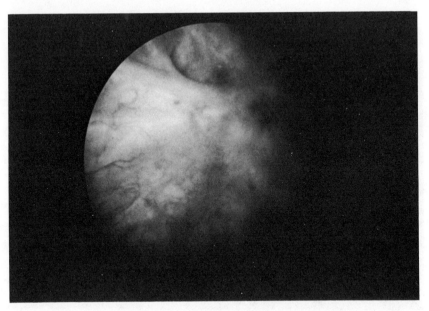

Fig. 6. Endoscopic findings 9 weeks after photoradiation therapy show complete remission of the tumor. This patient is disease free at 22 months now.

There were no significant complications except slight sunburn of the skin.

Discussion

We have performed laser photoradiation therapy in 11 bladder tumors and at present have obtained complete remission with no evidence of recurrence in 8 cases. They are disease free at from 10 to 22 months now. Therefore the effectiveness of laser photoradiation therapy with HpD administration for certain kinds of bladder carcinoma is clear.

In 1960, Lispon[4] reported the preparation of HpD which showed greater affinity for malignant tissue than normal tissue. Since then photoradiation therapy with HpD has received more attention. Dougherty et al.[5] reported encouraging results by administration of HpD and arc lamp hotoradiation of primary skin tumors and skin tumors metastatic from breast cancer. Hayata and Kato[6,7] showed that this method was effective in the treatment of early stage central type lung cancer. We have shown that it can be effective in certain bladder tumors.

Concerning the 3 cases of recurrence, it is important to know whether the cause was insufficient photoradiation therapy or whether these cases were not auitable indications for photoradiation therapy. Our conclusion is that this new therapeutic modality is absolutely indicated in cases of carcinoma in situ and T_1 tumors in the mucosal epithelium, and relatively indicated in cases of T_2 tumor invading areas of the muscular layer which can be reached by the laser beam. Advantages of this method include 1. it requires no anesthesia in women and only urethral anesthesia in men, 2. it can be repeated at short intervals, 3. it is tumor-specific and does not damage normal tissue, 4. no danger of hemorrhage or perforation, 5. great skill such as in transurethral resection is not required, 6. the quality of life of the patient is not impaired, and 7. it can be performed in inoperable or very elderly patients.

There are still some problems concerning this modality such as light delivery, laser power and dosimetry. The solution of these problems will provide improved results. This modality holds hope for the future treatment of malignant tumors.

ACKNOWLEDGEMENTS

The authors would like to express their appreciatin to Dr. T.J. Doughery and Mr. J.P. Barron for their cooperation. This study was supported in part by a Grant-in-Aid for Scientific Research from the Ministry of Education and a Cancer Research Grant from the Ministry of Welfare, Japan.

REFERENCES

1. T.J. Dougherty, G.B. Crindey, K.R. Weishaupt, and D.G. Boyle,
    Photoradiation therapy. II. Cure of animal tumors with
    Hematoporphyrin and light. J. Natl. Cancer Inst. 55:115
    (1975).
2. Y. Matsushima, Effect of Hematoporphyrin Derivative and laser
    photoradiation on cultured human lung cancer cells (PC-7)
    and transplanted mice tumors, Lung Cancer 22:549 (1982).
3. Y. Hayata, H. Kato, C. Konaka, N. Hayashi, M. Tahara, T. Saito,
    and J. Ono, Fiberoptic bronchoscopic photoradiation in ex-
    perimentally induced canine lung cancer, Cancer 51:50 (1983).
4. R.L. Lipson and J. Baldes, Photodynamic properties of a par-
    ticular Hematoporphyrin Derivative, Arch. Dermatol. 82:508
    (1960).
5. T.J. Dougherty, G. Lawrence, J.H. Kaufman, D. Boyle, K.R. Wei-
    shaupt, and A. Goldfarb, Photoradiation in the treatment of
    recurrent breast carcinoma, J. Natl. Cancer Inst. 62:231
    (1979).
6. Y. Hayata, H. Kato, C. Konaka, J. Ono, and N. Takizawa, Hema-
    toporphyrin Derivative and laser photoradiation in the treat-
    ment of lung cancer, Chest. 81:269 (1982).
7. H. Kato, C. Konaka, J. Ono, Y. Matsushima, K. Nishimiya, J.
    Lay, H. Sawa, H. Shinohara, K. Kinoshita, T. Tomono, M. Ai-
    da, and Y. Hayata, Effectiveness of Hpd and radiation the-
    rapy in lung cancer, in: "Porphyrin Photosensitization", D.
    Kessel and T.J. Dougherty, ed., Plenum Publishing Co, New
    York (1983).

PRECLINICAL EXAMINATION OF OCULAR PHOTORADIATION THERAPY

Charles J. Gomer, A. Linn Murphree, Daniel R. Doiron,
Bernard C. Szirth and Nicholas J. Razum

Clayton Center for Ocular Oncology, Childrens Hospital
of Los Angeles and Departments of Pediatrics (Division
of Hematology-Oncology) and Ophthalmology, USC School
of Medicine, Los Angeles, CA 90027, U.S.A.

INTRODUCTION

Hematoporphyrin derivative photoradiation therapy is an
effective therapeutic modality for several types of solid tumors
1,2 . One area of recent clinical interest is the exploitation
of HpD PRT for the treatment of ocular malignancies 3,4 . New
therapies which can provide effective tumor destruction and
minimal normal ocular tissue damage are needed since the current
modalities used for treating eye tumors (external beam radiation,
radioisotope plaques, photocoagulation and cryotherapy) are not
totally satisfactory 5,6 . HpD PRT may provide a modality
which can be utilized for the treatment of both retinoblastoma and
uveal melanoma. In addition, this procedure may be useful as both
a primary modality in selective instances as well as a secondary
modality following recurrence.

We have performed preclinical studies as a normal
prerequisite to the clinical application of ocular HpD PRT. This
paper describes the results obtained from preclinical studies
which were designed to determine the efficacy of ocular HpD PRT.
Specifically, acute and chronic toxicologic data as well as drug
localization and tumor response of ocular HpD PRT are described.

METHODS

Animal and Tumor Models

Pigmented rabbits (1.5-3 kg) were used in all experiments.
The tumor system employed in experimental studies consisted of an
amelanotic hamster melanoma heterotransplanted to the anterior

447

chamber of the rabbit eye. Single nodule tumors were obtained by placing a 1 mm^3 piece of viable tumor onto the iris through a radial cut made in the cornea.

Drugs

Sterile HpD (5 mg/ml) was obtained from ORD, Inc., Cheektowaga, N.Y. and was used without any modification. A combination of ketamine (30 mg/kg), acepromazine (3 mg/kg) and atropine sulfate (0.15 mg/kg) was used as an intramuscular injection to anesthetize all animals prior to experimental procedures. The ocular pupils were dilated in several experiments using 10% phenylephrine.

Light Sources

Monochromatic red light (630 nm or 635 nm) was generated with either a rhodamine-B or kiton-red dye laser pumped by a 5 watt argon laser (Spectra-Physics, Inc.). Violet light (407 and 413 nm) was generated using an 18 watt krypton laser (Coherent Radiation). The output from the laser systems was coupled to a quartz fiber (200 or 400 micron) for light delivery. A thermopile was used to measure light intensity and a scanning monochromator was used to document the output wavelength.

Normal Ocular Tissue Toxicity

A detailed description of the procedure utilized to examine normal ocular tissue toxicity has been published 3 . Briefly, rabbits received a single I.V. injection of HpD (0-10 mg/kg) and then 48 hours latered a 1 cm^2 area of the retina of each test eye was treated for 15 minutes with red light (635 nm, 40-400 mW/cm^2) via a trans-pupil illumination. A total of 45 eyes were treated and analyzed for acute (14 day) toxicity and 18 eyes were treated and analyzed for long term toxicity. Acute ocular toxicity was documented using fundus photography, fluorescein angiography and histological examination. Long term ocular toxicity has been documented using fundus photography, fluorescein angiography and slit lamp examination. Fundus photography and fluorescein angiograms were obtained using an Equator Plus camera. Histological specimens were fixed either in 1/2 strength Karnovsky´s fixative and embedded in glycol-methocylate or in 10% formalin and embedded in parafin. Specimens were routinely sectioned and then stained with hematoxylin and eosin.

HpD Localization

Levels of HpD in the aqueous and vitreous were measured using a spectrofluorometer (SLM Instruments). Animals received an I.V. injection of HpD (5 or 20 mg/kg) and then at various time periods following injection (1 to 72 hours) samples of aqueous and vitreous were removed from each eye and then the rabbit was sacrificed. Excitation and emission scans were obtained for each sample. In addition, known concentrations of HpD dissolved in control samples of aqueous were also examined.

Documentation of HpD fluorescence in various ocular tissue was obtained following injection of 5 mg HpD/kg in rabbits having anterior chamber tumors. Eyes were enucleated 24 hours following injection, and various ocular structures (tumor, cornea, lens, iris, retina, choroid, and sclera) were obtained. These structures were then photographed (first under white light and then under violet light). Qualitative assessment of HpD distribution was made from developed slides.

Photoradiation Treatment of Experimental Ocular Tumors

Rabbits with an anterior chamber tumor were entered into treatment studies when the tumor nodule measured at least 4.5 mm in diameter. Rabbits received an I.V. injection of HpD (1–10 mg/kg) and 48 hour later the entire tumor nodule (plus a 1 mm margin of normal iris) was irradiated with red light (630 nm). The light fluence ranged from 40 to 150 mW/cm^2 and the total delivered light doses ranged from 36 to 180 J/cm^2. When tumor cure was desired, it was occasionally necessary to retreat an eye. This was due to the development of secondary lesions resulting from tumor seeding at the time of initial implant. Photographic documentation of all tumors was obtained prior to treatment and at 24 hours post treatment (at the time of enucleation in histologic studies) and once a week in long term observation studies.

RESULTS

Results of HpD PRT induced normal ocular tissue toxicity have been recently published 3 . Clinically relevant doses of HpD PRT did induce ocular damage in the form of retinal edema, detachment and necrosis. The damage was visible within 24 hours of treatment and was limited to the treatment site in all but the highest doses of HpD PRT. It is important to note that 15 minute exposures of red light at intensities at or above 300 mW/cm^2 (in the absence of HpD) induced thermal damage to the retina.

The long term toxicity study is still in progress. The

observation period following single fraction HpD PRT is currently
20 months. The inital retinal damage which had been documented in
the acute toxicity studies was again observed and remained present
throughout the chronic observation period. The retina outside the
treatment field continued to appear normal as determined by fundus
examination and fluorescein angiography. No abnormalities have
been observed in the lens of any treated eye as determined by slit
lamp examination.

Photographic and visual documentation of HpD fluorescence in
various ocular structures were obtained 24 hours after a 5 mg/kg
dose of HpD. In these cases, HpD induced fluorescence has been
observed primarily in the tumor tissue and in areas of cornea
which were in contact with the tumor. No HpD fluorescence was
observed in the dissected lens.

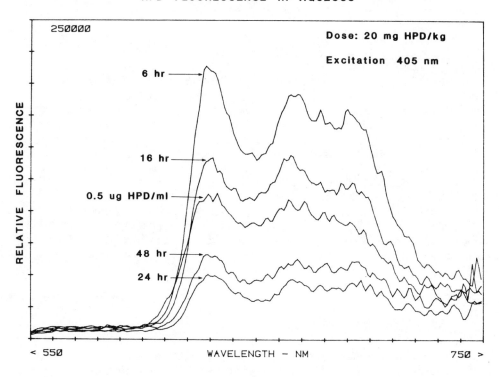

Figure 1.   Emission scans of HpD from the aqueous fluid of normal
            rabbit eyes at various time intervals following the
            I,V. injection of HpD (20 mg/kg). Excitation
            wavelength was 405 nm.

Figure 1 shows the emission spectra of HpD in the aqueous of rabbits as a function of time (6-48 hrs) after injection of HpD (20 mg/kg). The amount of HpD observed in the aqueous at 1 hour post injection was significantly greater than at 6 hours. A spectrum for 500 ng HpD/ml was also included on the graph. A rapid influx of porphyrin into the aqueous was observed following an I.V. injection of HpD. The level of HpD in the aqueous decreases with time following injection. Only minimal levels of HpD could be detected in the vitreous. The time dependent distribution of HpD in the aqueous was also observed at lower HpD doses (5 mg/kg).

The effect of HpD PRT on the anterior chamber amelanotic melanoma has been studied by visual, histological and long term documentation of tumor response. There was a rapid alteration in the appearance of the anterior chamber tumor following treatment. The tumor would characteristically appear blanched, swollen and hemorrhogic within 24 hours of treatment. The normally well organized and visible tumor microvasculature was completely destroyed. Massive tumor tissue necrosis and vascular hemorrhage were observed histologically following HpD treatments at doses which induced severe but well localized retinal damage in normal eyes. In addition to tumor tissue damage, HpD PRT of anterior chamber tumors also induced a transient haziness of the overlying cornea. In those eyes where a prolonged observation period was performed, the tumor continued to appear opaque and necrotic. The lesion decreased in size following treatment and usually disappeared by 20 days. Normally, a residual scar remained on the iris where the tumor had invaded and a small opaque area of cornea remained in the area of the original tumor. A total of 5 anterior tumors have been cured (no tumor recurrence for 150 days post treatment) using HpD doses of 5 or 10 mg/kg and light treatments of 90-180 J/cm^2 delivered at 150 mW/cm^2.

DISCUSSION

The use of HpD PRT may prove to be beneficial for the destruction of retinoblastoma and uveal melanoma patients in which conventional treatment modalities can not be used or have failed to produce cures. As a normal and necessary prerequisite to the clinical application of ocular HpD PRT, it was necessary to determine and document potential side effects of this modality on normal ocular structures. Our preclinical studies demonstrated that ocular damage to normal eyes, could be induced by HpD PRT [3]. This damage was characterized by circumscribed areas of retinal edema, detachment and necrosis. The retinal damage was permanent (visible for up to 20 months) but did not increase in size. Fortunately, no damage (either acute or chronic) has been observed in the lens following single fraction HpD PRT.

The observations of HpD fluorescence in experimental ocular amelanotic melanoma are in agreement with a previous study examining HpD uptake in this tumor when transplanted to the choroid 7 . The lack of any observable HpD fluorescence at 24 hours post injection in the lens was expected since this structure is avascular and no HpD PRT induced damage has been observed in the lens. Of potential significance for all clinical applications of HpD PRT was the finding that relatively large levels of HpD could be detected in the aqueous at short intervals following administration of HpD. While it is not known whether the levels of HpD achieved in the aqueous of humans are large enough to cause injury it would not be advisable to perform ocular examinations on any patient within the first few hours of drug injection. The lack of significant levels of HpD in the vitreous would suggest that vitreous seeds arising in retinoblastoma will not accumulate sufficient levels of HpD to respond to light treatment. However, there may be leakage of HpD out of tumors and this may influence levels of HpD in the vitreous. The fact that HpD PRT has not induced any cataract formation (during the 20 month observation period) is an important finding as it relates to the clinical usefulness of ocular HpD PRT. However, our study has demonstrated that HpD does accumulate in the aqueous and a previous study has shown that photosensitization using 8-methyoxypsoralen can induce lens damage 8 . Therefore, it will be mandatory to continue observations (preclinical and clinical) as they relate to potential lens damage resulting from HpD PRT.

One area which has major importance in ocular HpD PRT is the subject of light dosimetry. Two published studies in this area are directly relevant to ocular HpD PRT. One study examined light transmission through normal human lens from individuals with an age range of 6 months to 82 years 9 . The results demonstrated that while greater than 90% of red light is transmitted through the lens of a 6 month old, there is a significant decrease in red light transmission with increasing age. At ages greater than 25 years, there is less than 50% transmission of 630 nm light through the lens. This information indicates that the total level of light reaching the retina (via transpupil illumination) in HpD PRT will differ by at least a factor of 2 for infants with retinoblastoma (less than 2 years of age) and adults with choroidal melanoma (averaging 60 years of age). The second aspect of light penetration deals with trans-scleral illumination 10 . In this case it is observed that approximately 35 percent of red light (696 nm) would be transmitted through the sclera. This finding also has major implications for calculating delivered levels of light from trans-scleral probes in treating choroidal melanomas.

Finally, our preclinical ocular tumor treatment studies are

significant from two aspects.   First, we have been able to demonstrate that HpD PRT (at doses which would produce a localized area of normal retinal damge) could completely destroy this rapidly growing tumor.   Tumor cures have been obtained and have led to the realization that human iris melanomas may be successfully treated with HpD PRT.   The second aspect of the preclinical tumor study which requires comment deals with the documentation of the visual appearance of the treated lesion. Observations of tumor blanching, swelling and hemorrhage which were documented in experimental tumors were also observed following HpD PRT in patients with uveal melanoma and retinoblastoma (A.L. Murphree, unpublished results).   While the appearance of tumor blanching, edema and hemorrhage can be taken to indicate that HpD PRT has induced tumor destruction, these observations should not be used to evaluate the extent of tumor response.   A characteristic visual cytotoxic response (blanching, edema and hemorrhage) was observed in the experimental anterior chamber tumor when the corresponding histological evaluation showed partial or full thickness tumor necrosis.   Factors such as tumor thickness and tissue pigmentation will influence the dose of HpD PRT needed to produce satisfactory clinical responses.

ACKNOWLEDGEMENTS

This investigation was performed in conjunction with the Clayton Foundation for Research and was supported in part by USPHS Grants CA 31230 and CA 31885, awarded by the NCI, DHHS. We thank Albert L. Castorena for assistance in the preparation of this manuscript.

REFERENCES

1.   T.J. Dougherty, J.B. Kaufman, A. Goldfarb, K.R. Weishaupt, D.G. Boyle, and A. Mittleman, Photoradiation therapy for the treatment of malignant tumors,   Cancer Res. 38:2628-2635. (1978).

2.   T.J. Dougherty, K.R. Weishaupt, and D.G. Boyle, "Photosensitizers" in: (eds., De Vita, V., S., Helman, and S. Rosenberg), Cancer, Principles and Practices of Oncology, pp. 1836-1844, Philadelphia: J.B. Lippincott Co., (1982).

3.   C.J. Gomer, D.R. Doiron, J.V. Jester, B.C. Szirth, and A.L. Murphree, Hematoporphyrin derivative photoradiation therapy for the treatment of intraocular tumors: Examination of acute ocular tissue toxicity. Cancer Res.   43:721-727, (1983).

4.   C.J. Gomer, D.R. Doiron, L. White, J.V. Jester, S. Dunn, B.C. Szirth, N.J. Razum, and A.L. Murphree,

Hematoporphyrin derivative photoradiation induced damage to
normal and tumor tissue of the pigmented rabbit eye.
Current Eye Res., (In Press).

5.   L.W. Brady, J.A. Shields, J.J. Augsburger, and J.L. Day,
      Malignant intraocular tumor. Cancer (Phila.) 49:578-585,
      (1982).

6.   J.A. Shields, and J.J. Augsburger, Current approaches to
      the diagnosis and management of retinoblastoma. Surv.
      Ophthalmol. 25:347-372, (1981).

7.   D.L. Krohn, R. Jacobs, and D.A. Morris, Diagnosis of model
      choroid malignant melanoma by hematoporphyrin derivative
      fluorescence in rabbits. Invest. Ophthalmol. 13:244-255,
      (1974).

8.   S. Lerman, M. Jocoy, and R.F. Borkman, Photosensitization
      of the lens by 8-methoxypsoralen. Invest. Ophthalmol.
      16:1065-1068, (1977).

9.   S. Lerman, and R.F. Borkman, Spectroscopic evaluation and
      classification of the normal, aging and cataractous lens.
      Ophthalmic. Res. 8:335-353, (1976).

10.   R.S. Smith, and M.N. Stein, Ocular hazards of transcleral
      laser radiation. Am. J. Ophthalmol. 66:21-31, (1968).

PHOTORADIATION FOR CHOROIDAL MALIGNANT MELANOMA

Robert A. Bruce Jr.

Assistant Professor
Department of Ophthalmology
The Ohio State University
Columbus, Ohio 43210

INTRODUCTION

Photoradiation therapy is the pretreatment of tissue with a photo sensitizing substance followed by exposure to light energy, resulting in a photodynamic reaction that causes cell death. This concept has been investigated since the early 1900s without success until the 1970s. At this time, Dougherty (1978; 1979; 1981) and his group at Roswell Park, New York developed a derivative of hematoporphyrin (HpD) that appears to meet the necessary criteria of a photoradiation therapy. It is well known that the HpD, when given to patients, is concentrated in neoplastic tissue to a greater extent than in normal tissues. Exposure of the sensitized tissue to red light (630 nm) results in a photodynamic reaction, causing oxidation of cross linkages in the cell wall resulting in cell lysis (Moan et al., 1979; Weishaupt et al., 1976). To date, many types of human and animal neoplasms have been responsive to this mode of therapy (McBride, 1979).

Following the initial reports of positive response in choroidal malignant melanoma to photoradiation therapy (PRT), a project to evaluate PRT on this tumor was initiated through the Laser Medical Research Foundation in Columbus, Ohio, in July, 1982. Since that time, 19 patients with choroidal melanoma have undergone PRT. This paper will discuss our preliminary data.

PATIENT EVALUATION

All patients included in this series were initially evaluated at The Ohio State University Department of Ophthalmology and

455

treated at Grant Hospital in Columbus, Ohio with the cooperation
of the Laser Medical Research Foundation of Columbus, Ohio.

All patients were referred by a general ophthalmologist to the
retinal service at The Ohio State University. Each patient underwent an ophthalmic examination including visual acuity, slit lamp
examination, tonometry, and a complete retinal examination to determine the location and size of the mass lesion. This examination was followed by diagnostic fluorescein angiography, photographic documentation, and quantitative ultrasonography to verify the
clinical diagnosis and obtain exact measurements of the size of the
melanomas being considered for treatment. The ophthalmologic examination has been followed by a medical work-up to evaluate the
presence or absence of metastatic disease. Testing includes: a
complete physical examination; chest x-ray, liver spleen scan, CT
scan, and bone scan; and hematologic evaluations. If all of the
testing in this evaluation program reveals no evidence of metastatic disease or other primary neoplasia, photoradiation therapy
has been offered to the patient.

TREATMENT REGIMEN

Hematoporphyrin derivative is administered intravenously in a
dose of 2.5 mg/Kg. Seventy-two hours following the administration
of the hematoporphyrin derivative, the tumor mass is exposed to red
light generated by a Spectra-Physics Rhodamine B tunable dye laser.
The time of exposure has varied from 10 to 40 minutes. The light
has been delivered to the tumor masses transcorneally, trans-
sclerally, or via a combination of both of these approaches. Post-
operatively, patients' responses have been evaluated by the measurement of visual acuity, fluorescein angiography, ultrasonography,
photography and clinical examination.

POWER LEVELS

The amount of energy delivered to each tumor is outlined in
Table 1. The calculation of these energy levels is shown with a
sample calculation in Figure 1. The distance measurements in
these calculations are approximate values. They reflect the power
density delivered to the area of the tumor if the fiberoptic probes
were held in the same position throughout the duration of the
treatment. In reality, the probes have been hand held, and the
beam has been moved deliberately to cover all treated areas of the
tumor mass. I believe that this results in lower power densities
being delivered to the tumor masses than are reflected in the calculations shown in the table. A more exact method of controlling
the distance of the probes from the tumor mass is being developed.

Table 1: Amount of Energy Delivered to Each Tumor

PT	AGE	SIZE(mm)	TR.CORN. (watts)	TRSCL*** (watts)	TIME (min)	POWER DNSTY (J/cm^2)	PREOP VA	POSTOP VA	TIME FROM Tx (mos)	DECREASED TUMOR SIZE
EH	59	10.5x6x3	1.00	.500	40	3060	20/25	20/50	10	Total
LM	35	7x7x3.6	1.00	.300	40	6800	20/20	20/20	5	80%
NS	35	12x9x3	1.00	.500	40	2880	20/30	FC	5	50%
RT	53	7.5x7.5x2	1.00	—	40	2600	20/30	20/200	5	Total
LJ	83	6x6x1	1.00	.300	40	1500	20/60	LP	5	Total
ED	55	10x6x1	1.00	.300	40	1920	20/300	HM	5	**
CS	77	10x6x5	1.00	.250	40	3060	LP	LP	3	--
MH	57	7.5x7.5x2	1.00	—	20	614	20/100	HM	1	--
HB	67	12x6x7.5	1.00	.500	40	1700	20/70	20/400	1	--
DB	35	6x7.5x4	1.00	—	10	293	20/70	20/200	1	--
JH	66	12x10x6	1.00	.275	30	3050	FC	HM	1	--

*Approximate measurement by ultrasonography
**Patient has been retreated after 4 months
LP=Light perception; FC=Finger counting
***70% loss of power through sclera

F=Reading, Coherent fiber tip (mW)
A=Distance tip to lens (mm); lens = 2 mm thick
X=Estimated distance surface of eye to tumor (mm)
Z=Distance fiber tip to tumor (mm)
R_Z=Coherent radiometer reading at distance Z with lens in
   place (mW)
D_Z=Diameter spot size at distance Z (cm)
A_S=Area spot size at distance Z (cm^2)
A_T=Estimated area of tumor (cm^2)

Sample: F=1000 mW, A=12 mm, lens=2 mm, X=10 mm
          Z=24 mm, R_Z=850 mW, D_Z=.8 cm, A_S=π(.8) (.8)=.5 cm^2
          A_T=15 mmx20 mm = 30 cm^2 ―――――
                                                             4

          TIME = 30 min

$$\underline{\text{FOR SPOT SIZE}}: R_Z = \frac{850}{A_S} = \frac{850}{.5} = \frac{1700 \text{ mW}}{\text{cm}^2}$$

$$\frac{R_Z \text{ (mW)}}{A_S \text{(cm}^2)} \times \frac{30 \text{ min}}{\text{min.}} \times \frac{60 \text{ sec.}}{mW} \times \frac{10^{-3}w}{} = \frac{\text{watt sec.}}{\text{cm}^2} = \frac{\text{Joules}}{\text{cm}^2}$$

$$= \frac{1700 \text{ mW}}{\text{cm}^2} \times 1800 \text{ sec} \times \frac{10^{-3}W}{mW} = \frac{3060 \text{ Joules}}{\text{cm}^2}$$

$$\underline{\text{FOR TUMOR SIZE}}: \frac{R_Z \times 30 \times 60 \times 10^{-3}}{A_T} = \frac{850mW}{3cm^2} \times 30 \text{ min} \times \frac{60sec}{min} \times$$

$$\frac{10^{-3}}{mW} = \frac{\text{Joules}}{\text{cm}^2} = \frac{510 \text{ Joules}}{\text{cm}^2}$$

$$\underline{\text{RETROBULBAR}}: \frac{R_B}{A_B} = \frac{\text{Coherent Reading}}{\text{Area Spot}} \quad \frac{mW}{cm^2} = \frac{275}{1.3} = \frac{211 \text{ mW}}{\text{cm}^2} \times$$

$$\frac{275 \text{ mW}}{1.3cm^2} \times 30min \times \frac{60 \text{ sec}}{min} = \frac{380 \text{ Joules}}{\text{cm}^2}$$

Fig. 1. Sample calculation of dosage.

REACTION TO TREATMENT

In all of the patients treated to date, the administration of
hematoporphyrin derivative intravenously has not revealed any adverse systemic side effects. The drug is administered intravenously, and the patients are kept in a dark room to eliminate discomfort from sunlight, which results from the generalized photosensitivity caused by the drug. The photosensitivity of the skin
appears to be persistent for 8 to 12 weeks after the administration
of the dye. This information has been documented by patient experience within our series.

Changes in the appearance of the tumor mass are noted within
minutes after they are exposed to the laser light. These changes
include a blanching of the tumor mass, causing it to turn white.
Additionally, the overlying retina becomes edematous with pinpoint
intraretinal hemorrhaging. The adjacent uninvolved retina does not
appear to become acutely involved with this edematous/hemorrhagic
change in the retina overlying the tumor.

Alterations in the vascular supply to the tumors have been
noted in the immediate post-treatment fluorescein angiograms. This
is dramatic and has been a persistent change in the studies carried
out in the follow-up period of all but one of our patients.

Reduction in tumor mass has been observed in all patients who
are five months or longer post-treatment. Shrinkage has been identified initially 10 to 12 weeks after treatment. This clinical
observation is one of a gradual change from the initial postoperative white color of the tumor mass to a mottled appearance which
is seen in a typical chorioretinal scar. As this occurs, dimpling
on the surface of the tumor can be identified. The loss of the
tumor tissue volume requires several weeks to months to occur.
This loss of tumor mass is easily verified by ultrasonography. The
final appearance is that of a large chorioretinal scar.

Post-treatment complications in the treated eyes are listed
in Table 2. All patients have experienced some degree of chemosis,
iritis and lid swelling, which have been treated with cycloplegics
and corticosteroid drops. The chemosis usually clears within seven
days. The iritis lasts up to six weeks. The lid swelling can be
eliminated by careful draping of the eyelids with an opaque material.

Exudative retinal detachment has developed in 9 of our 11 cases.
This occurs usually within three days of treatment. In those cases
in which preoperative detachment existed (3/11), the detachment
worsened after treatment. In all but three cases, the detachment
of the retina resolved within six weeks of treatment.

Other clinical changes which have been noted include choroidal

Table 2.   Post-Treatment Complications

Complications	No. Cases (11 Total Cases)
Photosensitivity of skin	11
Iritis	11
Exudative retinal detachment	9
Reduced visual acuity	11
Vitreous reaction	1
Vitreous hemorrhage	2
Chemosis	11
Cataract	1
Choroidal detachment	1

detachment, cataract, vitreous hemorrhage, vitreous inflammatory reaction, and reduced visual acuity. These changes all appear to be transitory except for the reduction in visual acuity. The final visual acuity appears to be related to the location and the size of the tumor mass. If the tumor has undermined the macular area, central vision is sacrificed. In the case of the larger melanomas, the exudative retinal detachments are more extensive and have resulted in macular involvement. This may be a contributing factor to reduced postoperative visual acuity.

DISCUSSION

Initial short-term results from this series of patients with choroidal malignant melanoma treated with photoradiation therapy are very encouraging. Several aspects of our treatment regimen and results may vary a great deal from the experience of other investigators. The greatest difference is the amount of tumor mass destruction that our series has demonstrated when compared to other series. L'Esperance (personal communication) found little if any reduction in the size of the tumor mass after 18 months of follow-up. Our results are most likely due to the large power density that we have employed, which may produce a thermal effect in addition to the phototoxic effect of hematoporphyrin derivative plus red light.

Other side effects from the exposure of the retina to the intense light, which may affect the ultimate visual acuity in the involved eyes, have yet to be identified. Electrophysiologic testing pre- and post-treatment may supply many of these answers.

CONCLUSION

Photoradiation therapy as described by Dougherty, et al is a

viable alternative to enucleation in the treatment of choroidal
malignant melanoma. This conclusion is drawn from our initial im-
pressions from our series of patients. Photoradiation therapy
offers a noninvasive form of therapy that may provide a more acceptable mode of therapy to the patient than enucleation. Moreover, it
appears to surpass the results obtained with other alternative
treatment methods currently being employed.

REFERENCES

Dougherty T.J., 1981, Photoradiation therapy for cutaneous and
    subcutaneous malignancies, J Invest Derm, 77:122.
Dougherty T.J., Kaufman J.E., Goldfarb A., Weishaupt K.R., Boyle
    D., Mittleman A., 1978, Photoradiation therapy for the treat-
    ment of malignant tumors, Cancer Research 38:2628.
Dougherty T.J., Lawrence G., Kaufman J.H., Boyle D., Weishaupt
    K.R., Goldfarb A., 1979, Photoradiation in the treatment of
    recurrent breast carcinoma, J Natl Cancer Inst 62:231.
McBride G., 1979, New treatment for cancer under development, JAMA
    242:403.
Moan J., Peteersen E.O., Christensen T., 1979, The mechanism of
    photodynamic inactivation of human cells in vitro in the
    presence of haematoporphyrin. Br J Cancer 39:398.
Weishaupt K.R., Gomer C.J., Dougherty T.J., 1976, Identification
    of singlet oxygen as the cytotoxic agent in photo-inactivation
    of a murine tumor, Cancer Research 36:2326.